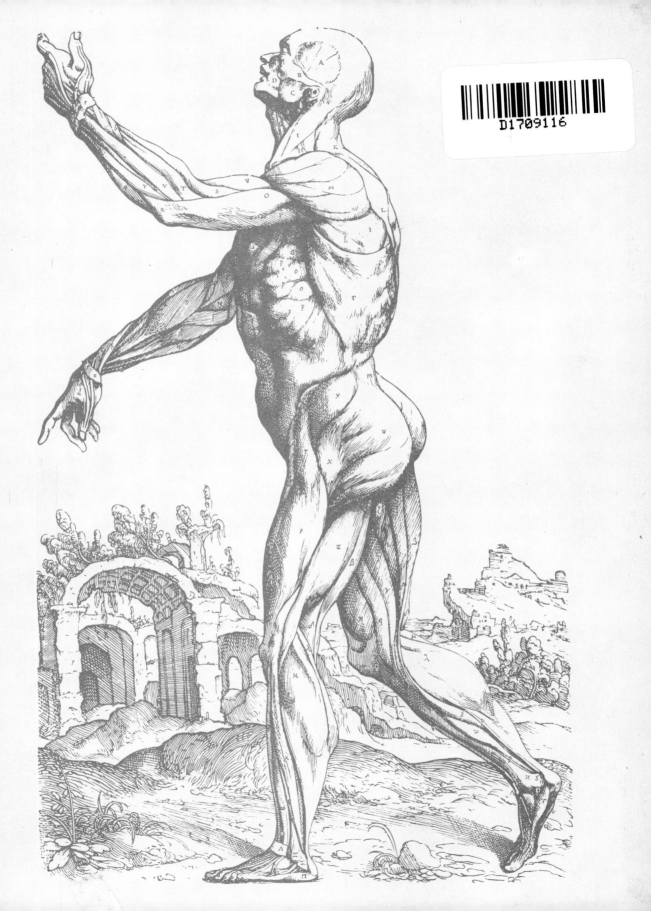

Sobotta/Figge

# Atlas of Human Anatomy

Original Author Dr. med. Johannes Sobotta †, Professor and Director of the Anatomical Institute, University of Bonn, Germany

9th English Edition by Frank H. J. Figge †, Ph.D., Sc.D. (hon.), Professor Emeritus of Anatomy, School of Medicine, University of Maryland

Walther J. Hild, M.D., Professor and Chairman, Department of Anatomy
The University of Texas Medical Branch, Galveston, Texas

Based upon the 17th German Edition, edited by

Prof. Dr. med. Helmut Ferner, Director of the Anatomical Institute, University of Vienna, Austria
Prof. Dr. med. Jochen Staubesand, Director of the Anatomical Institute, University of Freiburg, Germany

Vol. 1: Regions, Bones, Ligaments, Joints and Muscles
Vol. 2: Visceral Anatomy
Vol. 3: Central Nervous System, Autonomic Nervous System
Sense Organs and Skin, Peripheral Nerves and Vessels

Urban & Schwarzenberg · München-Berlin-Wien 1974

Sobotta/Figge

# Atlas of Human Anatomy

9th English Edition by Frank H. J. Figge †, Ph.D., Sc.D. (hon.), Professor Emeritus of Anatomy, School of Medicine, University of Maryland

Based upon the 17th German Edition, edited by

Prof. Dr. med. Helmut Ferner, Director of the Anatomical Institute, University of Vienna, Austria
Prof. Dr. med. Jochen Staubesand, Director of the Anatomical Institute, University of Freiburg, Germany

Vol. 1

Regions, Bones, Ligaments, Joints and Muscles

365 Illustrations, mostly in color

Urban & Schwarzenberg · München-Berlin-Wien 1974

The Original Author, Professor Dr. med. Johannes Sobotta, was born on January 31, 1869 in Berlin. He died on April 20, 1945 in Bonn, where he was Professor and Director of the Anatomical Institute, University of Bonn, Germany.

Addresses of the English editors:

Mrs. Frank H. J. Figge, 4 Maryland Avenue, Towson, Maryland 21204

Walther J. Hild, M.D., Professor and Chairman, Department of Anatomy,
The University of Texas Medical Branch, Galveston, Texas 77550

Addresses of the German editors:

Professor Dr. med. Helmut Ferner, Vorstand der I. Anatomischen Lehrkanzel der Universität,
A-1090 Wien, Währingerstraße 13, Austria

Professor Dr. med. Jochen Staubesand, Direktor des Anatomischen Instituts der Universität,
7800 Freiburg, Albertstraße 17, Germany

The pictures on the end leaves of the present volume show reproductions of the work of "Andreae Vesalii de corporis humani fabrica libri septem", which appeared in Basle in 1542. ANDREAS VESALIUS (* Brussels 1514, † 1564) urged and practised the dissection of human bodies and may be considered to be the Founder of Modern Anatomy.

This Atlas is also available in the following languages:

17th German Edition, Urban & Schwarzenberg, München–Berlin–Wien 1972.

9th English Edition (with Nomenclature in Latin), Urban & Schwarzenberg, München–Berlin–Wien 1975.

14th Italian Edition, USES, Utet – Sansoni Edizioni Scientifiche, Firenze 1974.

2nd Japanese Edition, Igaku Shoin Ltd., Tokyo 1974.

Spanish Edition, Ediciones Toray, S.A. – Barcelona 1974.

Turkish Edition, Urban & Schwarzenberg, München–Berlin–Wien 1973.

Greek Edition, Gregory Parisianos, Athens: in preparation.

Portuguese Edition, Editora Guanabara Koogan, Rio de Janeiro/Brasil: in preparation.

ISBN 3-541-06869-8

Printed in Germany by Kastner & Callwey, Buch- und Offsetdruckerei, München.

# American Editor's Preface to the 9th Edition in English

During the revision of the Atlas for the 9th English Edition and after he had completed the work for the first and second volumes, Professor Frank H. J. Figge died suddenly. It was his wish, conveyed to me by Mrs. Rosalie Yerkes Figge and Mr. Michael Urban, that I should continue his work and arrange the translation of Volume III. I followed this request without hesitation because I felt that I owed this duty to my dear friend Frank who, together with his wife, had shown me so many personal and professional favors when I came to this country as an immigrant.

I welcome the decision by the publishers and Frank Figge to depart radically from previous English editions and to replace the Latin with anglicized nomenclature because education in classical languages of the prospective medical student today is minimal. However, the etymology appropriate for each volume is conveniently included to further the understanding of anatomical terms.

Due to the close cooperation of Mr. Michael Urban and Mr. Klaus Gullath of Urban & Schwarzenberg, the guaranteed publication at the scheduled time was possible, even in the face of delays caused by Professor Figge's untimely death. However, this schedule could not have been observed without the unflagging efforts of Mrs. Rosalie Yerkes Figge who, with her daughters, Rosalie Ann Figge Beasley and Barbara Figge Fox, continued to be responsible for the myriad technical details of preparing the manuscripts for Volumes I and II for publication, including the meticulous proofreading and indexing. I also wish to thank my colleagues in the Department of Anatomy for many valuable suggestions for my revision of Volume III.

It is my hope and expectation that all this concerted and time-consuming work by many people will make Sobotta's unsurpassed illustrations even more useful to future students of anatomy.

Galveston, Texas, July 1974

Walther J. Hild

# Part of the Author's Preface to the First Edition

This anatomical atlas is intended to serve in the first place the practical needs of medical students and physicians; it is not intended for the professional anatomist. For this reason I have restricted myself to those essentials which I considered necessary in obtaining a general knowledge of the anatomy of the human body. The present volume which is the first of a total of three volumes, is organized in the form of an atlas to be used in the first place as a guide during the dissection in the anatomical student laboratory. Keeping in mind this purpose I have presented the material strictly in accordance with the method customary in the dissecting rooms of our medical schools. As a matter of principle I have avoided using for the illustrations such dissections which show the parts in unusual positions as they make orientation very difficult for the beginner.

For the purpose of ready reference during the dissection the student will find on the pages opposite the plates, in addition to the explanation of the plate, a brief descriptive text. The description of the muscles is presented for the most part in the form of convenient tables in which origin, insertion, innervation and function are listed.

In order to enable the reader to differentiate at the first glance between different parts, many different colors were employed in the illustrations. A yellowish tone was used for the bones in the pictures of the joints, a red color for the muscles, and several different colors for individual cranial bones in pictures illustrating the whole skull and topographical relations of parts of the skull. The terminology is the "Basel Anatomical Nomenclature". The publishers took great pains to make this volume superior to most of the existing works in point of quality of reproduction and at least equal in regard to the number of illustrations.

Würzburg, October 1903

The Author

## Foreword to the 17th German Edition

Sobotta's concept of the Atlas has remained the guiding principle for the new editors. In order to emphasize the Atlas character of the work, they have eliminated all text passages. Only the valuable tables on muscles, their origins, insertions, innervation and functions have been retained and – wherever possible – have been coordinated with the corresponding figures.

The planning of a large portion of the new illustrations has still been done by Professor Dr. H. Becher. The accurate execution of the illustrations has been accomplished by the scientific artist, Professor E. Lepier of Vienna.

The repeated request by many students to coordinate figures and captions could be honored in the interest of improved usability by the accommodating attitude of the publishers. To this end, also, the index has been simplified. The nomenclature has been consequently based upon the Nomina Anatomica (Paris 1955) with reference to the latest additional recommendations (New York 1960 and Wiesbaden 1965); (compare: Nomina Anatomica, 3rd Ed. Excerpta Medica Foundation, Amsterdam–New York–London–Paris–Milan–Tokyo–Buenos Aires 1968).

Medical student Miss G. Adelmann has given valuable help with proofreading. The editors express their appreciation to Mrs. M. Engler for the arrangement of the index.

Special appreciation is due to the publishing house of Urban and Schwarzenberg and their coworkers – especially Dr. R. Degkwitz and Mr. K. Gullath – for the thoughtful consideration of the wishes of the editors.

Heidelberg and Freiburg i. Br.
February 1972

H. Ferner
J. Staubesand

# Table of Contents

# The human body, corpus humanum

The human body is subdivided into these main sections:
– Head *(caput)*
– Trunk *(truncus)*
– Upper extremities or limbs *(membra superiora)* and
– Lower extremities or limbs *(membra inferiora)*.

In these main sections one can distinguish the following:
– Face *(facies)*, the anterior or ventral part of the head,
– Neck *(collum* or *cervix)*, tapering or constricted area of the body (or organ).
– Back *(dorsum)*, the entire posterior or dorsal surface of the trunk; its most cranial part bordering the head is designated nape *(nucha)*
– Thorax *(pectus)*
– Abdomen *(abdomen* or *venter)*
– Perineum, the small region between anus and the external genitalia.

The freely movable extremities *(membra libera)* are so intimately connected to the trunk that their proximal portions cannot be immediately distinguished by inspection from outside.

The free part of the upper extremity *(membrum superius)* consists of:
– Arm *(brachium)*
– Forearm *(antebrachium)* and
– Hand *(manus)*.

The lower extremity *(membrum inferius)* consists of:
– Thigh *(femur)*
– Leg *(crus)* and
– Foot *(pes)*.

The entire outer surface of the human body is covered by the external skin *(integumentum commune)* which serves as a protective cover, organ of excretion (cutaneous glands) and receptive organ for external stimuli (most nervous receptors are located immediately beneath the epidermis). One distinguishes between true and false openings of the body. True openings are the following: the mouth *(os* or *rima oris)* ; the two nostrils *(nares)* ; the anal opening *(anus)* ; the opening of the vagina in the female *(ostium vaginae)* ; the orifice of the female urethra *(ostium urethrae externum)*. In the female six true ostia are present. In the male body there are only five, since in the male the ostium urethrae externum serves as the outlet for the urine as well as of the semen. Apparent body openings are the openings between the eyelids *(rimae palpebrarum)* and the openings of the external ears *(pori acustici externi)*.

The extremities consist only of skeletal parts (bones) with their corresponding joints and ligaments and of muscles (to which are added blood vessels and nerves). Inside the head and trunk are located the body cavities, walled in by bones and (usually) muscles as well, these cavities housing inner organs *(viscera)*. These viscera are the organs of digestion, respiration, and urinary and reproductive functions and, furthermore the heart (center of the vascular system) and the central organs of the nervous system, brain and spinal cord.

In each of the parts of the body, described above, there are distinguished again smaller areas or regions (regiones corporis humani). Regions with triangular borders are called trigones (trigona). In cases of distinctly depressed areas the term region is replaced by the term fossa. Some regions are denoted by special terms: palm of the hand *(palma manus)*, back of the hand *(dorsum manus)*, sole of the foot *(planta pedis)*, upper surface of the foot *(dorsum pedis)*. Concerning location, boundaries and names of individual regions see Figs. 1 to 5.

# General Terms of Direction and Position

The following terms designate the position of organs and parts of the body in their relationship to each other, sometimes irrespective of the position of the body in space. These designations are used not only in human anatomy, but also in medical practice and in comparative anatomy.

## A. General designations

*Anterior – posterior* = in front – behind (e.g., anterior and posterior tibial arteries)

*ventral – dorsal* = toward the belly – toward the back

*superior – inferior* = above – below

*cranial – caudal* = toward the head – toward the tail

*dexter – sinister* = right – left (e.g., right and left common iliac arteries)

*internal – external* = located inside – located outside

*superficial – deep* = located superficially – located deeply (e.g., superficial and deep flexores digitorum muscles)

*medius* or *intermedius* = middle (in the middle between two other structures) (e.g., the middle nasal concha is located between the superior and inferior nasal concha)

*medianus* = located in the midline, median (e.g., median fissure of the spinal cord)
A "median sagittal section" divides the body into two mirror image-like portions.

*medial – lateral* = located toward the middle of the body – located toward the side of the body (e.g., medial and lateral inguinal fossae)

*frontal* = located in a frontal plane, also located toward the forehead (e.g., frontal process of maxilla)

*longitudinal* = parallel to the long axis (e.g., superior longitudinal muscle)

*sagittal* = in a plane perpendicular to the frontal plane (e.g., sagittal suture of the cranium)

*transversal* = in a transversal plan, at right angles to the long axis of the body or organ (e.g., transversus abdominis muscle)

*transverse* = running transversely (e.g., transverse process of a thoracic vertebra)

## B. Designations for Directions and Positions of the Extremities

*proximal – distal* = located toward the root of the extremity – located toward the free end of the extremity (e.g., proximal and distal radioulnar joints)

For the upper extremity:
*radial – ulnar* = on the radial side – on the ulnar side (e.g., ulnar and radial arteries)

For the hand:
*palmar – dorsal* = toward the palm of the hand – toward the back of the hand (e.g., palmar aponeurosis)

For the lower extremity:
*tibial – fibular (peroneal)* = on the tibial side – on the fibular side

For the foot:
*plantar – dorsal* = toward the sole of the foot – toward the upper surface of the foot (e.g., lateral and medial plantar arteries, dorsal artery of the foot)

# Abbreviations

| | | |
|---|---|---|
| ant. | = | anterior |
| a. or aa. | = | artery or arteries |
| art. | = | articulation |
| br. | = | branch |
| caud. | = | caudal |
| cran. | = | cranial |
| dist. | = | distal |
| dors. | = | dorsal |
| ext. | = | external |
| exten. | = | extensor |
| flex. | = | flexor |
| inf. | = | inferior |
| int. | = | interior |
| inteross. | = | interosseous |
| lat. | = | lateral |
| lig. or ligg. | = | ligament or ligaments |
| m. or mm. | = | muscle or muscles |
| med. | = | medial |
| n. or nn. | = | nerve or nerves |
| obl. | = | oblique |
| post. | = | posterior |
| prot. | = | protuberance |
| prox. | = | proximal |
| r. or rr. | = | ramus or rami |
| sup. | = | superior |
| superf. | = | superficial |
| surf. | = | surface |
| sut. | = | suture |
| transv. | = | transverse |
| tuberc. | = | tubercle |
| tuberos. | = | tuberosity |
| v. or vv. | = | vein or veins |
| vent. | = | ventral |
| vert. | = | vertebra |

Terms are those of the Paris Nomenclature Anatomica (PNA) with a few exceptions: BNA indicates terms of the Basle Nomenclature Anatomica, 1895, and INA indicates Jena Nomenclature, 1936.

# Etymology of Anatomical Terms of Volume I

acetabulum ........ L. *acetum*, vinegar
-*bulum*, a small cup
Cup-shaped part of hip bone which resembles the Roman vinegar cruet.

acromion ........ Gr. *akron*, summit ⎫ Highest point
*ōmos*, shoulder ⎭ of shoulder

ala .............. L. wing

alveolus ......... L. dim. of *alveus*, a hollow, a cavity. Vesalius in 16th century called the tooth socket an *alveolus*; and Rossignol in 19th century applied the term to the minute parts of the lung.

anconeus ........ Gr. *ankon*, elbow

antebrachium ..... L. the forearm

anulus .......... L. a small ring, *annulus* with two n's is a medieval misspelling

anus ............ L. a ring, a circular form

apertura ......... L. an opening, a hole

arachnoidal ....... Gr. *arachnē*, spider
*eidos*, resemblance
Applied in mid-17th century to the thin, cobweb-like structures.

arcuate .......... L. *arcus*, arch or bow

articulation ....... L. *articulus*, dim. of *artus*, joint
-*atio*, suffix, meaning action

aspera .......... L. *asper, -era, -erum*, rough, *uneven*

atlas ............ Vesalius in 16th century gave this name to the 1st cervical vertebra which supported the head, naming it after the Greek god, who supported the heavens on his shoulders.

biceps .......... L. *bi*, double
*caput*, head

brachium ........ L. arm
Gr. *brachiōn*, arm

brachycephalic .... Gr. *brachy*, wide
*kephalē*, head

bregma .......... Gr. front of head

brevis .......... L. short

buccinator ....... L. *bucino*, to sound a trumpet
*bucinator*, a trumpeter
Buccinator muscles form the wall of the cheek.

calcaneus ........ L. *calx, calcis,* heel

calvaria.......... L. scalp without hair, roof of cranium

cancellus......... L. a grating, lattice, crisscross with lines, hence to disfigure. This gives rise to the term "to cancel" in modern usage.

canine .......... L. *caninus*, pertaining to dog, dog teeth, eye teeth. Canines are pointed teeth resembling those of a dog.

capitate.......... L. *capitatus*, having a head
*caput*, head

carpus .......... Gr. *karpos*, root of the hand, wrist. Found in writings of Galen.

ca ilaget ......... L. *cartilago*, gristle, cartilage

cerrvix........... L. neck or nape

cingulum ........ L. *cingo, -ere*, to surround, girdle. Shingles is the common name for Herpes zoster. The vesicles encircle the body like a girdle, following the intercostal nerves. The word shingles is a corruption of *cingulum*.

clavicle .......... L. *clavicula*, a small key, dim. of *clavis*, a key

coccyx........... Gr. *kokkyx*, cuckoo. An allusion to the resemblance to the cuckoo's bill. Herophilus applied this term about 300 B. C.

collum .......... L. neck

concha .......... Gr. *konchē*, shell of a mussel
L. *concha*, used for shell-shaped structures.

condyle ......... Gr. *kondylos* ⎫ knuckle
L. *condylus* ⎭
Expanded parts of bones at joints.

conoid .......... Gr. *konos*, cone
*eidos*, appearance, like

coracoid ......... Gr. *korakōdes* ⎫ *korax*, raven
⎭ *eidos*, resemblance
Evidently the curved coracoid process was supposed to resemble a raven's beak. Actually, no crow or raven has a hooked beak.

cornu .......... L. horn
cornua (pl.)

coronoid......... Gr. *korōnē*, crow
*eidos*, resembling
Shaped like the beak of a crow.

corrugator ....... L. *con* (cor-) together
*ruga*, wrinkle
*corrugo*, to make wrinkles

costal .......... L. *costa*, rib, a side, a wall

cranium ......... Gr. *kranion*, the skull

cremaster ........ Gr. *kremastēr*, a suspender
Galen used this for muscle that suspends the testicle.

cribriform ....... L. *cribrum*, sieve ⎫ sieve-like plate
*forma*, form ⎭ of ethmoid

crista galli ....... L. *crista*, ridge, crest ⎫ cock's
*gallus*, a cock ⎭ comb

cruciate.......... L. *crux, cruris*, a cross, cross-shaped

crus ............ L. leg
crura (pl.)

cubital .......... L. *cubitum*, elbow, cubit. An ancient measure, a cubit was equal to 18–22 inches.

cuneiform........ L. *cuneus*, wedge
*forma*, shape
Wedge-shaped bones in wrist and ankle.

decussate ........ L. *decussatio*, intersection of two lines
*decussis*, ten was represented by X which is the intersection of two lines in the form of a cross.

deltoid . . . . . . . . . . Gr. *delta*, Greek letter *Δ*
*eidos*, resembling

diaphragm . . . . . . . Gr. *dia*, across ⎱ a partition,
*phragma*, wall ⎰ wall

diaphysis . . . . . . . . Gr. *dia*, between ⎱ separates
*physis*, growth ⎰ growth areas

digit . . . . . . . . . . . . L. *digitus*, finger
Numbers are called digits because
counting was first done on fingers.

diploë . . . . . . . . . . . Gr. fem. of *diplous*, double, folded.
Ancient name for spongiosa of the
bones of the *calvaria*.

disc . . . . . . . . . . . . . Gr. *diskos*, the flat disc between
individual vertebrae

dolichocephalic . . . . Gr. *dolichos*, long
*kephalē*, head

dorsal . . . . . . . . . . . L. *dorsum*, the back

epiphysis . . . . . . . . Gr. *epi*, upon, on top ⎱ upon growth
*physis*, growth ⎰ areas

epistropheus . . . . . . Gr. *epi*, upon
(BNA) *strephein*, to turn
*ho epistropheys*, theturner,
pivot, axis (second cervical
vertebra)

ethmoid . . . . . . . . . Gr. *ethmos*, a sieve
*eidos*, resemblance

facies. . . . . . . . . . . . L. a surface

fascia . . . . . . . . . . . L. *fascia*, a band, girth

fasciculus . . . . . . . . L. dim. of *fascis*, a small bundle

femoral . . . . . . . . . L. *femur, femoris*, the thigh

fibula . . . . . . . . . . . L. clasp, brooch, that which fastens
two things together. The tibia and
fibula resemble a bar-pin. (see also
*peroneal*)

flava . . . . . . . . . . . . L. *flavus*, golden yellow

fontanel . . . . . . . . . L. *fons, fontis*, spring, fountain
Fr. *fontanelle*, dim. of *fontaine*, foun-
tain. The fontanels in the infant skull
are probably so-called because the
rhythmical pulsation, which is visible,
resembles a snall bubbling fountain.

foramen . . . . . . . . . L. a hole, an opening

fossa . . . . . . . . . . . . L. a pit or ditch; in anatomy,
a deep depression

fovea . . . . . . . . . . . L. a pit; in anatomy, a shallow depression

foveola . . . . . . . . . . L. dim. *fovea*, a small pit

frontal . . . . . . . . . . L. *frons, frontis*, forehead

gastrocnemius . . . . . Gr. *gaster*, belly
*kneme*, lower leg
A muscle belly resting upon the shin-
bone (the bulging belly of the calf)
Spigelius, in 17th century, coined
the term.

gemellus . . . . . . . . . L. dim. *geminus*, double, twins
paired

genioglossus. . . . . . . Gr. *geneion*, chin,
*glossa*, tongue

genu . . . . . . . . . . . . L. knee (genitive, *genus*)
Used for bent structures.

ginglymus. . . . . . . . .Gr. *ginglymos*, a hinge-joint

glabella . . . . . . . . . L. *glaber*, beardless, smooth, bald.
A smooth prominence more
pronounced in the male.

gladiolus . . . . . . . . . L. dim. of *gladius*, a sword. Middle
portion or body of the sternum was
formerly called gladiolus because of
its swordshape.

gluteus . . . . . . . . . . Gr. *gloutos*, rump,
pl., the buttocks

gracilis . . . . . . . . . . L. slender, thin, strap-like

hallux . . . . . . . . . . . L. *hallex*, great toe
*allex*, an older Latin term for
thumb or great toe

hamate . . . . . . . . . . L. *hamus*, hook, curved

hamulus . . . . . . . . . L. dim. of *hamus*, a small hook

hiatus . . . . . . . . . . . L. *hiatus*, an opening, a yawn,
aperture, cleft

humerus . . . . . . . . . L. shoulder

hyoid . . . . . . . . . . . Gr. *hy*, Gr. letter upsilon.
*eidos*, resemblance
Hyoid bone
resembles a Greek upsilon.

hypophysis . . . . . . . Gr. *hypo*, below, under
*physis*, growth
This gland grows under the brain.

ilium. . . . . . . . . . . . L. *ilia*, groin, flank

Inca Bone . . . . . . . . Occasionally exists as a separate
bone, separated from the rest of the
occipital by the *sutura mendosa* (INA).
Observed especially in the ancient
Peruvian skulls among the Incas.
(PNA, interparietal bone)

incisura. . . . . . . . . . L. *in*, into
*caedere*, to cut
*incido*, an incision, to cut into

incus . . . . . . . . . . . . L. *cudere*, to beat
*incus (incudis)*, an anvil.
Galen first noted the resemblance of
the ossicle to an anvil.

index . . . . . . . . . . . L. *indico*, to point out, inform, betray
*index, -icis*, a discoverer,
an informer

infundibulum. . . . . . L. *infundere*, to pour into, to wet,
moisten
*-bulum*, the vessels, small cup,
funnel
A funnel-shaped passage.

inguinal . . . . . . . . . L. *inguen*, groin, front part of body
between the hips

ischium . . . . . . . . . Gr. *ischion*, hip

juga (cerebralia) . . . L. *jugo*, to bind, to join (A crossbeam
or rail fastened horizontally to
perpendicular poles)

labium . . . . . . . . . . L. lip

labia (pl.) Applied to other liplike structures
besides the mouth.

lambdoidal. . . . . . . Gr. *lambda*, Gr. letter *λ*
*eidos*, resemblance
Applied to suture shaped like the
Gr. lambda *λ*

larynx . . . . . . . . . . Gr. voice box
First used in English in 16th century.

latus . . . . . . . . . . . L. broad, wide, extended, side or flank

levator . . . . . . . . . L. *levere*, to raise
*levator, -oris*, a lifter, a thief

lumbar . . . . . . . . . L. *lumbus*, loin

lumbrical ........ L. *lumbricus*, intestinal worm, earthworm-shaped

lunate .......... L. *luna*, the moon
*lunatus*, crescent-shaped

malar .......... L. *mala*, cheek bone, jaw

malleolar ........ L. *malleolus*, dim. *malleus*, a small hammer. The "little hammers" of the foot are much larger than those of the ear.

malleus .......... L. *malleus*, a hammer, mallet, maul.

mandibula ........ L. *mando, -onis*, a glutton ⎱ lower
*mandere*, to chew ⎰ jaw

manubrium ....... L. handle, from *manus*, a hand. Handle of a sword.

manus .......... L. the hand

masseter ......... Gr. *masētēr*, the chewer
One of the few muscles named by Galen.

mastoid ......... Gr. *mastos*, breast
*eidos*, resembling
Mastoid process resembles the nipple.

maxilla .......... L. dim. of *mala*, jaw bone
Now restricted to upper jaw.

meniscus......... Gr. *meniskos*, a crescent
L. *menis*, a little half-moon

mentalis ......... L. *mentum*, chin

mesaticephalic ..... Gr. *mesatius*, medium
*kephalē*, head

metacarpus ....... Gr. *meta*, after, between, over
*karpos*, the wrist

metatarsus ....... Gr. *meta*, after, between
*tarsos*, the flat of the foot

multangulum ...... L. *multus*, many ⎱ having
*angulus*, corner ⎰ many angles

multifidus ........ L. *multus*, many
*findo*, to split, to divide, cleft into many parts, diverse, manifold

musculus ........ L. dim. of *mus*, mouse; in old German texts actually called "*Mauslein*". A muscle resembles a little mouse running under the skin.

mylohyoid ....... Gr. *myle*, a mill, for posterior teeth meaning grinders
*hy*, ancient Gr. Y
*eidos*, resemblance

myology ......... Gr. *mys*, mouse or muscle
*logus*, word or study
The study or knowledge of muscles.

navicular ........ L. *navis*, boat ⎱ This bone resem-
*-cula*, dim. ⎰ bles a small boat.

nucha(l) ......... Latinized from the Arabic, means nape or dorsal region of the neck.

obturator ........ L. *obturare*, to stop up, to close. The membrane and muscles close the obturator foramen.

occipital .......... L. *occipitium* ⎱ *ob*, back
⎰ *caput*, head
Back part of head.

olecranon........ Gr. *olēnē*, elbow
*kranion*, skull or head
Head of the elbow.

orbicular ........ L. *orbiculus*, dim. *orbis*, circle or orb

orbital .......... L. *orbita*, wheel-rut, a circuit, orbit, but used since ancient times for the eye socket.

os .............. L. *os, oris*, mouth
ora (pl.)

os .............. L. *os, ossis*, bone
ossa (pl.)

osteology ........ Gr. *osteon*, bone
*logos*, study
The study of bones.

papyracea ....... Gr. *papyrus*, paper made from the bark of tree
L. *papyraceus*, made of papyrus, papery

parietal.......... L. *paries*, wall

parotid .......... Gr. *para*, beside
*ous*, ear
Parotid gland lies just in front of ear.

patella .......... L. dim. *patina*, a small pan, little plate, knee cap (an ancient word)

pecten........... L. *pecten, -inis*, comb, weaving. Anatomical structures with comb-like projections.

pectoral ......... L. *pectus, -oris*, chest, breast

pelvis L. basin

perineum ........ Gr. *peri*, around ⎱ *perinaeon*
*naiein*, to dwell ⎰
"The space between the sexual parts and the fundament".
Andrew's Latin-English Lexicon, 1850.

peroneal ......... Gr. *perone*, brooch, the fibula, small bone of leg

pes ............. L. *pes, pedis*, foot
pedes (pl.)

petros ........... L. *petrosus*, rocky, stony ⎱ Hard as
Gr. *petra*, stony ⎰ a rock
Petrous portion of temporal bone is most dense bone in the body.

phalanx ......... L. Because of their arrangement in
phalanges (pl.) rows, the bones of the fingers are compared with the Greek battle formation.

pharynx ......... Gr. *pharynx*, throat

piriform ......... L. *pirum*, a pear ⎱ pear-shaped
*forma*, form ⎰

pisiform ......... L. *pisum*, a pea
*forma*, form, shape

plantar .......... L. *planta*, sole of the foot

platysma ........ Gr. *platys*, a plate, broad, flat, Galen first called it the *platysma myoides*, because it resembled a muscle.
(*mys*, muscle and *eidos*, resemblance)

pollex ........... L. *pollex, pollicis*, thumb

popliteal.......... L. *poples, -itis*, ham of the knee

profundus ........ L. deep, bottomless, boundless

promontory ....... L. *promineo*, to jut out
*promontorium*, highest part of mountain ridge, a headland

pronate........... L. *pronare*, to bend forward, to bow. To turn palm or face downward.

psoas ........... Gr. *psoa*, muscle of the loin

pterygoid ........ Gr. *pteryx*, wing
*eidos*, resemblance
The pterygoid process resembles a wing in shape.

pubis............ L. *pubis*, grown up, adult, i.e., the hair
pubes (pl.) which appears on the body at the age of puberty.

pudendalis ........ L. *pudenda,* the parts of shame, the privy parts
     *pudere,* to be ashamed
     *pudendum,* external genitalia

pulp ............ L. *pulpa,* flesh. The softer part of a tooth. Cicero used the word for the soft flesh of the breasts and buttocks of young girls.

quadriceps ........ L. *quadri-* ⎱ four
     *quattuor* ⎰
     *caput,* head

radius ........... L. spoke of a wheel. Galen used this term.

rectus ........... L. *rego, rexi, rectum,* to keep straight
     *rectus, -a, -um,* straight, upright

retinaculum ....... L. *retineo,* to hold back, to restrain
     *retinaculum,* that which holds back or binds.

rostrum ......... L. beak, bill, mouth
The curved end of a ship's prow.

sacrum .......... L. *sacer,* sacred. A very ancient anatomical term. Applied to the pelvic keystone because it was thought this bone survived after death and became part of the body after resurrection.

sagittal .......... L. *sagitta,* shaft, arrow, arrow-shaped, such as the fontanelles on child's head

sartorius ......... L. *sartor,* a patcher, tailor
The sartorius muscle is the only muscle that flexes both knee and hip joints. It is used in crossing the legs in the tailor's position.

scalene .......... Gr. *skalēnos,* uneven, triangular with uneven sides. These muscles were named by Riolan in the mid-17th century.

scaphoid ......... Gr. *skaphe,* boat
     *eidos,* resemblance
The scaphoid bone is of this shape.

scapula .......... L. *scapula,* shoulder blade. In ancient times it was used in the plural to mean the back. This term was adopted in the 17th century from the Gr. *skaptein,* to dig, because the bone resembles a spade.

sciatic ........... L. *sciaticus,* corruption of *ischiadikos,* the hip

sella turcica ....... L. *sella,* saddle
     *turcica,* Turkish
A saddle-shaped depression on the sphenoid bone, lodging the hypophysis.

serratus ......... L. *serratus,* notched
     *serra,* a saw

sesamoid ........ Gr. *sesame,* an herb
     *eidos,* resemblance
Galen used this name for the little bones because they resembled sesame seeds.

sigmoid ......... Gr. *sigma,* the Greek letter *S* which was formerly written as a single curve like our letter C.
     *eidos,* resemblance
L. *sigma,* a semi-circular couch for reclining at meals. The curved part of the large bowel, the sigmoid colon, resembles the sigma.

sinus ........... L. *sinum,* a large round drinking vessel with swelling sides.

soleus .......... L. *solum,* lowest part of a thing, sole of foot or sandal. The soleus muscle moves the sole of the foot.

sphenoid ........ Gr. *sphen,* wedge
     *eidos,* resembling
Wedge-shaped from any view, but it resembles a butterfly.

spinalis .......... L. *spinalis,* of or belonging to the spine or vertebral column.

splenius ......... Gr. *splēnion,* plaster, bandage
Applied to any structure resembling a bandage.

squama.......... L. a fish scale

stapes ........... L. *stirrup.* Smallest ossicle resembles a stirrup. It is thought that the ancients used no stirrups, and that the term was adopted into Medieval Latin from Old High German, *stapf,* a step.

sternum ......... Gr. *sternon,* the male chest, until Galen limited the meaning to breast bone.

sulcus .......... L. groove, ditch, furrow made by a plow.

supercilium ....... L. *super,* above ⎱ eyebrow
     *cilium,* eyelid ⎰

supinate ......... L. *supinus, -a, -um,* bent backward, thrown backward, lying on the back, supine

sura............. L. calf of the leg

sustentaculum ..... L. *sub,* under ⎱ *sustento,* to hold
     *teneo,* to hold ⎰ upright, support

suture ........... L. *suo, sui, sutum,* to sew or stitch together
     *sutura,* a seam, a suture

symphysis ........ Gr. *syn,* with, together
     *physis,* growth
Grown together, not a true joint.

synchondrosis ..... Gr. *syn,* with, together
     *chondros,* cartilage

synovial ......... Gr. *syn,* with
     L. *ovum,* egg
Modern Latin word invented by Paracelsus in the 16th century. He evidently thought the joint synovial fluid resembled egg white.

talus ............ L. ankle or one of a set of dice. The Romans carved the heelbone or talus of horses for dice.

tarsus ........... Gr. *tarsos,* the flat of the foot (also edge of eyelid)

tegmen .......... L. *tego,* to cover, to shelter, protect
     *tegumen,* a covering, a roof

temporal ........ L. *tempus,* time
     *temporalis,* lasting but for a time, of or belonging to the temples of the head. The temporal region was so named because human hair first turns gray at temples, and this is one of the indications of the passage of time.

teres ............ L. round

thorax........... Gr. *thōrax,* chest, breast plate

thyroid .......... Gr. *thyreos,* a large oblong shield used by Greeks
     *eidos,* resemblance

Named by Wharton in the 17th century. However, Vesalius was the first person to accurately describe the thyroid.

tibia ............ L. an ancient flute, originally made from an animal's leg bone.

trabeculae ....... L. dim. of *trabs*, a beam

triceps........... L. *tri*, three
caput, head

triquetrum ....... L. *triquetrus*, having 3 corners, angles, or edges; triangular

trochanter ....... Gr. *trechein*, to run
*trochantēr*, runner
*trochos*, a wheel
Muscles used for running are attached to the trochanter.

trochlea ......... L. pulley

tuba ............ L. a straight trumpet

tuber............ L. a hump, a knot, or swelling (eminence)
L. *tumeo, -ere*, to swell

tuberculum ....... L. dim. *tuber*, a small swelling or protuberance

tuberosity........ L. dim. *tuber*
-*osity*, condition
*tuberosus*, full of lumps
Prominence for attachment of muscles.

tympanus........ Gr. *tympanon*, drum
L. *tympanum*, tambourine
The eardrum.

ulna ............ L. elbow, forearm. Now limited to the larger bone of the forearm.

umbilicus ........ L. the navel

uncinate ......... L. *uncus*, hooks
*uncinatus*, furnished with hooks or barbs.

unguis........... L. nail of a person's finger or toe

vagina........... L. scabbard or sheath

vastus ........... L. huge, immense

vertebra ......... L. *vertero*, to turn
*vertebra*, joint
This term adopted in early 17th century.

vomer ........... L. plowshare
Vomer resembles this in shape.

Wormian ........ Small irregularly shaped bones sometimes found along the cranial sutures. These were named for Ole Worm, Danish anatomist, 1599–1654. They are now called sutural bones.

xiphoid.......... Gr. *xiphos*, sword
*eidos*, resemblance
The name for the tip of the sternum, due to its swordshape.

zygomatic ....... Gr. *zygon*, yoke
*zygoma*, bolt or bar
Cheek bone yokes or joins several bones together.

# Regions of the Human Body

2

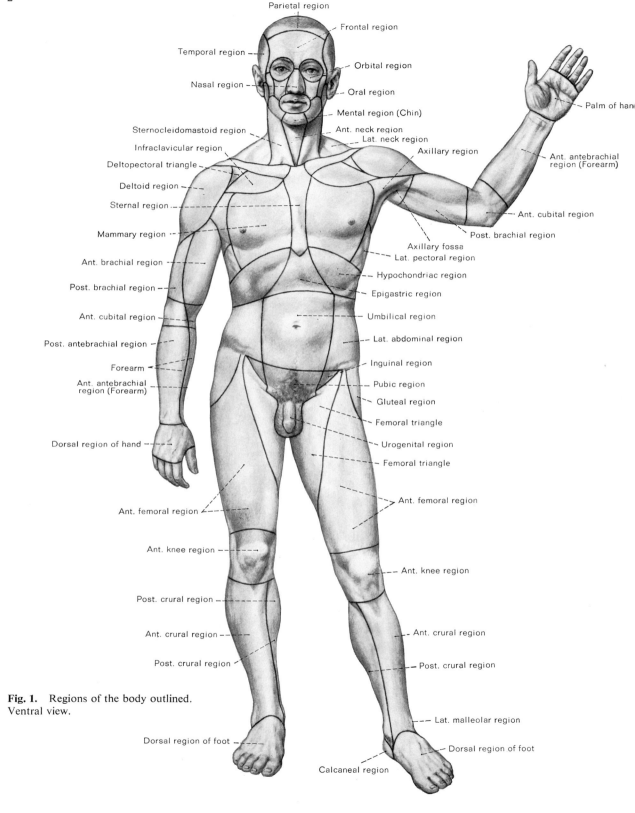

Parietal region
Frontal region
Temporal region —
Orbital region
Nasal region —
Oral region
Mental region (Chin)
Ant. neck region
Sternocleidomastoid region
Lat. neck region
Infraclavicular region
Axillary region
Deltopectoral triangle
Deltoid region —
Sternal region
Palm of han[
Ant. antebrachial
region (Forearm)
Mammary region
Ant. cubital region
Post. brachial region
Axillary fossa
Lat. pectoral region
Ant. brachial region —
Hypochondriac region
Post. brachial region —
Epigastric region
Ant. cubital region —
Umbilical region
Post. antebrachial region —
Lat. abdominal region
Forearm
Inguinal region
Ant. antebrachial
region (Forearm)
Pubic region
Gluteal region
Femoral triangle
Urogenital region
Dorsal region of hand —
Femoral triangle
Ant. femoral region
Ant. femoral region
Ant. knee region —
Ant. knee region
Post. crural region —
Ant. crural region —
Ant. crural region
Post. crural region —
Post. crural region
Lat. malleolar region
Dorsal region of foot —
Dorsal region of foot
Calcaneal region

**Fig. 1.** Regions of the body outlined.
Ventral view.

3

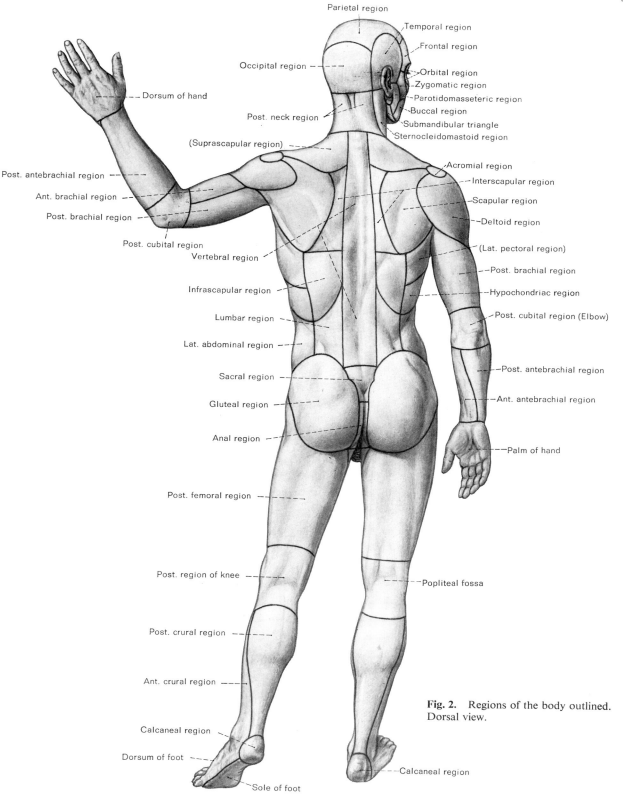

Parietal region

Temporal region

Frontal region

Occipital region

Orbital region

Zygomatic region

Parotidomasseteric region

Buccal region

Post. neck region

Submandibular triangle

Sternocleidomastoid region

(Suprascapular region)

Acromial region

Post. antebrachial region

Interscapular region

Ant. brachial region

Scapular region

Post. brachial region

Deltoid region

Post. cubital region

(Lat. pectoral region)

Vertebral region

Post. brachial region

Infrascapular region

Hypochondriac region

Lumbar region

Post. cubital region (Elbow)

Lat. abdominal region

Dorsum of hand

Post. antebrachial region

Sacral region

Ant. antebrachial region

Gluteal region

Anal region

Palm of hand

Post. femoral region

Post. region of knee

Popliteal fossa

Post. crural region

Ant. crural region

Calcaneal region

Dorsum of foot

Calcaneal region

Sole of foot

**Fig. 2.** Regions of the body outlined. Dorsal view.

4

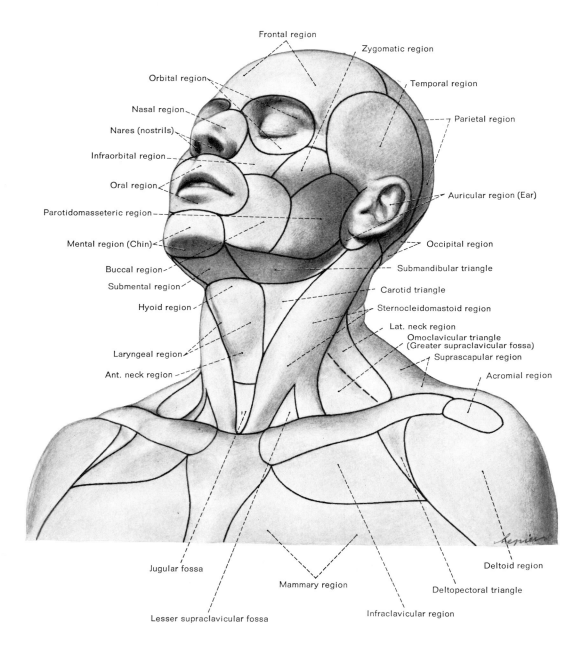

**Fig. 3.** Regions of the head, neck, and upper body outlined. Ventral view.

Frontal region
Zygomatic region
Orbital region
Temporal region
Nasal region
Parietal region
Nares (nostrils)
Infraorbital region
Oral region
Auricular region (Ear)
Parotidomasseteric region
Mental region (Chin)
Occipital region
Buccal region
Submandibular triangle
Submental region
Carotid triangle
Hyoid region
Sternocleidomastoid region
Lat. neck region
Omoclavicular triangle
(Greater supraclavicular fossa)
Suprascapular region
Laryngeal region
Acromial region
Ant. neck region
Jugular fossa
Deltoid region
Mammary region
Deltopectoral triangle
Lesser supraclavicular fossa
Infraclavicular region

5

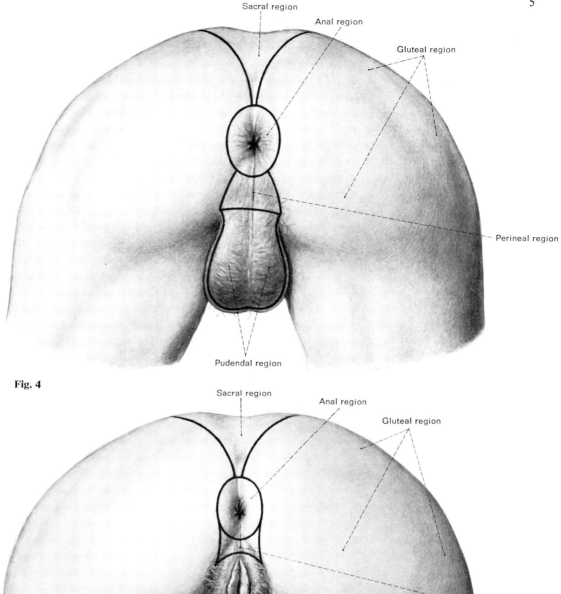

Fig. 4

Fig. 5

**Figs. 4 and 5.** Perineal regions of the body outlined, male and female.

# Osteology

## General Characteristics and Classifications of Bones

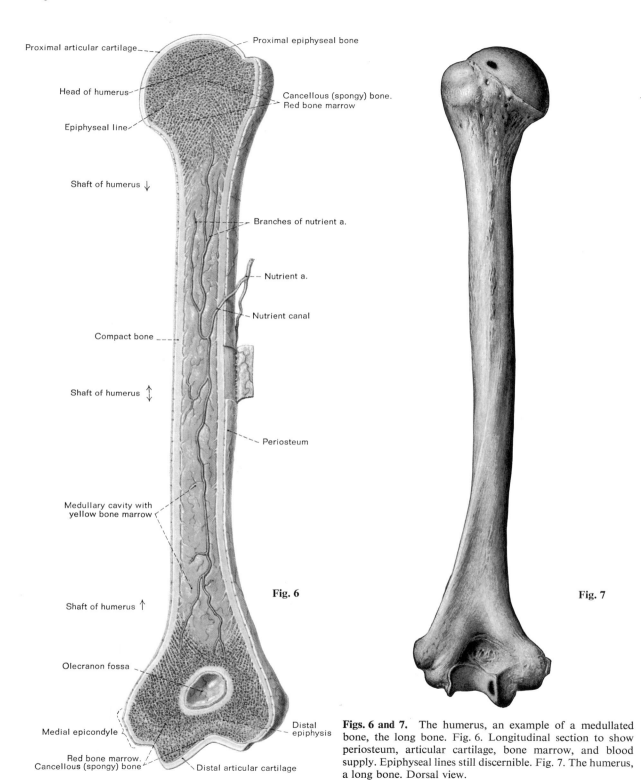

Proximal articular cartilage

Proximal epiphyseal bone

Head of humerus

Cancellous (spongy) bone.
Red bone marrow

Epiphyseal line

Shaft of humerus ↓

Branches of nutrient a.

Nutrient a.

Nutrient canal

Compact bone

Shaft of humerus ↕

Periosteum

Medullary cavity with
yellow bone marrow

Shaft of humerus ↑

**Fig. 6**

Olecranon fossa

Medial epicondyle

Distal
epiphysis

Red bone marrow.
Cancellous (spongy) bone

Distal articular cartilage

**Fig. 7**

**Figs. 6 and 7.** The humerus, an example of a medullated bone, the long bone. Fig. 6. Longitudinal section to show periosteum, articular cartilage, bone marrow, and blood supply. Epiphyseal lines still discernible. Fig. 7. The humerus, a long bone. Dorsal view.

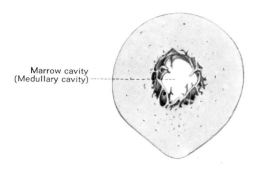

Marrow cavity
(Medullary cavity)

**Fig. 8.** Cross section of the shaft of a long bone, showing the medullary cavity.

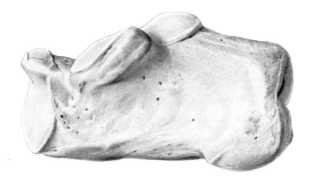

**Fig. 9.** The calcaneus, an example of a short bone.

**Fig. 10.** The sternum, an example of a flat bone.

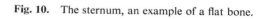

**Fig. 11.** The temporal bone. An example of a pneumatic bone, sectioned to show mastoid air cells.

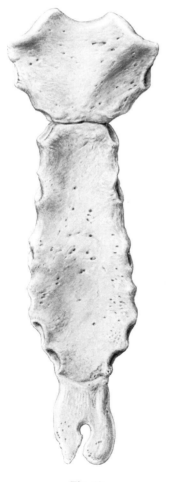

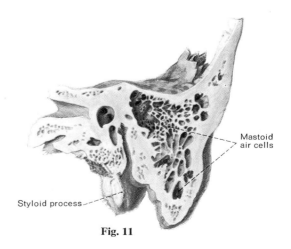

Mastoid air cells

Styloid process

**Fig. 10**

**Fig. 11**

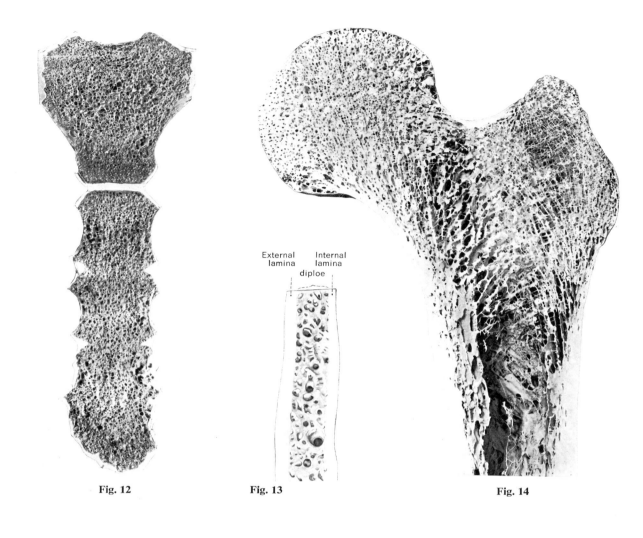

External lamina    Internal lamina
diploe

**Fig. 12**           **Fig. 13**           **Fig. 14**

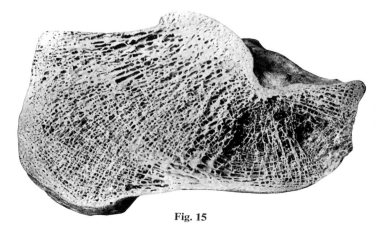

**Fig. 15**

**Fig. 12.** Sectioned surface of the sternum. The manubriosternal synchondrosis is the fibrocartilage which appears clear between the manubrium and the body of the sternum.

**Fig. 13.** A sectioned flat cranial bone (slightly enlarged).

**Fig. 14.** Frontal longitudinal section of the proximal end of the femur.

**Fig. 15.** Sagittal longitudinal section of the calcaneus. The trabeculae are oriented to give maximum strength and elasticity with minimal weight.

11

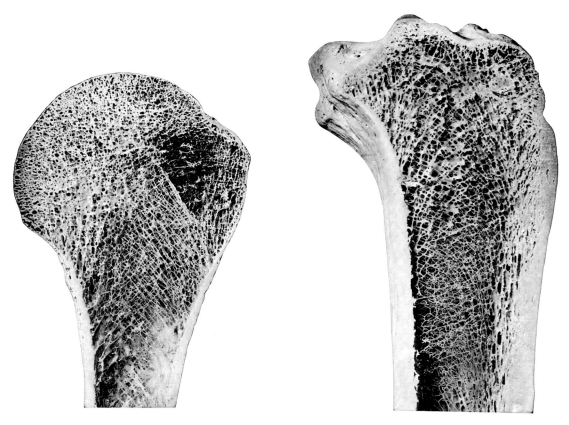

**Fig. 16.** Frontal longitudinal section through the proximal end of the humerus.

**Fig. 17.** Sagittal longitudinal section through the proximal end of the tibia.

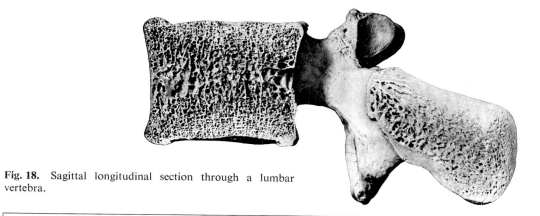

**Fig. 18.** Sagittal longitudinal section through a lumbar vertebra.

Note: The structure of the trabeculae in the cancellous bones gives rise to the "trajectorial theory", i.e., the bony trabeculae follow the lines of maximal internal stress. (Figs. 14, 15, 16)

# Osteology

*The Trunk*

## Summary of the Structural Characteristics of the Typical Vertebra

|  | 7 Cervical* | 12 Thoracic | 5 Lumbar | Sacrum 5 Vertebrae |
|---|---|---|---|---|
| Terminal surfaces of the body of the vertebrae | rectangular small | somewhat triangular | bean-shaped large | fused |
| Vertebral foramen | triangular large | round | triangular small | sacral canal |
| Articular surfaces (articular processes) | oblique, sloping toward dorsal | frontal | sagittal | intermediate sacral crest |
| Transverse processes | transverse process | club-shaped with transverse costal facet | mammillary and accessory processes | lateral sacral crest |
| Spinous processes | horizontal short divided | directed steeply caudalward | horizontal, lateral, large flattened | median sacral crest |
| Rib rudiments | ventral part transverse process and dorsal tubercle | none, since the ribs are developed | costal process | lateral parts |
| Characteristic differentiations | transverse foramen | inf. and sup. costal facets | mammillary and accessory processes | synostosis of the vertebrae |

* The first two cervical vertebrae, the atlas and axis, are not typical cervical vertebrae. They have special characteristics.

**Figs. 19–21.** Spinal columns. Fig. 19. Ventral view. Fig. 20. Dorsal view. Fig. 21. Left lateral view. The transverse costal ▶ facet is missing on the 10th thoracic vertebra.

15

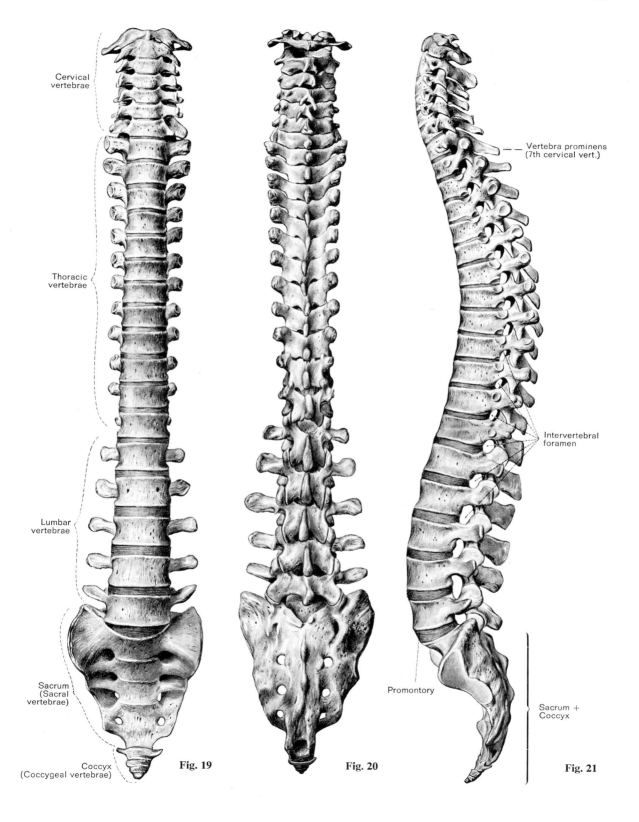

Cervical
vertebrae

Thoracic
vertebrae

Lumbar
vertebrae

Sacrum
(Sacral
vertebrae)

Coccyx
(Coccygeal vertebrae)

Vertebra prominens
(7th cervical vert.)

Intervertebral
foramen

Promontory

Sacrum +
Coccyx

**Fig. 19**

**Fig. 20**

**Fig. 21**

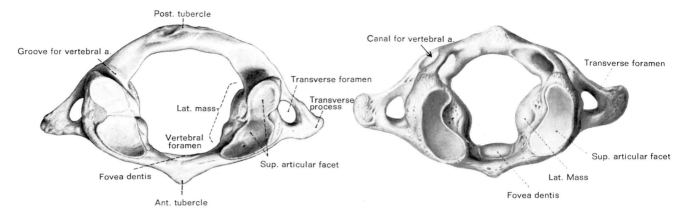

**Fig. 22.** Atlas. Cranial view.

**Fig. 23.** Atlas. Cranial view, with closed sulcus for vertebral artery.

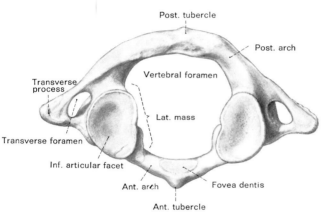

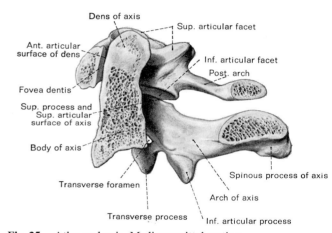

**Fig. 24.** Atlas. Caudal view.

**Fig. 25.** Atlas and axis. Median sagittal section.

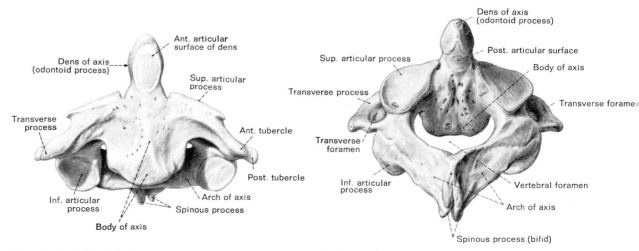

**Fig. 26.** Axis. Ventral view.

**Fig. 27.** Axis. Dorsal view.

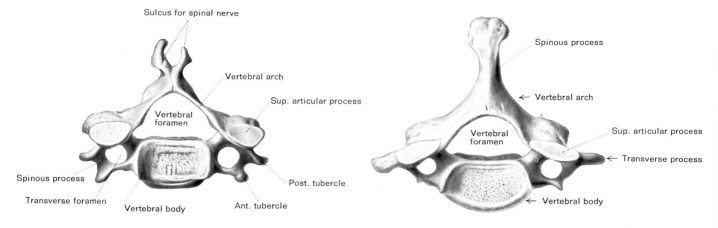

**Fig. 28.** Fifth cervical vertebra. Cranial view.

**Fig. 29.** Seventh cervical vertebra (vertebra prominens). Cranial view.

**Fig. 30.** Cervical spinal column. Dorsal view, somewhat from right side. Roman numerals indicate the number of the cervical vertebra.

**Fig. 31.** Lower cervical spinal column. Ventral view. * Cranial flanges of lateral borders of vertebral bodies.

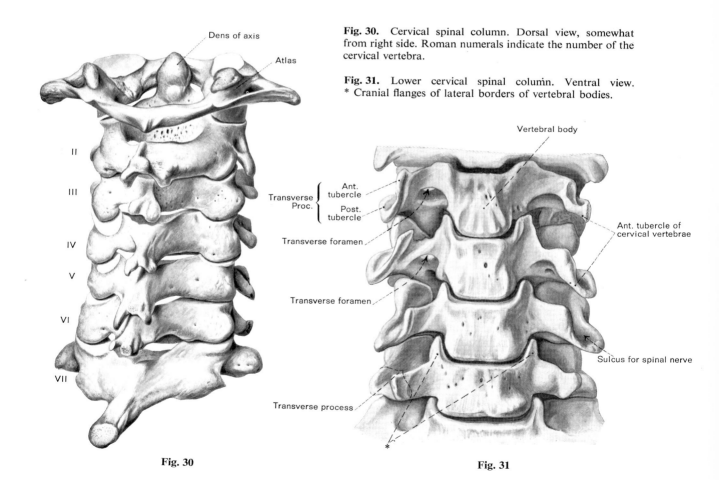

**Fig. 30**

**Fig. 31**

18

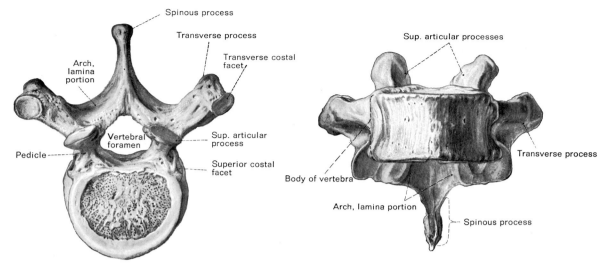

**Fig. 32.** Sixth thoracic vertebra. Cranial view.

**Fig. 33.** Tenth thoracic vertebra. Ventral view.

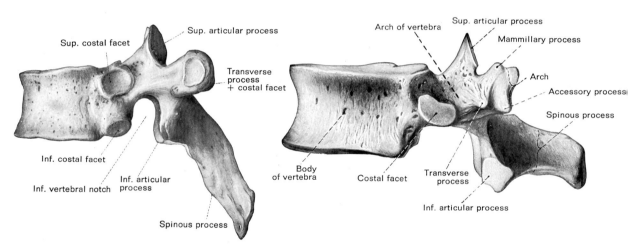

**Fig. 34.** Sixth thoracic vertebra. Left lateral view.

**Fig. 35.** Twelfth thoracic vertebra. Left lateral view.

Note: The sixth thoracic vertebra has three articular surfaces for the ribs: an upper, on the body for the 6th rib; a lower, on the body for the 7th rib; and one on the transverse process for the 6th rib. On the 12th thoracic vertebra, there is only one articular surface present, which is for the 12th rib.

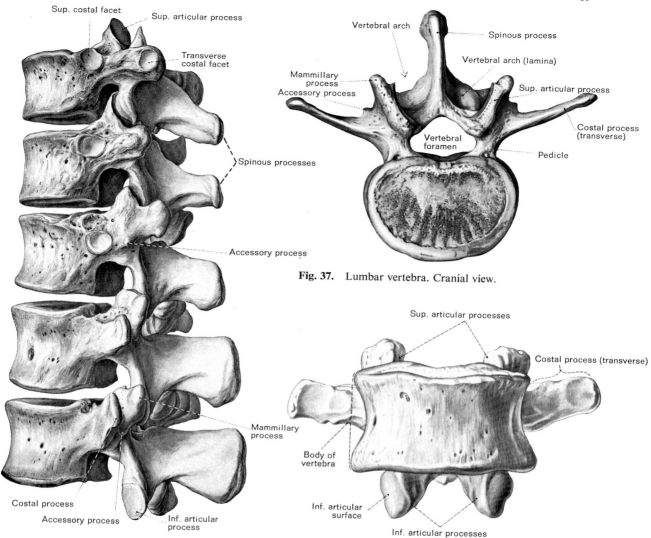

Fig. 37. Lumbar vertebra. Cranial view.

Fig. 36. The last three thoracic vertebrae, X–XII, and the first two lumbar vertebrae, I and II. Left lateral view.

Fig. 38. Lumbar vertebra. Ventral view.

Note: The increase in size of the body of the more caudal vertebrae. The two lower vertebrae of Fig. 36 are lumbar. They have no articular surfaces for ribs, but the rib rudiments, costal processes, are present. The transverse process is divided into an upper mammillary and a small lower process called the accessory. The articular surfaces of the articular processes are, on the thoracic vertebrae, directed ventrally and dorsally; on the lumbar vertebrae, sagittally (ante- and retroflexion are possible). The spinous processes of the lumbar vertebrae are massive and somewhat quadrilateral and extend more horizontal than those of the thoracic.

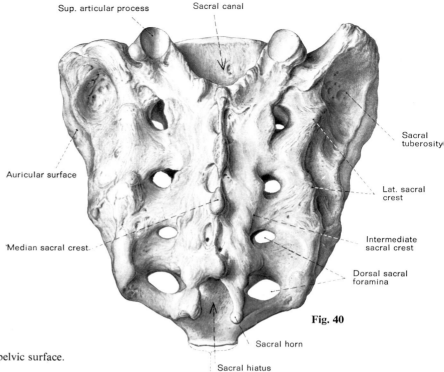

Sup. articular process

Sacral canal

Sacral
tuberosity

Auricular surface

Lat. sacral
crest

Median sacral crest

Intermediate
sacral crest

Dorsal sacral
foramina

**Fig. 40**

Sacral horn

Sacral hiatus

Apex of sacrum

**Fig. 39.** The sacrum. Ventral view, pelvic surface.

**Fig. 40.** The sacrum. Dorsal view.

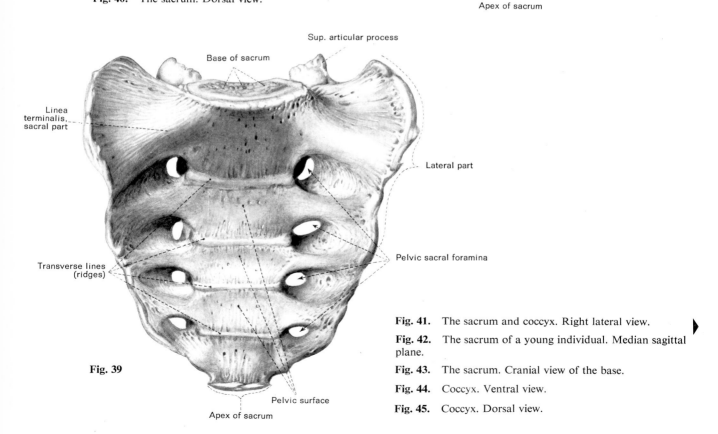

Base of sacrum

Sup. articular process

Linea
terminalis,
sacral part

Lateral part

Transverse lines
(ridges)

Pelvic sacral foramina

**Fig. 39**

Pelvic surface

Apex of sacrum

**Fig. 41.** The sacrum and coccyx. Right lateral view.

**Fig. 42.** The sacrum of a young individual. Median sagittal plane.

**Fig. 43.** The sacrum. Cranial view of the base.

**Fig. 44.** Coccyx. Ventral view.

**Fig. 45.** Coccyx. Dorsal view.

21

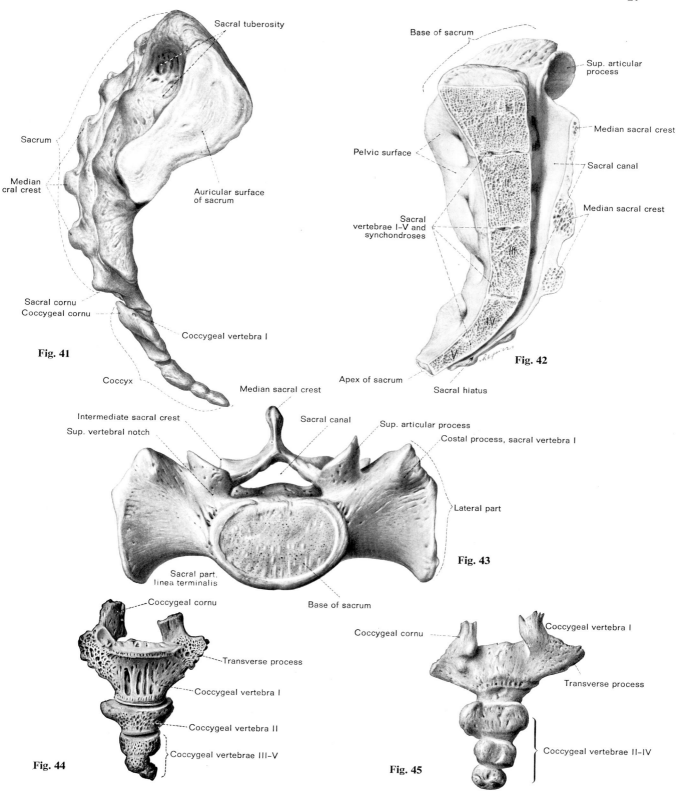

Sacral tuberosity

Base of sacrum

Sup. articular process

Sacrum

Median sacral crest

Median cral crest

Pelvic surface

Sacral canal

Auricular surface of sacrum

Sacral vertebrae I–V and synchondroses

Median sacral crest

Sacral cornu
Coccygeal cornu

Coccygeal vertebra I

**Fig. 41**

Coccyx

Apex of sacrum

Sacral hiatus

**Fig. 42**

Median sacral crest

Intermediate sacral crest

Sacral canal

Sup. vertebral notch

Sup. articular process

Costal process, sacral vertebra I

Lateral part

**Fig. 43**

Sacral part, linea terminalis

Base of sacrum

Coccygeal cornu

Transverse process

Coccygeal cornu

Coccygeal vertebra I

Coccygeal vertebra I

Transverse process

Coccygeal vertebra II

Coccygeal vertebrae III–V

Coccygeal vertebrae II–IV

**Fig. 44**

**Fig. 45**

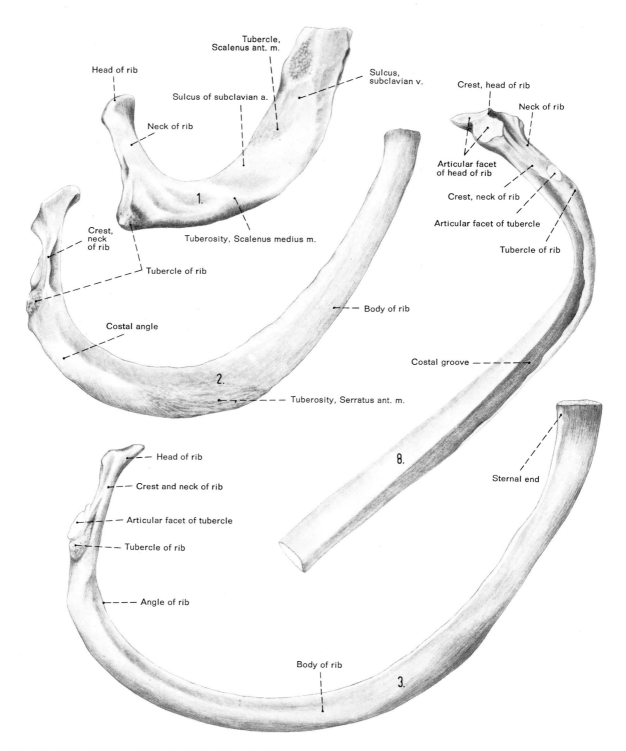

**Fig. 46.** 1st, 2nd, 3rd, and 8th ribs of the right side of the thorax, without costal cartilages. Seen from above. The shortened 8th rib is seen from below.

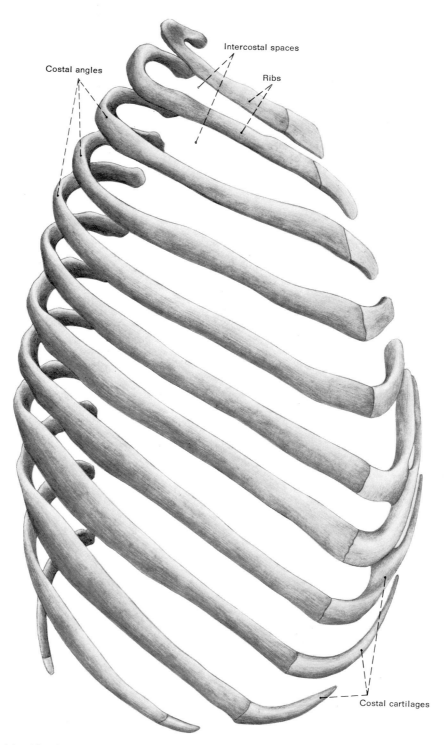

**Fig. 47.** The ribs of the right side of the thorax, in the natural position.

24

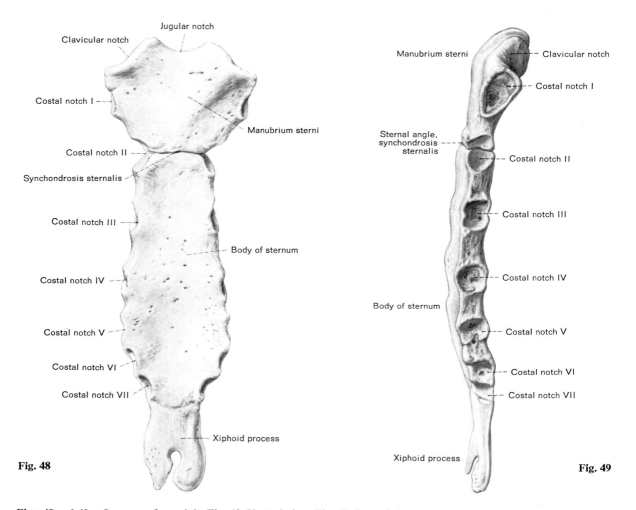

Clavicular notch

Jugular notch

Costal notch I

Costal notch II

Synchondrosis sternalis

Costal notch III

Costal notch IV

Costal notch V

Costal notch VI

Costal notch VII

Manubrium sterni

Body of sternum

Xiphoid process

**Fig. 48**

Manubrium sterni

Clavicular notch

Costal notch I

Sternal angle,
synchondrosis
sternalis

Costal notch II

Costal notch III

Body of sternum

Costal notch IV

Costal notch V

Costal notch VI

Costal notch VII

Xiphoid process

**Fig. 49**

**Figs. 48 and 49.** Sternum of an adult. Fig. 48. Ventral view. Fig. 49. Lateral view.

**Fig. 50.** Skeleton of the trunk with shoulder and pelvic girdles and the proximal part of the femur in blue. Left median half viewed from the lateral side.
**Fig. 51.** Skeleton of the trunk, with shoulder and pelvic girdles in blue. Left median half viewed from median aspect.

25

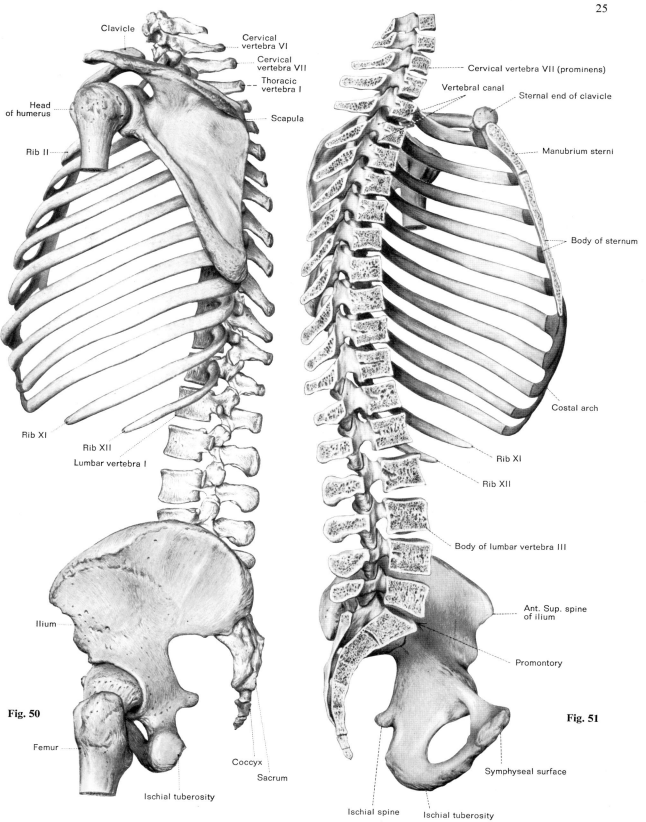

Clavicle

Cervical vertebra VI

Cervical vertebra VII

Thoracic vertebra I

Head of humerus

Scapula

Rib II

Rib XI

Rib XII

Lumbar vertebra I

Ilium

Femur

Ischial tuberosity

Coccyx

Sacrum

Fig. 50

Cervical vertebra VII (prominens)

Vertebral canal

Sternal end of clavicle

Manubrium sterni

Body of sternum

Costal arch

Rib XI

Rib XII

Body of lumbar vertebra III

Ant. Sup. spine of ilium

Promontory

Symphyseal surface

Ischial spine

Ischial tuberosity

Fig. 51

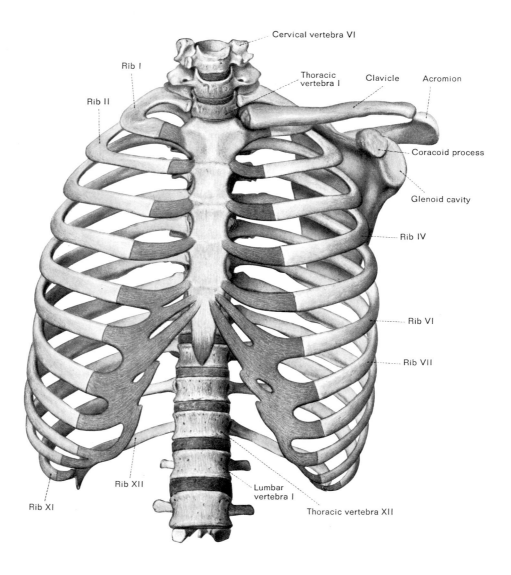

**Fig. 52.** Thorax. Ventral view (moderate inspiration). Left shoulder girdle blue.

Note: The insertion of the second rib meets the sternal angle, i.e., where the manubrium meets the body of the sternum (synchondrosis). This bulge across the sternum is always palpable under the skin as an indication of the ending of the second rib.

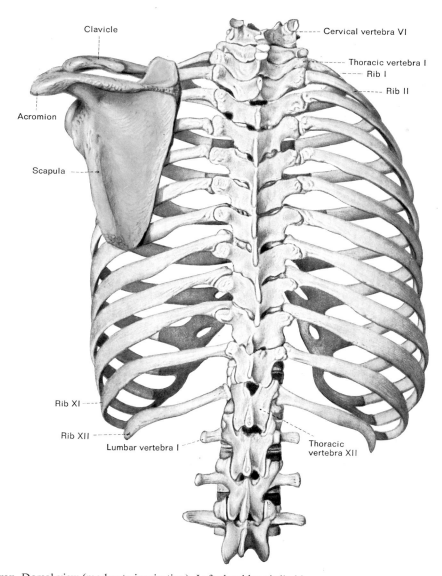

Clavicle

Acromion

Scapula

Rib XI

Rib XII

Lumbar vertebra I

Cervical vertebra VI

Thoracic vertebra I

Rib I

Rib II

Thoracic
vertebra XII

**Fig. 53.** Thorax. Dorsal view (moderate inspiration). Left shoulder girdle blue.

Note: The superior thoracic aperture is bounded by the first thoracic vertebra, the first rib, the manubrium sterni with its jugular notch. The inferior thoracic aperture is bounded by the 12th thoracic vertebra, the 12th rib, and the cartilaginous costal arch. The upper seven ribs are called true ribs because they are attached by cartilage to the sternum. The remaining 5 are called false ribs because they are not directly attached to the sternum. Three of them form the costal arch; and the 11th and 12th are referred to as floating ribs.

# Osteology

*The Skull*

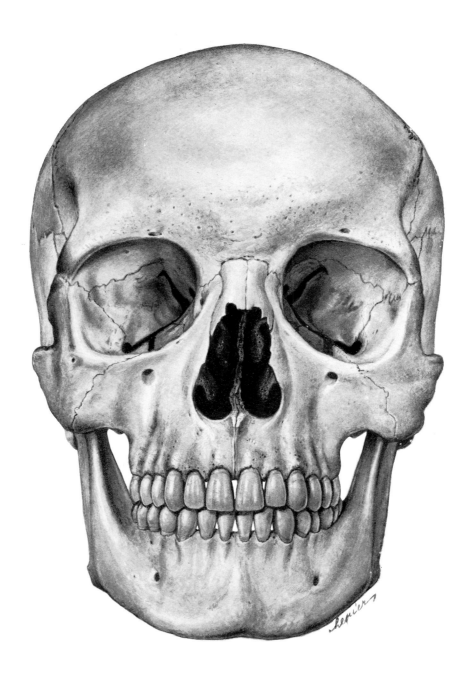

**Fig. 54.** The skull. Anterior aspect.

31

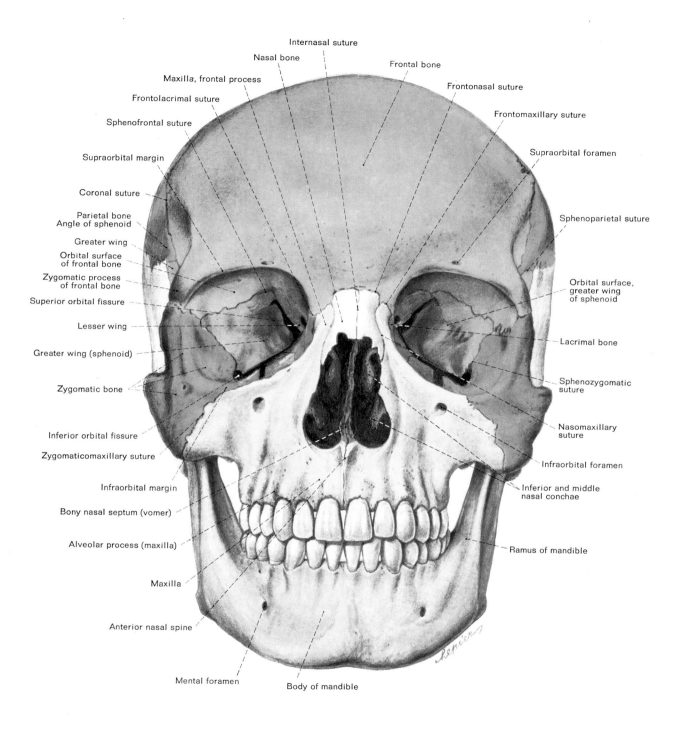

**Fig. 55.** The skull. Anterior aspect. The bones are set apart by different colors.

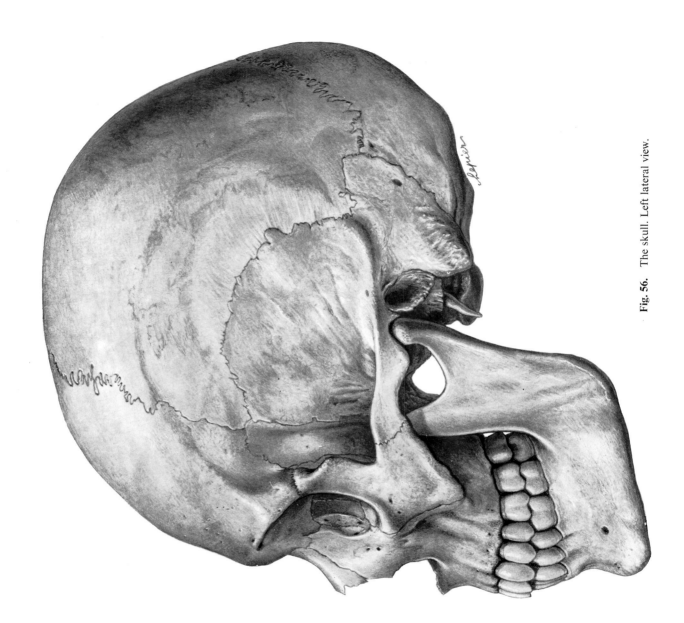

**Fig. 56.** The skull. Left lateral view.

33

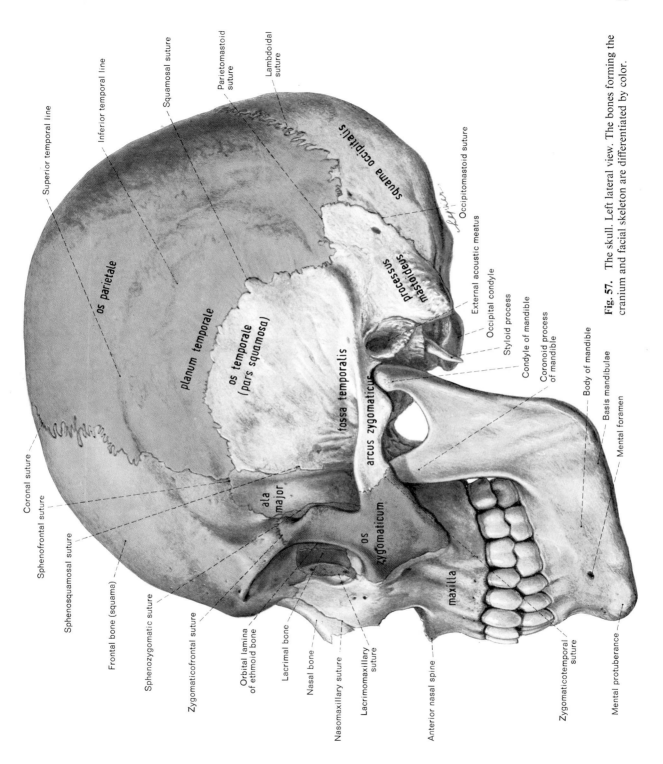

Superior temporal line

Inferior temporal line

Squamosal suture

Parietomastoid suture

Lambdoidal suture

os parietale

planum temporale

squama occipitalis

Occipitomastoid suture

External acoustic meatus

processus mastoideus

Occipital condyle

os temporale (pars squamosa)

Styloid process

Condyle of mandible

fossa temporalis

Coronoid process of mandible

arcus zygomaticus

Body of mandible

Basis mandibulae

ala major

Mental foramen

os zygomaticum

maxilla

Coronal suture

Sphenofrontal suture

Sphenosquamosal suture

Frontal bone (squama)

Sphenozygomatic suture

Zygomaticofrontal suture

Orbital lamina of ethmoid bone

Lacrimal bone

Nasal bone

Nasomaxillary suture

Lacrimomaxillary suture

Anterior nasal spine

Zygomaticotemporal suture

Mental protuberance

**Fig. 57.** The skull. Left lateral view. The bones forming the cranium and facial skeleton are differentiated by color.

34

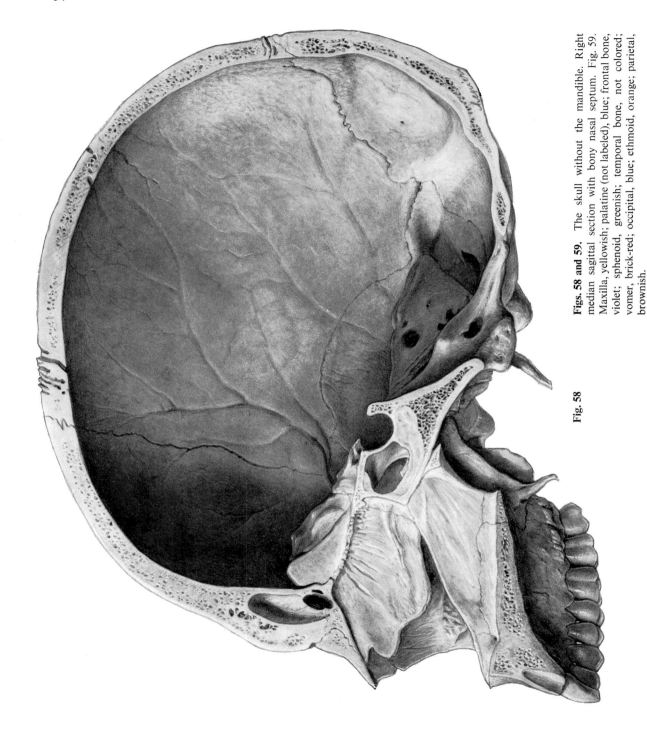

Fig. 58

**Figs. 58 and 59.** The skull without the mandible. Right median sagittal section with bony nasal septum. Fig. 59. Maxilla, yellowish; palatine (not labeled), blue; frontal bone, violet; sphenoid, greenish; temporal bone, not colored; vomer, brick-red; occipital, blue; ethmoid, orange; parietal, brownish.

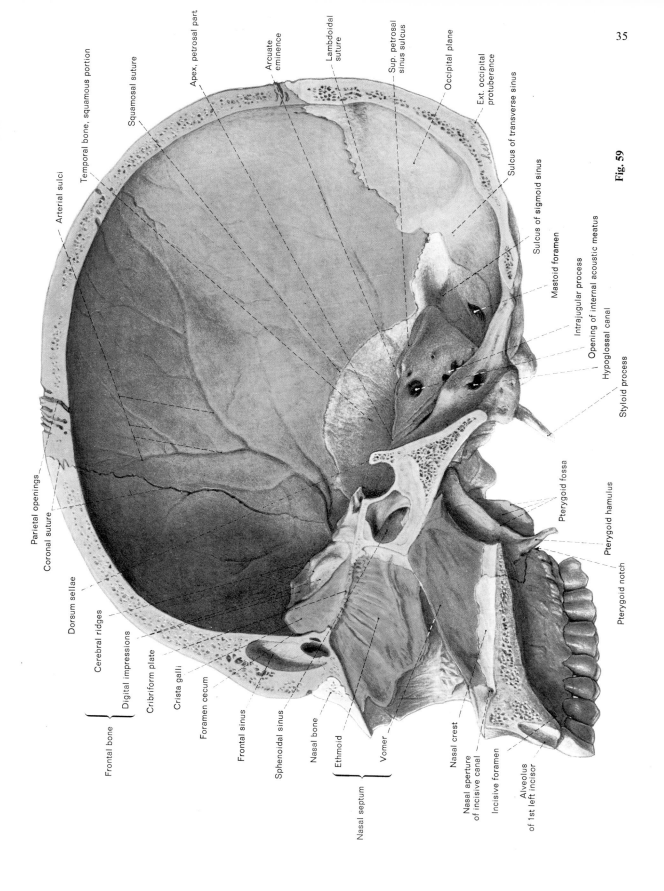

35

Fig. 59

Arterial sulci

Temporal bone, squamous portion

Squamosal suture

Apex, petrosal part

Arcuate eminence

Lambdoidal suture

Sup. petrosal sinus sulcus

Occipital plane

Ext. occipital protuberance

Sulcus of transverse sinus

Sulcus of sigmoid sinus

Mastoid foramen

Intrajugular process

Opening of internal acoustic meatus

Hypoglossal canal

Styloid process

Pterygoid fossa

Pterygoid hamulus

Pterygoid notch

Parietal openings

Coronal suture

Dorsum sellae

Cerebral ridges

Digital impressions

Cribriform plate

Crista galli

Foramen cecum

Frontal sinus

Sphenoidal sinus

Nasal bone

Ethmoid

Vomer

Nasal crest

Nasal aperture of incisive canal

Incisive foramen

Alveolus of 1st left incisor

Nasal septum

Frontal bone

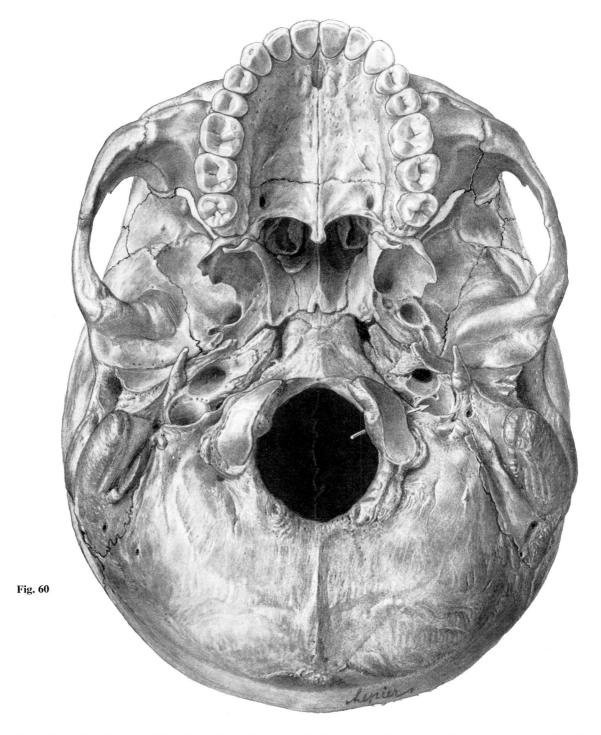

**Fig. 60**

**Figs. 60 and 61.** The base of the skull, without the mandible, from below. Arrow in the hypoglossal canal in Fig. 61.

37

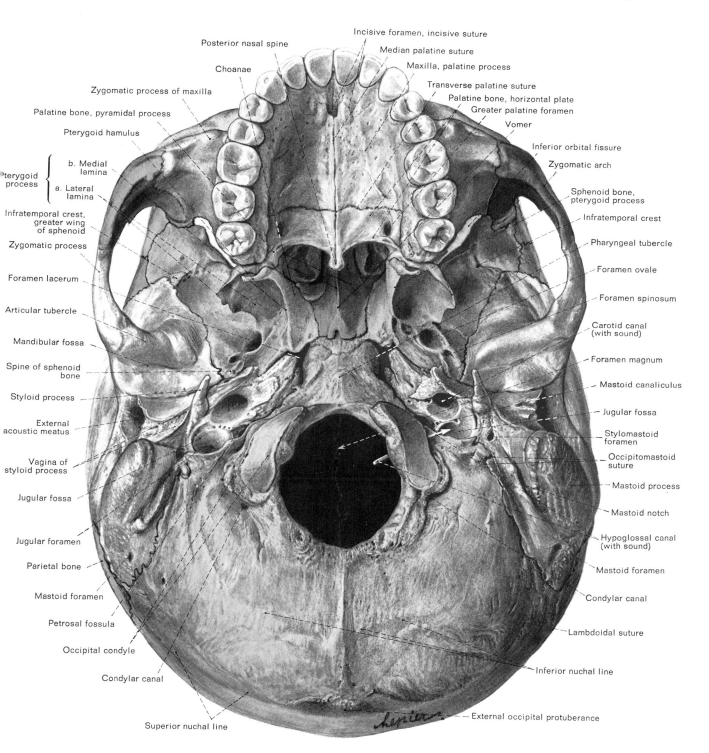

Posterior nasal spine

Choanae

Zygomatic process of maxilla

Palatine bone, pyramidal process

Pterygoid hamulus

b. Medial lamina

Pterygoid process

a. Lateral lamina

Infratemporal crest, greater wing of sphenoid

Zygomatic process

Foramen lacerum

Articular tubercle

Mandibular fossa

Spine of sphenoid bone

Styloid process

External acoustic meatus

Vagina of styloid process

Jugular fossa

Jugular foramen

Parietal bone

Mastoid foramen

Petrosal fossula

Occipital condyle

Condylar canal

Superior nuchal line

Incisive foramen, incisive suture

Median palatine suture

Maxilla, palatine process

Transverse palatine suture

Palatine bone, horizontal plate

Greater palatine foramen

Vomer

Inferior orbital fissure

Zygomatic arch

Sphenoid bone, pterygoid process

Infratemporal crest

Pharyngeal tubercle

Foramen ovale

Foramen spinosum

Carotid canal (with sound)

Foramen magnum

Mastoid canaliculus

Jugular fossa

Stylomastoid foramen

Occipitomastoid suture

Mastoid process

Mastoid notch

Hypoglossal canal (with sound)

Mastoid foramen

Condylar canal

Lambdoidal suture

Inferior nuchal line

External occipital protuberance

**Fig. 61**

38

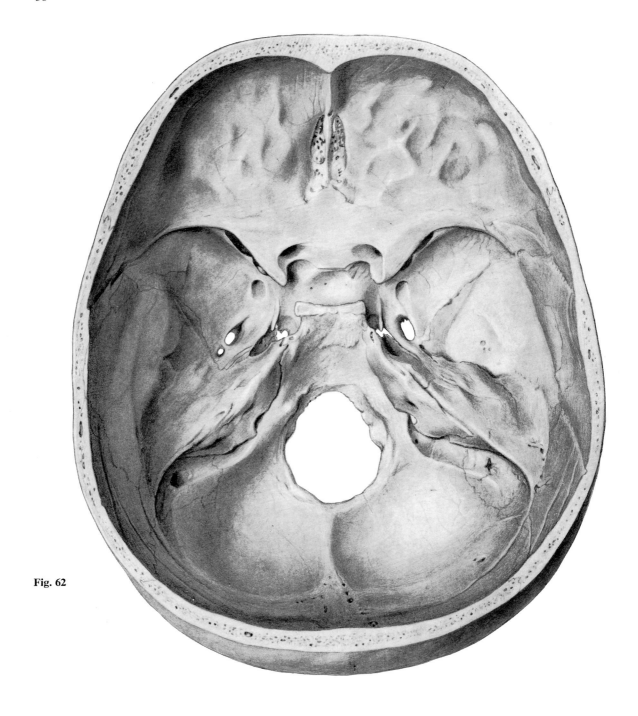

**Fig. 62**

**Figs. 62 and 63.** The base of the skull. Interior surfaces. Eight bones form the cranium; two are paired, so there are only six names to remember.

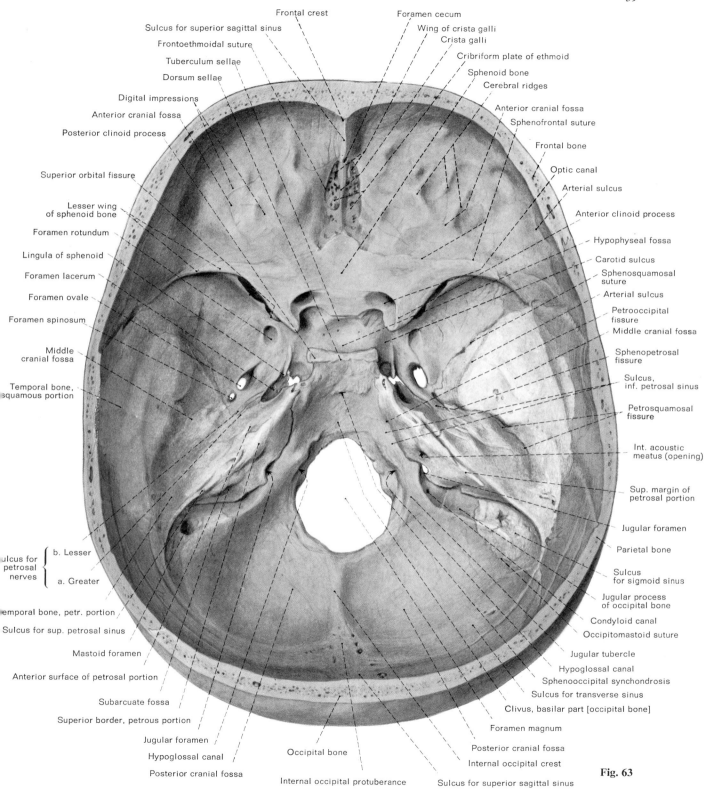

Frontal crest

Foramen cecum

Sulcus for superior sagittal sinus

Wing of crista galli

Frontoethmoidal suture

Crista galli

Tuberculum sellae

Cribriform plate of ethmoid

Dorsum sellae

Sphenoid bone

Cerebral ridges

Digital impressions

Anterior cranial fossa

Sphenofrontal suture

Anterior cranial fossa

Posterior clinoid process

Frontal bone

Superior orbital fissure

Optic canal

Arterial sulcus

Lesser wing
of sphenoid bone

Anterior clinoid process

Foramen rotundum

Hypophyseal fossa

Lingula of sphenoid

Carotid sulcus

Foramen lacerum

Sphenosquamosal
suture

Foramen ovale

Arterial sulcus

Foramen spinosum

Petrooccipital
fissure

Middle
cranial fossa

Middle cranial fossa

Temporal bone,
squamous portion

Sphenopetrosal
fissure

Sulcus,
inf. petrosal sinus

Petrosquamosal
fissure

Int. acoustic
meatus (opening)

Sup. margin of
petrosal portion

Jugular foramen

Parietal bone

b. Lesser
ulcus for
petrosal
nerves

Sulcus
for sigmoid sinus

a. Greater

Jugular process
of occipital bone

emporal bone, petr. portion

Condyloid canal

Sulcus for sup. petrosal sinus

Occipitomastoid suture

Mastoid foramen

Jugular tubercle

Anterior surface of petrosal portion

Hypoglossal canal

Sphenooccipital synchondrosis

Subarcuate fossa

Sulcus for transverse sinus

Superior border, petrous portion

Clivus, basilar part [occipital bone]

Jugular foramen

Foramen magnum

Hypoglossal canal

Posterior cranial fossa

Posterior cranial fossa

Occipital bone

Internal occipital crest

**Fig. 63**

Internal occipital protuberance

Sulcus for superior sagittal sinus

40

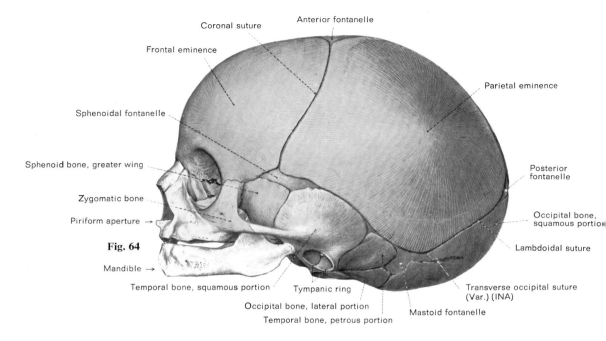

Coronal suture
Anterior fontanelle
Frontal eminence
Parietal eminence
Sphenoidal fontanelle
Sphenoid bone, greater wing
Zygomatic bone
Piriform aperture →
Posterior fontanelle
Occipital bone, squamous portion
Lambdoidal suture
Transverse occipital suture (Var.) (INA)
Mastoid fontanelle
Temporal bone, petrous portion
Occipital bone, lateral portion
Tympanic ring
Temporal bone, squamous portion
Mandible →

Fig. 64

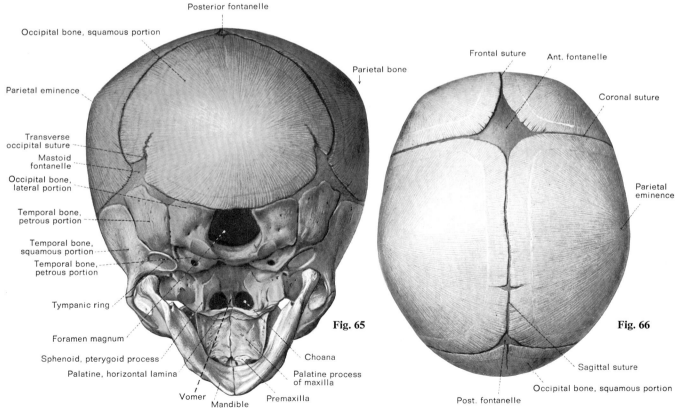

Posterior fontanelle
Occipital bone, squamous portion
Parietal bone
Parietal eminence
Transverse occipital suture
Mastoid fontanelle
Occipital bone, lateral portion
Temporal bone, petrous portion
Temporal bone, squamous portion
Temporal bone, petrous portion
Tympanic ring
Foramen magnum
Sphenoid, pterygoid process
Palatine, horizontal lamina
Vomer
Mandible
Premaxilla
Palatine process of maxilla
Choana

Fig. 65

Frontal suture
Ant. fontanelle
Coronal suture
Parietal eminence
Sagittal suture
Occipital bone, squamous portion
Post. fontanelle

Fig. 66

**Figs. 64–66.** The skull at birth. Fig. 64. Lateral view. Fig. 65. View from below and dorsally. Fig. 66. View from above.

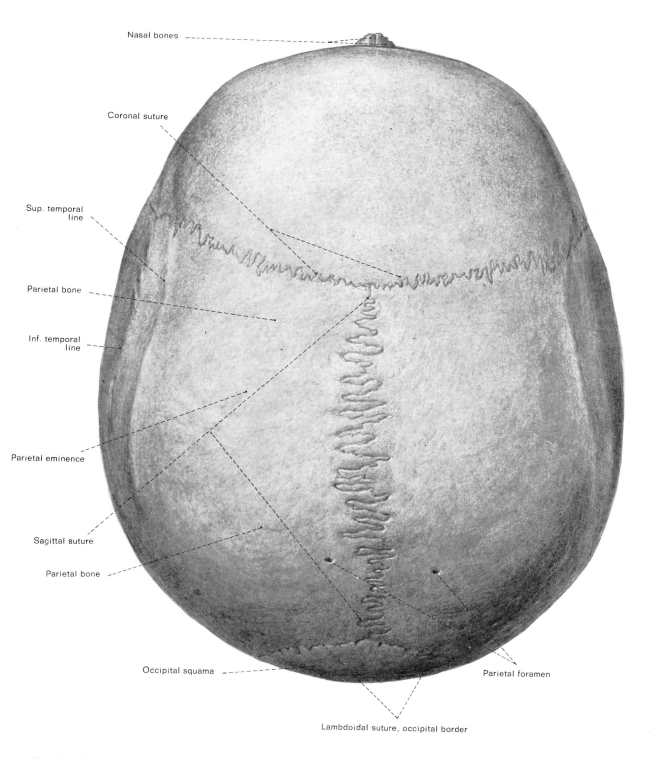

Nasal bones

Coronal suture

Sup. temporal line

Parietal bone

Inf. temporal line

Parietal eminence

Sagittal suture

Parietal bone

Parietal foramen

Occipital squama

Lambdoidal suture, occipital border

**Fig. 67.** The calvarium. Sutures of the neurocranium from above.

42

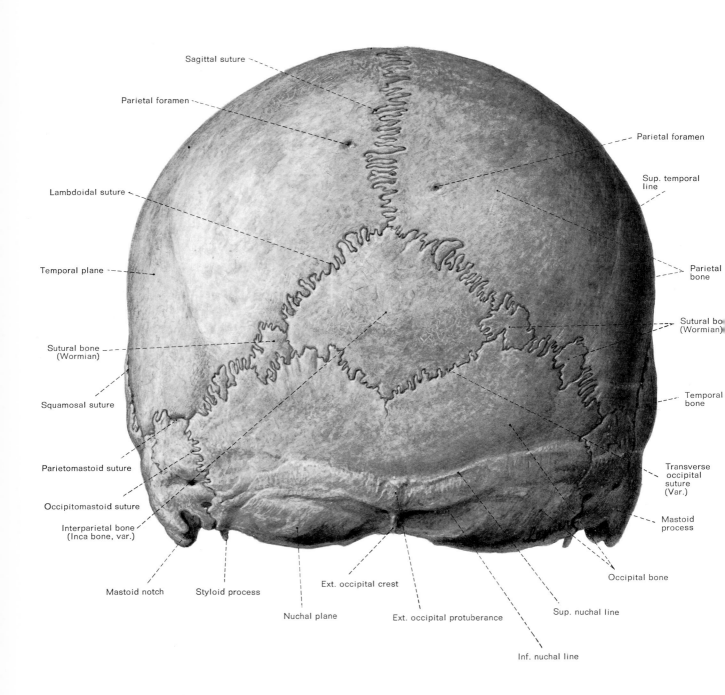

Sagittal suture

Parietal foramen

Parietal foramen

Sup. temporal line

Lambdoidal suture

Temporal plane

Parietal bone

Sutural bone (Wormian)

Sutural bone (Wormian)

Temporal bone

Squamosal suture

Parietomastoid suture

Transverse occipital suture (Var.)

Occipitomastoid suture

Mastoid process

Interparietal bone (Inca bone, var.)

Occipital bone

Mastoid notch    Styloid process    Ext. occipital crest

Sup. nuchal line

Nuchal plane    Ext. occipital protuberance

Inf. nuchal line

**Fig. 68.** Sutures of the cranium. Dorsal view. Sutural bones (Wormian) and interparietal bone formerly called the Inca bone.

43

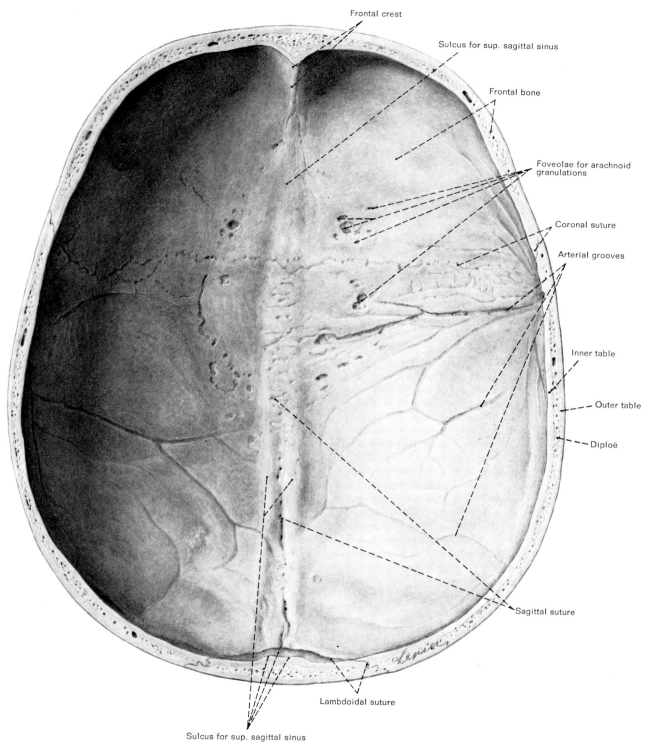

Frontal crest

Sulcus for sup. sagittal sinus

Frontal bone

Foveolae for arachnoid granulations

Coronal suture

Arterial grooves

Inner table

Outer table

Diploë

Sagittal suture

Lambdoidal suture

Sulcus for sup. sagittal sinus

**Fig. 69.** The calvarium, the neurocranial roof. Inner or cerebral surface.

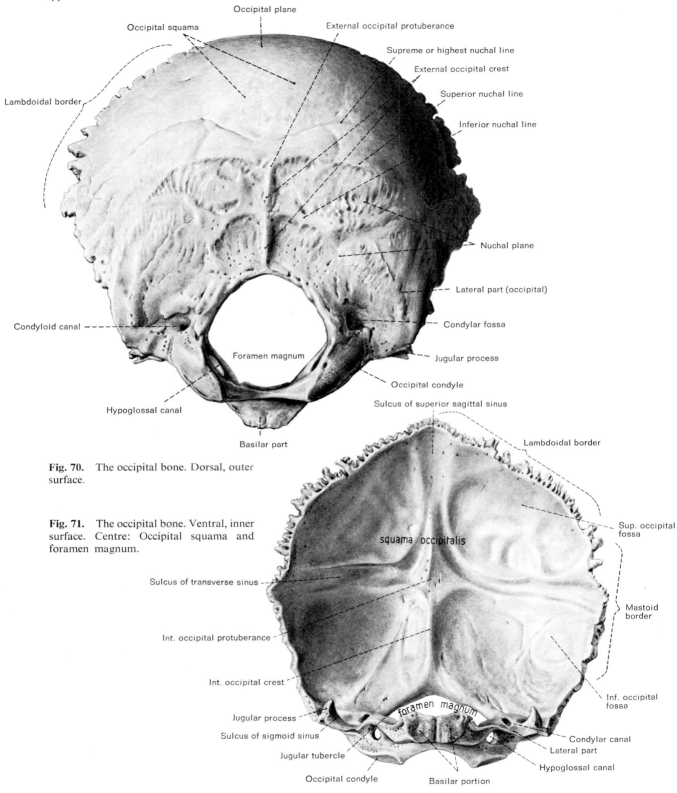

Occipital plane

Occipital squama

External occipital protuberance

Supreme or highest nuchal line

External occipital crest

Superior nuchal line

Inferior nuchal line

Lambdoidal border

Nuchal plane

Lateral part (occipital)

Condyloid canal

Condylar fossa

Jugular process

Occipital condyle

Hypoglossal canal

Foramen magnum

Basilar part

**Fig. 70.** The occipital bone. Dorsal, outer surface.

**Fig. 71.** The occipital bone. Ventral, inner surface. Centre: Occipital squama and foramen magnum.

Sulcus of superior sagittal sinus

Lambdoidal border

squama occipitalis

Sup. occipital fossa

Sulcus of transverse sinus

Int. occipital protuberance

Int. occipital crest

Mastoid border

Inf. occipital fossa

Jugular process

Sulcus of sigmoid sinus

Jugular tubercle

foramen magnum

Condylar canal

Lateral part

Hypoglossal canal

Occipital condyle

Basilar portion

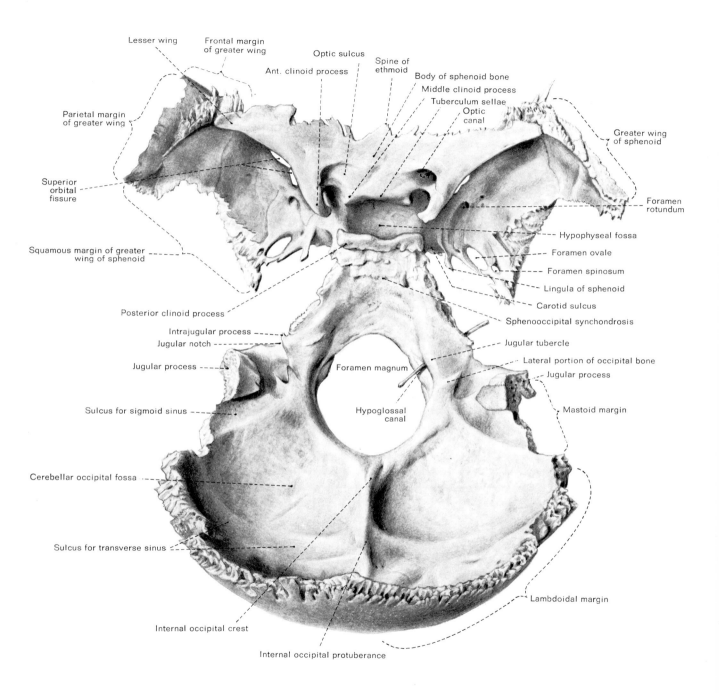

**Fig. 72.** Occipital and sphenoid bones. Seen from inside the skull. These are the bones of a growing youth, so the spheno-occipital synchondrosis is still present. The petrous part of the temporal bone in the space between the occipital and sphenoid bones is not shown.

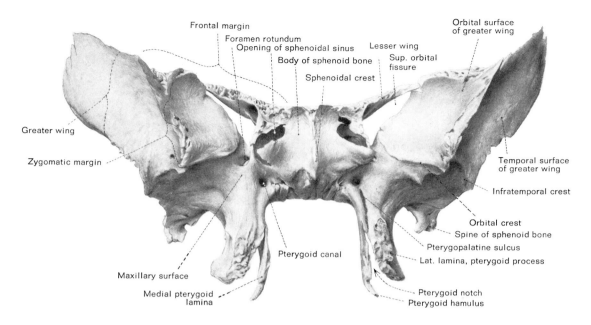

**Fig. 73.** Sphenoid bone. Ventral view.

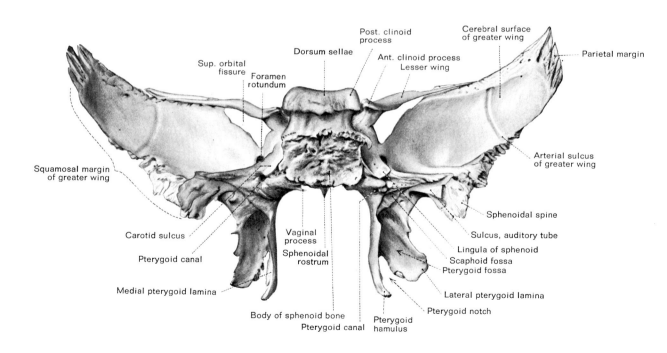

**Fig. 74.** Sphenoid bone. Dorsal view. A young person with an unossified sphenooccipital synchondrosis.

47

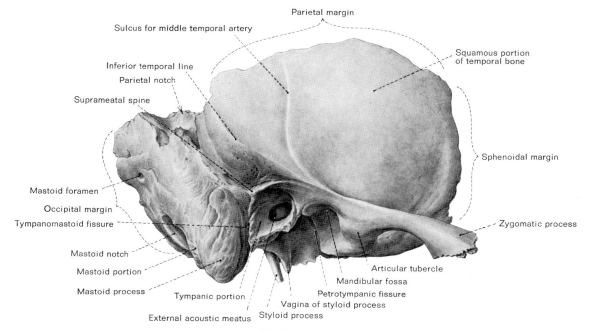

Parietal margin

Sulcus for middle temporal artery

Inferior temporal line

Parietal notch

Suprameatal spine

Squamous portion
of temporal bone

Sphenoidal margin

Mastoid foramen

Occipital margin

Tympanomastoid fissure

Mastoid notch

Mastoid portion

Mastoid process

Zygomatic process

Articular tubercle

Mandibular fossa

Petrotympanic fissure

Vagina of styloid process

Tympanic portion

External acoustic meatus

Styloid process

**Fig. 75**

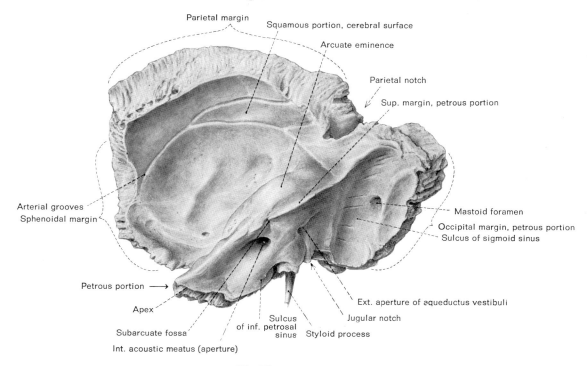

Parietal margin

Squamous portion, cerebral surface

Arcuate eminence

Parietal notch

Sup. margin, petrous portion

Arterial grooves

Sphenoidal margin

Mastoid foramen

Occipital margin, petrous portion

Sulcus of sigmoid sinus

Petrous portion →

Apex

Subarcuate fossa

Int. acoustic meatus (aperture)

Sulcus
of inf. petrosal
sinus

Styloid process

Ext. aperture of aqueductus vestibuli

Jugular notch

**Fig. 76**

**Figs. 75 and 76.**   Right temporal bone. Fig. 75. Lateral view. Fig. 76. Medial view.

48

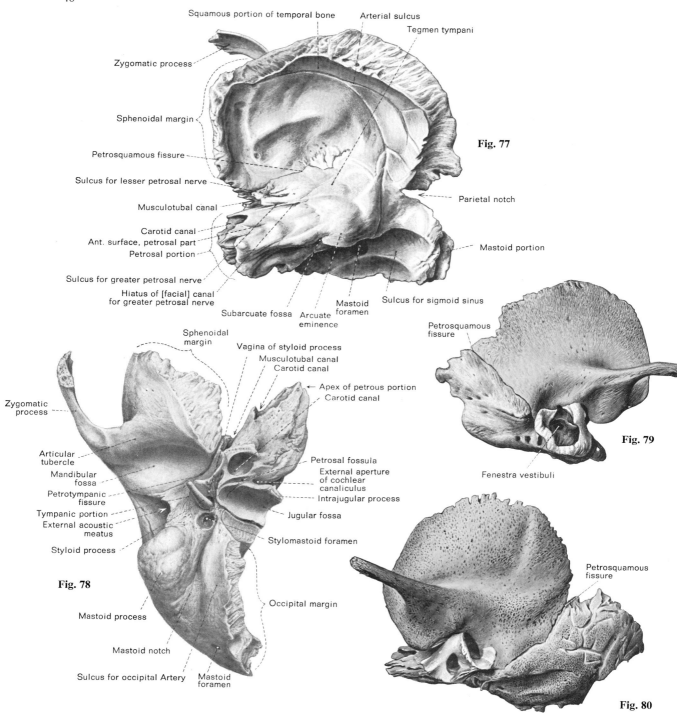

Squamous portion of temporal bone

Arterial sulcus

Tegmen tympani

Zygomatic process

Sphenoidal margin

Petrosquamous fissure

Sulcus for lesser petrosal nerve

Musculotubal canal

Carotid canal
Ant. surface, petrosal part
Petrosal portion

Sulcus for greater petrosal nerve

Hiatus of [facial] canal
for greater petrosal nerve

Subarcuate fossa

Arcuate eminence

Mastoid foramen

Sulcus for sigmoid sinus

Parietal notch

Mastoid portion

**Fig. 77**

Sphenoidal margin

Vagina of styloid process

Musculotubal canal
Carotid canal

Apex of petrous portion
Carotid canal

Zygomatic process

Articular tubercle

Mandibular fossa

Petrotympanic fissure

Tympanic portion

External acoustic meatus

Styloid process

**Fig. 78**

Mastoid process

Mastoid notch

Sulcus for occipital Artery

Mastoid foramen

Petrosal fossula

External aperture of cochlear canaliculus

Intrajugular process

Jugular fossa

Stylomastoid foramen

Occipital margin

Petrosquamous fissure

**Fig. 79**

Fenestra vestibuli

Petrosquamous fissure

**Fig. 80**

Fig. 77.   Right temporal bone. Inner cranial surface, displaying apex of petrous portion.
Fig. 78.   Right temporal bone. Caudal view, from below.
Figs. 79 and 80.   Right and left temporal bones of newborn. Squamous portion, green; petrosal portion, yellow; tympanic portion, not colored.

49

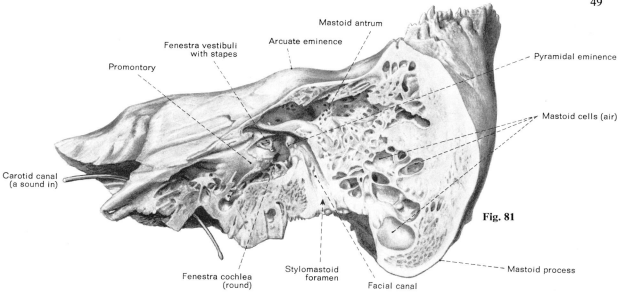

Mastoid antrum

Fenestra vestibuli
with stapes

Arcuate eminence

Promontory

Pyramidal eminence

Mastoid cells (air)

Carotid canal
(a sound in)

Fig. 81

Mastoid process

Fenestra cochlea
(round)

Stylomastoid
foramen

Facial canal

**Figs. 81–84.** Sawcuts through the temporal bone. Fig. 81. Left medial half, with probe in the carotid canal. Fig. 82. Lateral half.

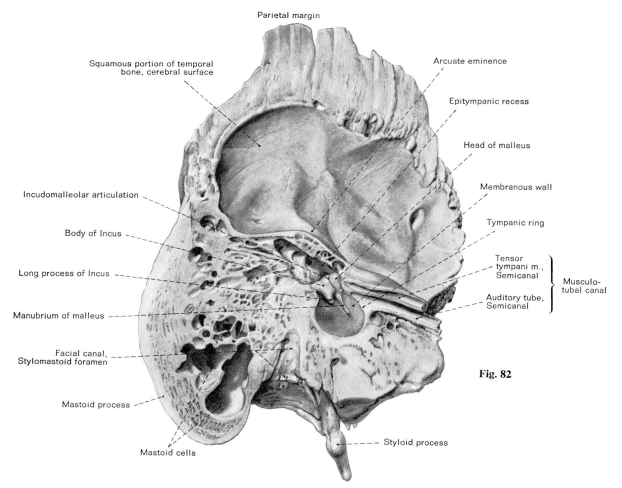

Parietal margin

Squamous portion of temporal
bone, cerebral surface

Arcuate eminence

Epitympanic recess

Head of malleus

Incudomalleolar articulation

Membranous wall

Body of Incus

Tympanic ring

Long process of Incus

Tensor
tympani m.,
Semicanal

Musculo-
tubal canal

Auditory tube,
Semicanal

Manubrium of malleus

Facial canal,
Stylomastoid foramen

Fig. 82

Mastoid process

Styloid process

Mastoid cells

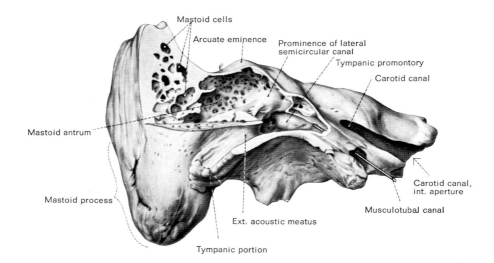

**Fig. 83.** Right temporal bone, from ventral. Mastoid cells, antrum, tympanic cavity, and outer auditory meatus, as well as a part of the musculotubal canal (with probe) were exposed by a sawcut.

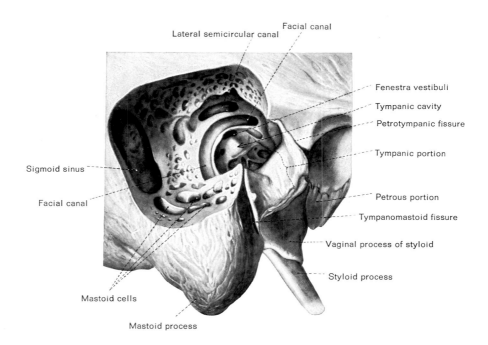

**Fig. 84.** Right temporal bone. Opened and dissected from lateral side, revealing the inner space with the relative positions between the sigmoid sinus, facial canal, and bony configuration of the organs of equilibrium and hearing.

51

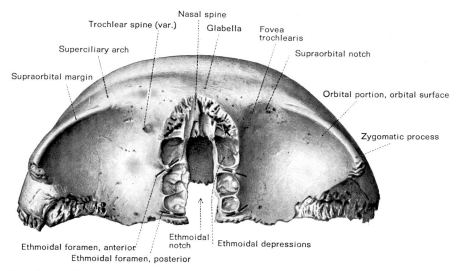

Nasal spine
Trochlear spine (var.)
Glabella
Superciliary arch
Fovea trochlearis
Supraorbital notch
Supraorbital margin
Orbital portion, orbital surface
Zygomatic process
Ethmoidal foramen, anterior
Ethmoidal notch
Ethmoidal depressions
Ethmoidal foramen, posterior

**Fig. 85.** Frontal bone. Seen from below.

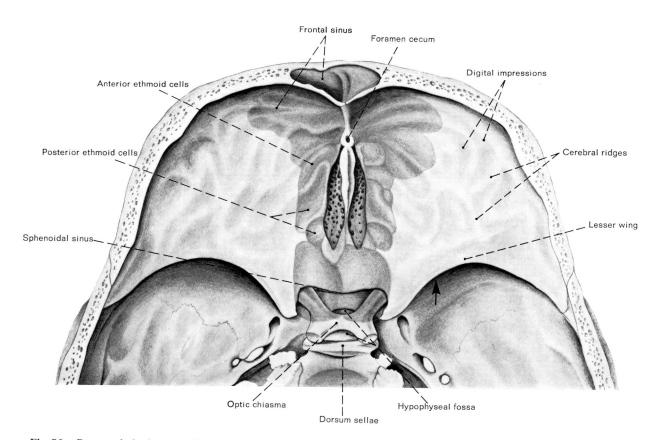

Frontal sinus
Foramen cecum
Anterior ethmoid cells
Digital impressions
Posterior ethmoid cells
Cerebral ridges
Sphenoidal sinus
Lesser wing
Optic chiasma
Hypophyseal fossa
Dorsum sellae

**Fig. 86.** Paranasal air sinuses and their projection on the anterior cranial fossa from which they are separated by only thin bony plates. The arrow points to the entrance of the superior orbital fissure.

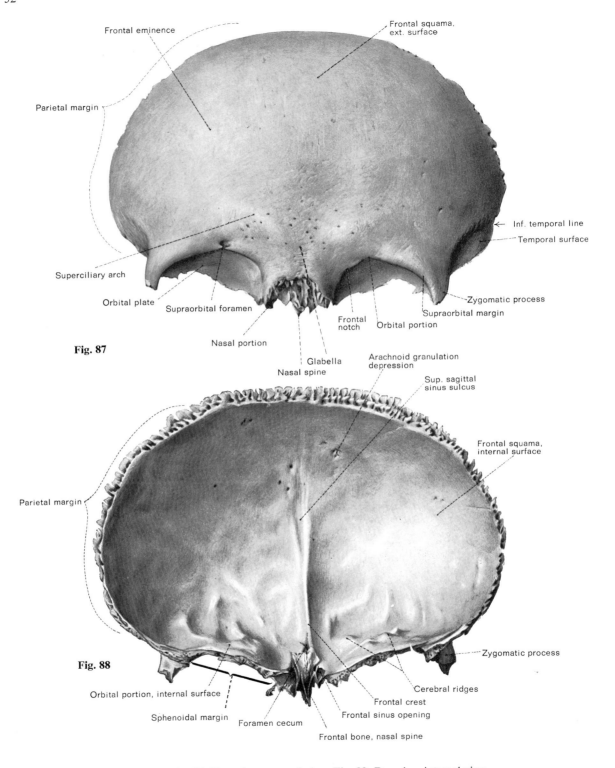

Frontal eminence

Frontal squama, ext. surface

Parietal margin

Inf. temporal line

Temporal surface

Superciliary arch

Orbital plate

Supraorbital foramen

Zygomatic process

Supraorbital margin

Nasal portion

Frontal notch

Orbital portion

**Fig. 87**

Glabella

Nasal spine

Arachnoid granulation depression

Sup. sagittal sinus sulcus

Frontal squama, internal surface

Parietal margin

Zygomatic process

**Fig. 88**

Orbital portion, internal surface

Sphenoidal margin

Foramen cecum

Cerebral ridges

Frontal crest

Frontal sinus opening

Frontal bone, nasal spine

**Figs. 87 and 88.** Frontal bone. Fig. 87. Ventral or external view. Fig. 88. Dorsal or internal view.

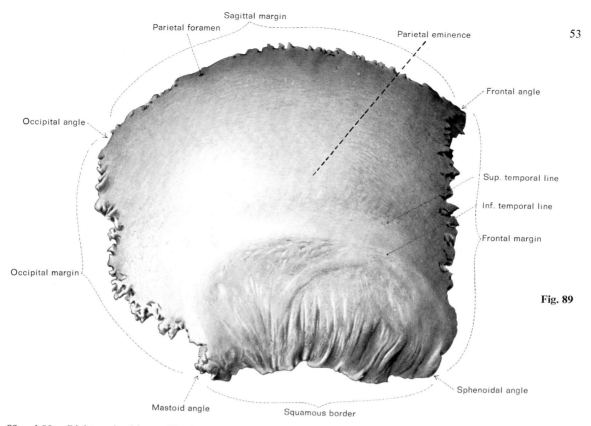

Sagittal margin
Parietal foramen
Parietal eminence
Frontal angle
Occipital angle
Sup. temporal line
Inf. temporal line
Frontal margin
Occipital margin
Fig. 89
Sphenoidal angle
Mastoid angle
Squamous border

**Figs. 89 and 90.** Right parietal bone. Fig. 89. External view. Fig. 90. Internal view.

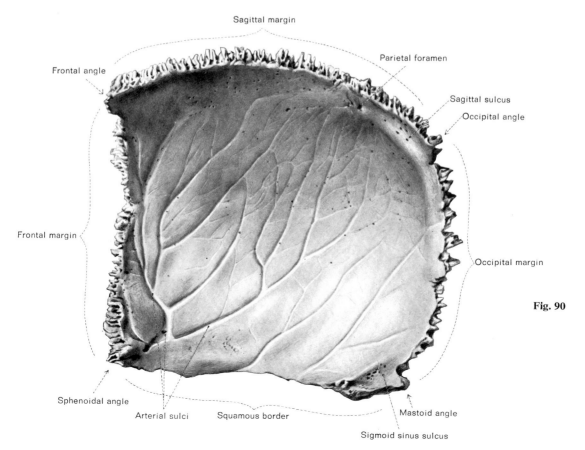

Sagittal margin
Parietal foramen
Frontal angle
Sagittal sulcus
Occipital angle
Frontal margin
Occipital margin
Fig. 90
Sphenoidal angle
Arterial sulci
Squamous border
Mastoid angle
Sigmoid sinus sulcus

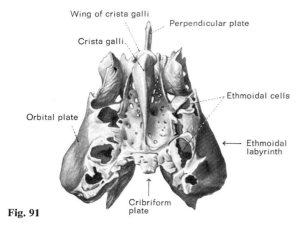

Fig. 91

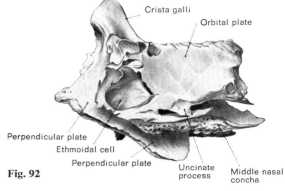

Fig. 92

**Figs. 91 and 92.** Ethmoid bone.
Fig. 91. Cranial view, from above. Fig. 92. Left lateral view.

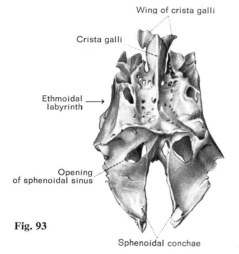

Fig. 93

**Fig. 93.** Ethmoid bone and sphenoidal concha. From above and dorsal.

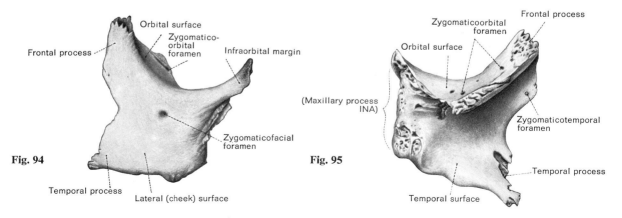

Fig. 94

Fig. 95

**Figs. 94 and 95.** Right zygomatic bone. Fig. 94. Lateral, external surface. Fig. 95. Temporal surface.

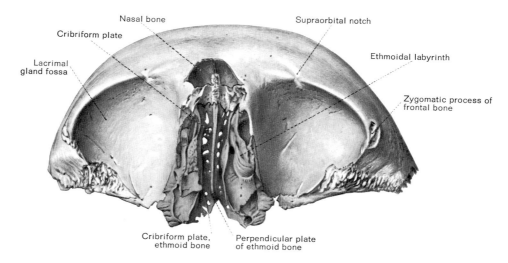

**Fig. 96.** Frontal bone with a large part of the ethmoid and nasal bones attached. Caudal view: Frontal bone, not colored; ethmoid, orange; nasal bone, reddish.

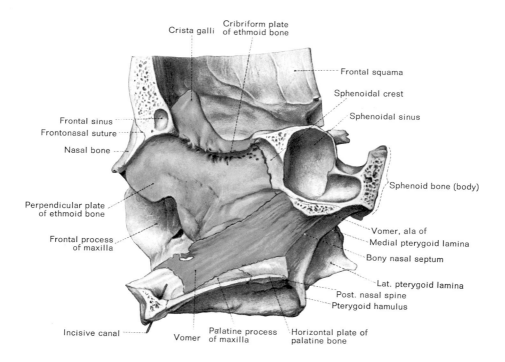

**Fig. 97.** Bony portion of the nasal septum. Seen from the left side. Ethmoid, orange; vomer, reddish.

56

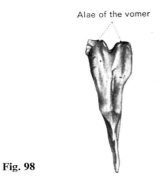

Alae of the vomer

**Fig. 98**

**Fig. 98.** Vomer. Dorsal view.

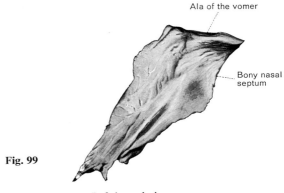

Ala of the vomer

Bony nasal
septum

**Fig. 99**

**Fig. 99.** Vomer. Left lateral view.

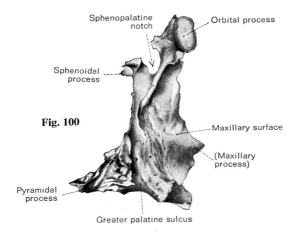

Sphenopalatine
notch

Orbital process

Sphenoidal
process

**Fig. 100**

Maxillary surface

(Maxillary
process)

Pyramidal
process

Greater palatine sulcus

**Figs. 100–102.** Right palatine bone.
Fig. 100. Lateral. Fig. 101. Dorsal. Fig. 102. Medial views.

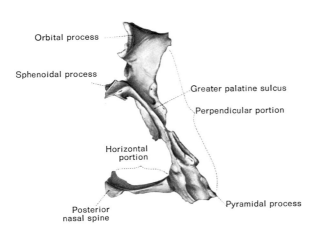

Orbital process

Sphenoidal process

Greater palatine sulcus

Perpendicular portion

Horizontal
portion

Posterior
nasal spine

Pyramidal process

**Fig. 101**

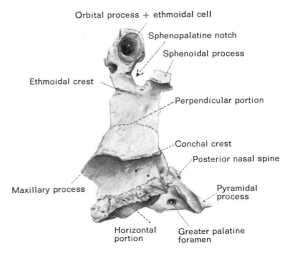

Orbital process + ethmoidal cell

Sphenopalatine notch

Sphenoidal process

Ethmoidal crest

Perpendicular portion

Conchal crest

Posterior nasal spine

Maxillary process

Pyramidal
process

Horizontal
portion

Greater palatine
foramen

**Fig. 102**

57

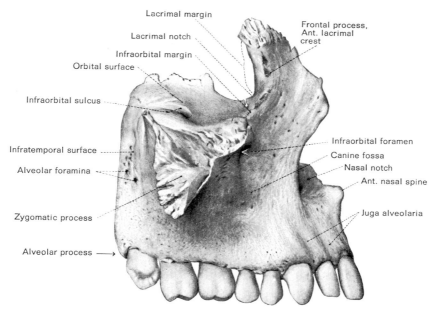

**Fig. 103.** Right maxilla. Lateral view.

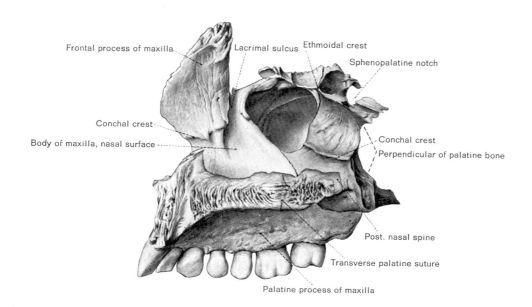

**Fig. 104.** Right maxilla and palatine bones. Palatine, blue.

58

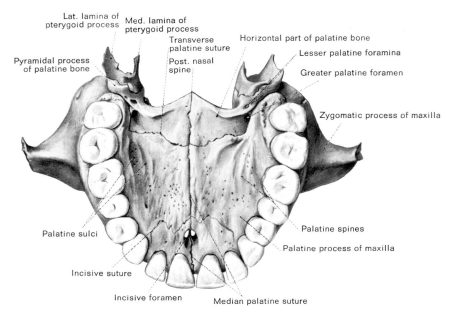

Lat. lamina of pterygoid process
Med. lamina of pterygoid process
Transverse palatine suture
Post. nasal spine
Horizontal part of palatine bone
Lesser palatine foramina
Greater palatine foramen
Pyramidal process of palatine bone
Zygomatic process of maxilla
Palatine spines
Palatine process of maxilla
Palatine sulci
Incisive suture
Incisive foramen
Median palatine suture

**Fig. 105**

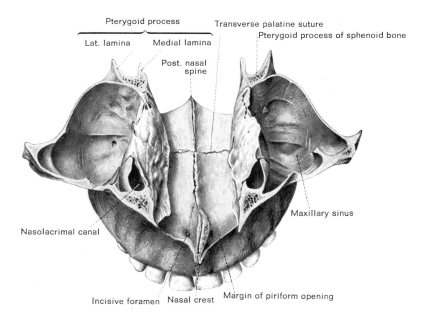

Pterygoid process
Transverse palatine suture
Lat. lamina
Medial lamina
Pterygoid process of sphenoid bone
Post. nasal spine
Maxillary sinus
Nasolacrimal canal
Incisive foramen
Nasal crest
Margin of piriform opening

**Fig. 106**

**Figs. 105 and 106.** Hard palate. Fig. 105. Oral view, from below. Fig. 106. With inferior nasal concha (not labeled nor colored) and maxillary sinus, from above. Maxilla, yellow; palatine, blue; sphenoid, green.

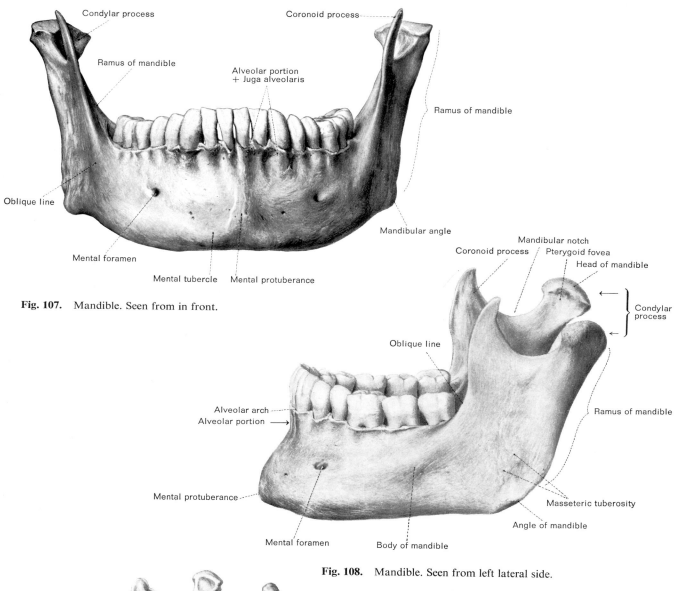

**Fig. 107.** Mandible. Seen from in front.

**Fig. 108.** Mandible. Seen from left lateral side.

**Fig. 109.** Mandible of an aged woman.

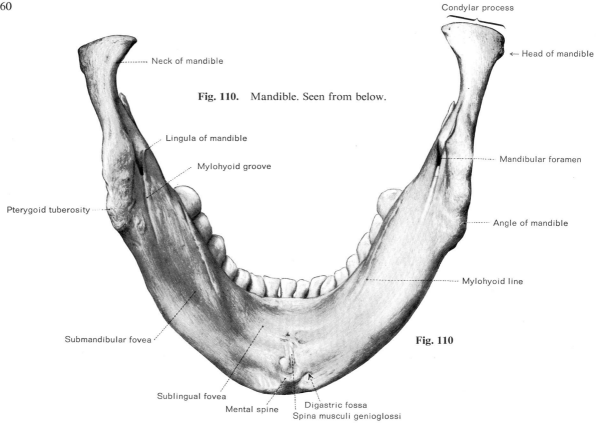

Condylar process

Head of mandible

Neck of mandible

**Fig. 110.** Mandible. Seen from below.

Lingula of mandible

Mylohyoid groove

Mandibular foramen

Pterygoid tuberosity

Angle of mandible

Mylohyoid line

Submandibular fovea

**Fig. 110**

Sublingual fovea

Digastric fossa

Mental spine

Spina musculi genioglossi

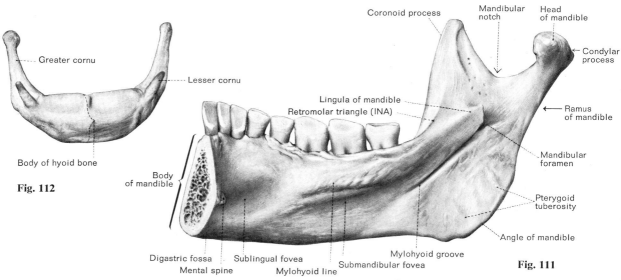

Coronoid process

Mandibular notch

Head of mandible

Condylar process

Greater cornu

Lesser cornu

Lingula of mandible

Retromolar triangle (INA)

Ramus of mandible

Mandibular foramen

Body of hyoid bone

Body of mandible

Pterygoid tuberosity

**Fig. 112**

Angle of mandible

Digastric fossa

Mental spine

Sublingual fovea

Mylohyoid line

Submandibular fovea

Mylohyoid groove

**Fig. 111**

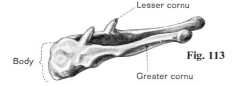

Lesser cornu

Body

**Fig. 113**

Greater cornu

**Fig. 111.** Right half of mandible. Medial view.
**Fig. 112.** Hyoid bone. Cranial and frontal view.
**Fig. 113.** Hyoid bone. Seen from left lateral side.

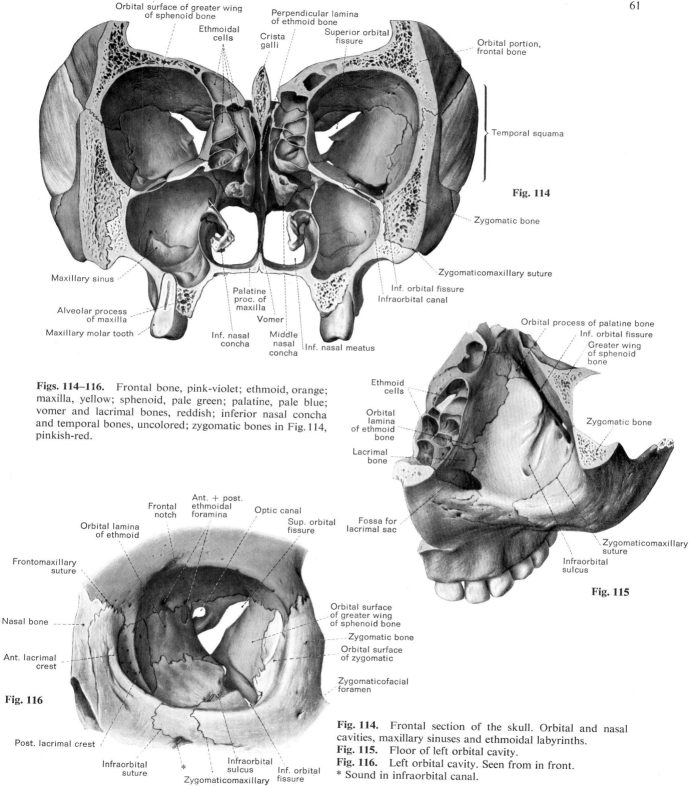

Orbital surface of greater wing of sphenoid bone

Ethmoidal cells

Perpendicular lamina of ethmoid bone

Crista galli

Superior orbital fissure

Orbital portion, frontal bone

Temporal squama

**Fig. 114**

Zygomatic bone

Zygomaticomaxillary suture

Inf. orbital fissure

Infraorbital canal

Maxillary sinus

Alveolar process of maxilla

Maxillary molar tooth

Palatine proc. of maxilla

Vomer

Inf. nasal concha

Middle nasal concha

Inf. nasal meatus

**Figs. 114–116.** Frontal bone, pink-violet; ethmoid, orange; maxilla, yellow; sphenoid, pale green; palatine, pale blue; vomer and lacrimal bones, reddish; inferior nasal concha and temporal bones, uncolored; zygomatic bones in Fig. 114, pinkish-red.

Orbital process of palatine bone

Inf. orbital fissure

Greater wing of sphenoid bone

Ethmoid cells

Orbital lamina of ethmoid bone

Lacrimal bone

Zygomatic bone

Fossa for lacrimal sac

Zygomaticomaxillary suture

Infraorbital sulcus

**Fig. 115**

Frontal notch

Ant. + post. ethmoidal foramina

Optic canal

Sup. orbital fissure

Orbital lamina of ethmoid

Frontomaxillary suture

Nasal bone

Ant. lacrimal crest

**Fig. 116**

Orbital surface of greater wing of sphenoid bone

Zygomatic bone

Orbital surface of zygomatic

Zygomaticofacial foramen

Post. lacrimal crest

Infraorbital suture

*

Infraorbital sulcus

Zygomaticomaxillary suture

Inf. orbital fissure

**Fig. 114.** Frontal section of the skull. Orbital and nasal cavities, maxillary sinuses and ethmoidal labyrinths.
**Fig. 115.** Floor of left orbital cavity.
**Fig. 116.** Left orbital cavity. Seen from in front.
* Sound in infraorbital canal.

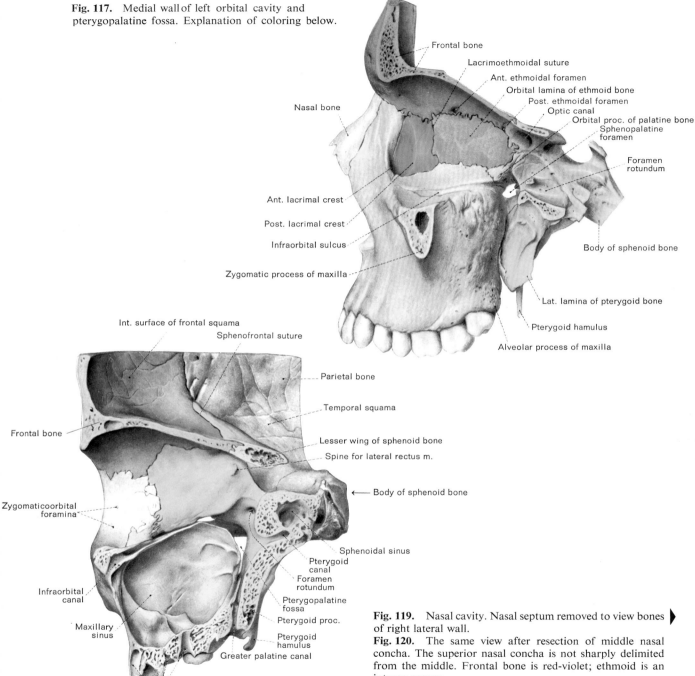

**Fig. 117.** Medial wall of left orbital cavity and pterygopalatine fossa. Explanation of coloring below.

Frontal bone

Lacrimoethmoidal suture

Ant. ethmoidal foramen

Orbital lamina of ethmoid bone

Post. ethmoidal foramen

Optic canal

Orbital proc. of palatine bone

Sphenopalatine foramen

Foramen rotundum

Body of sphenoid bone

Lat. lamina of pterygoid bone

Pterygoid hamulus

Alveolar process of maxilla

Nasal bone

Ant. lacrimal crest

Post. lacrimal crest

Infraorbital sulcus

Zygomatic process of maxilla

Int. surface of frontal squama

Sphenofrontal suture

Parietal bone

Temporal squama

Lesser wing of sphenoid bone

Spine for lateral rectus m.

Body of sphenoid bone

Frontal bone

Zygomaticoorbital foramina

Infraorbital canal

Maxillary sinus

Dental alveoli

Sphenoidal sinus

Pterygoid canal

Foramen rotundum

Pterygopalatine fossa

Pterygoid proc.

Pterygoid hamulus

Greater palatine canal

**Fig. 118.** Lateral wall of right orbital cavity, maxillary sinus, and the pterygopalatine fossa.

**Fig. 119.** Nasal cavity. Nasal septum removed to view bones of right lateral wall.
**Fig. 120.** The same view after resection of middle nasal concha. The superior nasal concha is not sharply delimited from the middle. Frontal bone is red-violet; ethmoid is an intense orange.
**Fig. 121.** Pterygopalatine fossa. Left lateral view. The zygomatic arch was removed.
Figs. 119–121. Frontal bone, pale violet; lacrimal, reddish; ethmoid, peach-orange; maxilla, yellow; palatine, pale blue; sphenoid, pale green.

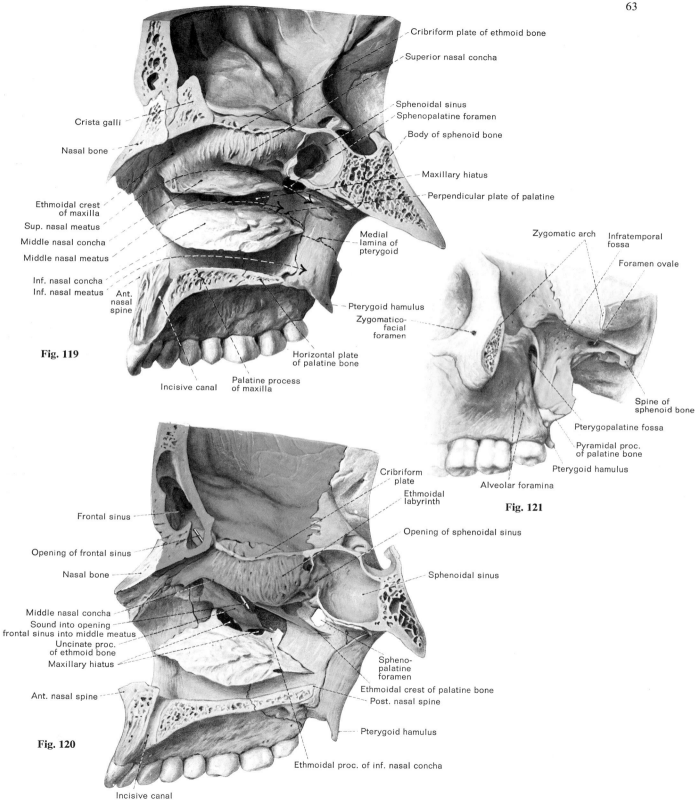

Fig. 119

Crista galli

Nasal bone

Ethmoidal crest of maxilla

Sup. nasal meatus

Middle nasal concha

Middle nasal meatus

Inf. nasal concha
Inf. nasal meatus

Ant. nasal spine

Incisive canal

Palatine process of maxilla

Horizontal plate of palatine bone

Cribriform plate of ethmoid bone

Superior nasal concha

Sphenoidal sinus
Sphenopalatine foramen

Body of sphenoid bone

Maxillary hiatus

Perpendicular plate of palatine

Medial lamina of pterygoid

Pterygoid hamulus

Fig. 121

Zygomatic arch

Infratemporal fossa

Foramen ovale

Zygomaticofacial foramen

Spine of sphenoid bone

Pterygopalatine fossa

Pyramidal proc. of palatine bone

Pterygoid hamulus

Alveolar foramina

Fig. 120

Frontal sinus

Opening of frontal sinus

Nasal bone

Middle nasal concha

Sound into opening frontal sinus into middle meatus

Uncinate proc. of ethmoid bone

Maxillary hiatus

Ant. nasal spine

Incisive canal

Cribriform plate

Ethmoidal labyrinth

Opening of sphenoidal sinus

Sphenoidal sinus

Sphenopalatine foramen

Ethmoidal crest of palatine bone

Post. nasal spine

Pterygoid hamulus

Ethmoidal proc. of inf. nasal concha

# Osteology

---

*The Pelvic Girdle and Upper Limb*

---

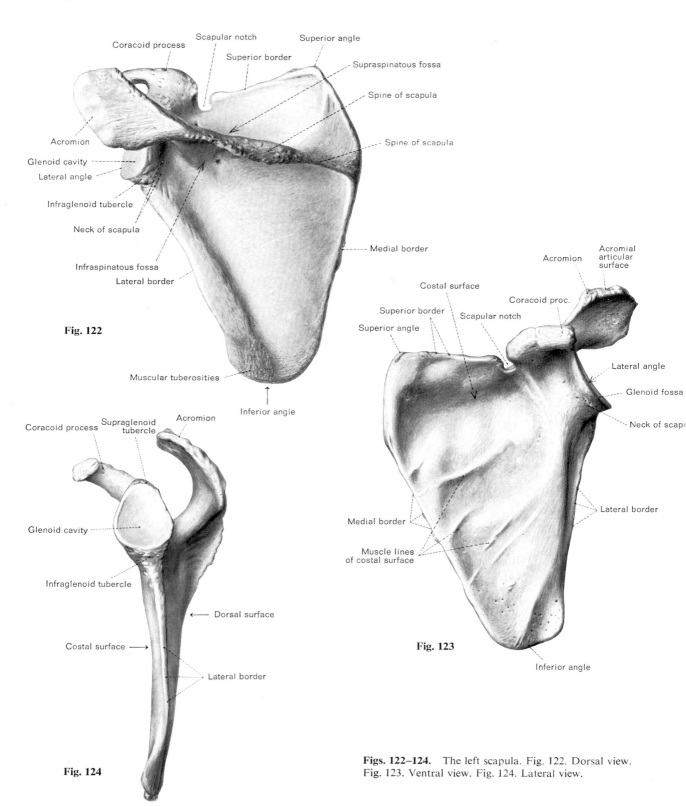

Coracoid process
Scapular notch
Superior angle
Superior border
Supraspinatous fossa
Spine of scapula
Acromion
Spine of scapula
Glenoid cavity
Lateral angle
Infraglenoid tubercle
Neck of scapula
Medial border
Infraspinatous fossa
Lateral border

**Fig. 122**

Muscular tuberosities

Inferior angle

Coracoid process
Supraglenoid tubercle
Acromion

Glenoid cavity

Infraglenoid tubercle

Dorsal surface

Costal surface

Lateral border

**Fig. 124**

Acromion
Acromial articular surface
Costal surface
Coracoid proc.
Superior border
Scapular notch
Superior angle
Lateral angle
Glenoid fossa
Neck of scap

Medial border

Lateral border

Muscle lines of costal surface

**Fig. 123**

Inferior angle

**Figs. 122–124.** The left scapula. Fig. 122. Dorsal view. Fig. 123. Ventral view. Fig. 124. Lateral view.

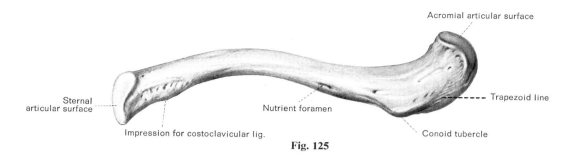

Acromial articular surface

Trapezoid line

Sternal
articular surface

Nutrient foramen

Conoid tubercle

Impression for costoclavicular lig.

**Fig. 125**

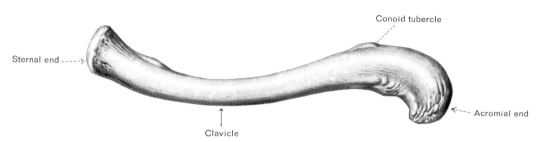

Conoid tubercle

Sternal end

Acromial end

Clavicle

**Fig. 126**

**Fig. 125 and 126.** The left clavicle.
Fig. 125. Caudal view. Fig. 126. Cranial view.

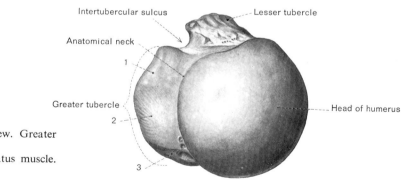

Intertubercular sulcus

Lesser tubercle

Anatomical neck

1

Greater tubercle

2

Head of humerus

3

**Fig. 127.** Head of left humerus. Proximal view. Greater
tubercle facets for:
1. the Supraspinatus muscle. 2. the Infraspinatus muscle.
3. the Teres minor muscle.

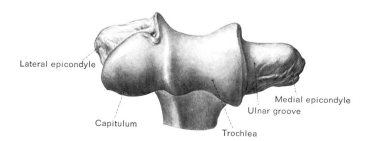

Lateral epicondyle

Medial epicondyle

Ulnar groove

Capitulum

Trochlea

**Fig. 128.** Distal end of the left humerus.

68

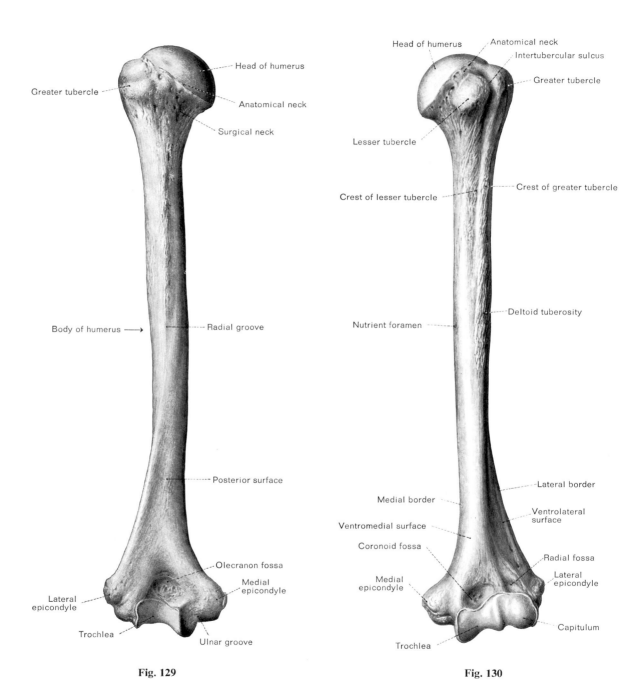

Greater tubercle

Head of humerus

Anatomical neck

Surgical neck

Body of humerus →

Radial groove

Posterior surface

Olecranon fossa

Medial
epicondyle

Lateral
epicondyle

Trochlea

Ulnar groove

**Fig. 129**

Head of humerus

Anatomical neck

Intertubercular sulcus

Greater tubercle

Lesser tubercle

Crest of lesser tubercle

Crest of greater tubercle

Nutrient foramen

Deltoid tuberosity

Medial border

Lateral border

Ventromedial surface

Ventrolateral
surface

Coronoid fossa

Radial fossa

Medial
epicondyle

Lateral
epicondyle

Capitulum

Trochlea

**Fig. 130**

**Figs. 129 and 130.**   Left humerus. Fig. 129. Dorsal view. Fig. 130. Ventral view.

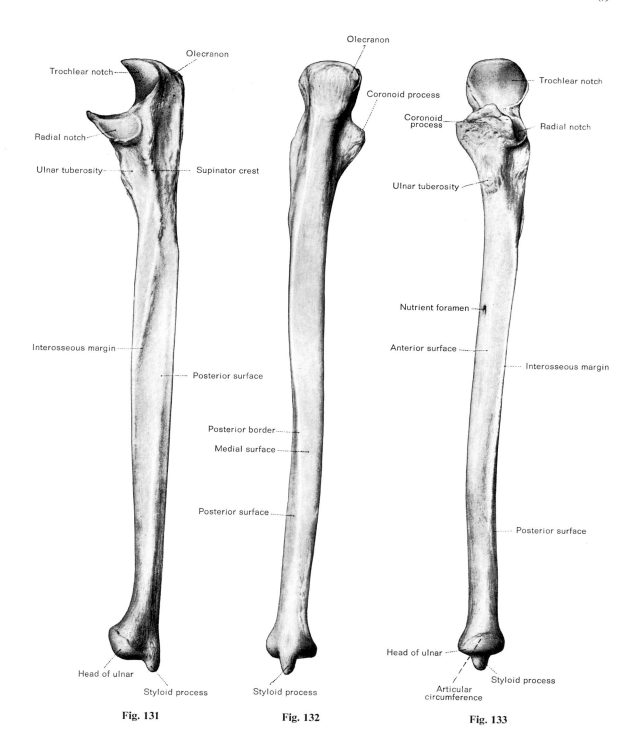

Olecranon

Trochlear notch

Olecranon

Radial notch

Coronoid process

Trochlear notch

Coronoid process

Ulnar tuberosity

Supinator crest

Radial notch

Ulnar tuberosity

Nutrient foramen

Interosseous margin

Anterior surface

Interosseous margin

Posterior surface

Posterior border

Medial surface

Posterior surface

Posterior surface

Head of ulnar

Head of ulnar

Styloid process

Styloid process

Styloid process

Articular circumference

**Fig. 131**            **Fig. 132**            **Fig. 133**

**Figs. 131–133.**   The left ulna. Fig. 131. Lateral (radial) aspect. Fig. 132. Dorsal aspect. Fig. 133. Palmar or anterior aspect.

70

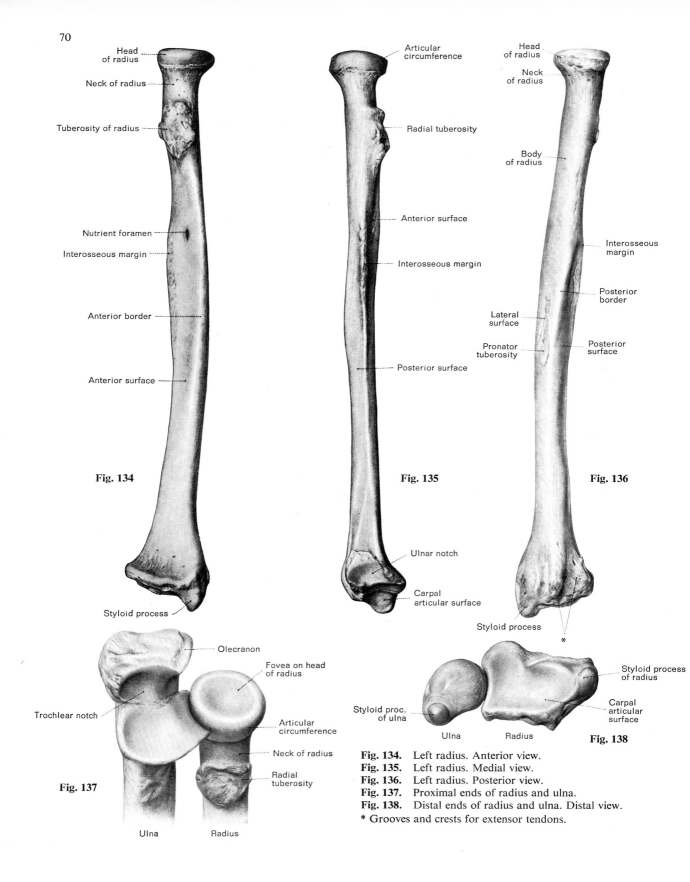

Head of radius
Neck of radius
Tuberosity of radius
Nutrient foramen
Interosseous margin
Anterior border
Anterior surface
Styloid process

**Fig. 134**

Articular circumference
Radial tuberosity
Anterior surface
Interosseous margin
Posterior surface
Ulnar notch
Carpal articular surface

**Fig. 135**

Head of radius
Neck of radius
Body of radius
Interosseous margin
Posterior border
Lateral surface
Pronator tuberosity
Posterior surface
Styloid process
*

**Fig. 136**

Olecranon
Fovea on head of radius
Trochlear notch
Articular circumference
Neck of radius
Radial tuberosity

**Fig. 137**

Ulna          Radius

Styloid proc. of ulna
Styloid process of radius
Carpal articular surface
Ulna          Radius

**Fig. 138**

Fig. 134.   Left radius. Anterior view.
Fig. 135.   Left radius. Medial view.
Fig. 136.   Left radius. Posterior view.
Fig. 137.   Proximal ends of radius and ulna.
Fig. 138.   Distal ends of radius and ulna. Distal view.

* Grooves and crests for extensor tendons.

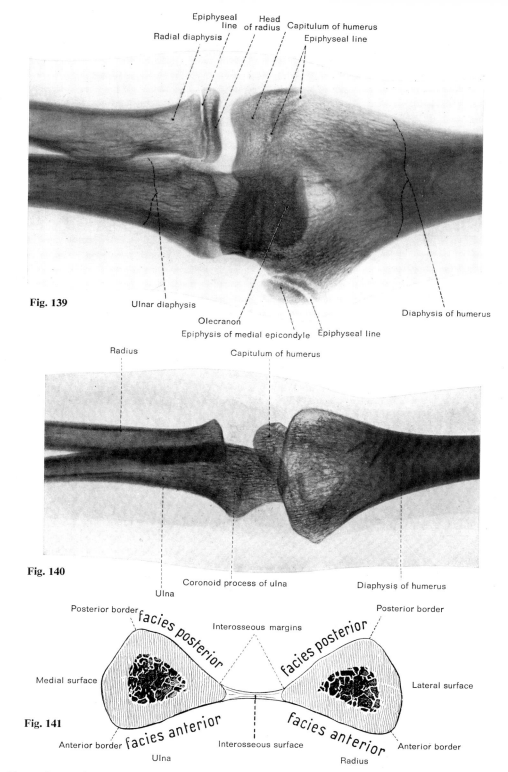

Epiphyseal line

Head of radius

Capitulum of humerus

Radial diaphysis

Epiphyseal line

Fig. 139

Ulnar diaphysis

Olecranon

Epiphysis of medial epicondyle

Epiphyseal line

Diaphysis of humerus

Radius

Capitulum of humerus

Fig. 140

Coronoid process of ulna

Ulna

Diaphysis of humerus

Posterior border

facies posterior

Interosseous margins

facies posterior

Posterior border

Medial surface

Lateral surface

Fig. 141

facies anterior

facies anterior

Anterior border

Ulna

Interosseous surface

Radius

Anterior border

**Fig. 139.** X-ray picture of the elbow (cubital region) of a 17 year old boy.
**Fig. 140.** X-ray picture of the elbow (cubital region) of a 5½ year old boy.
**Fig. 141.** Surfaces and borders of the bones of the left forearm. Diagrammatic section near the middle of its length. Facies anterior = Anterior surface; facies posterior = Posterior surface.

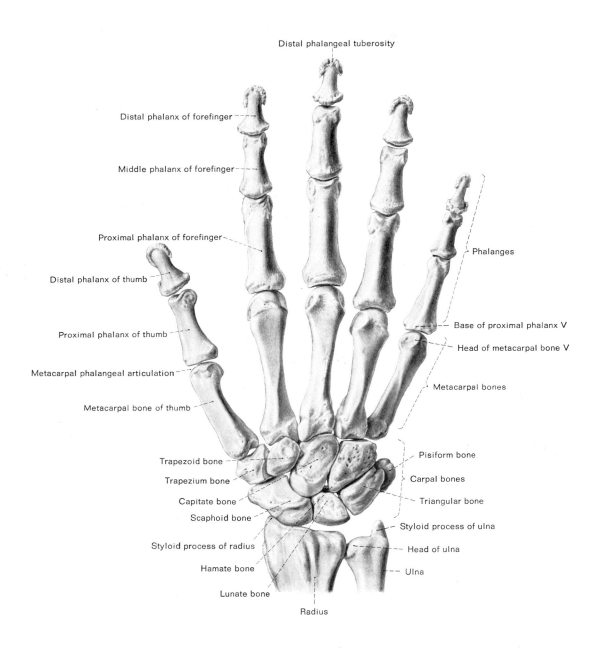

Distal phalangeal tuberosity

Distal phalanx of forefinger

Middle phalanx of forefinger

Proximal phalanx of forefinger

Distal phalanx of thumb

Proximal phalanx of thumb

Metacarpal phalangeal articulation

Metacarpal bone of thumb

Trapezoid bone

Trapezium bone

Capitate bone

Scaphoid bone

Styloid process of radius

Hamate bone

Lunate bone

Radius

Phalanges

Base of proximal phalanx V

Head of metacarpal bone V

Metacarpal bones

Pisiform bone

Carpal bones

Triangular bone

Styloid process of ulna

Head of ulna

Ulna

**Fig. 142.**   Skeleton of right hand with extended, slightly spread fingers, and the distal end of the forearm with bones in their natural position. Dorsal view.

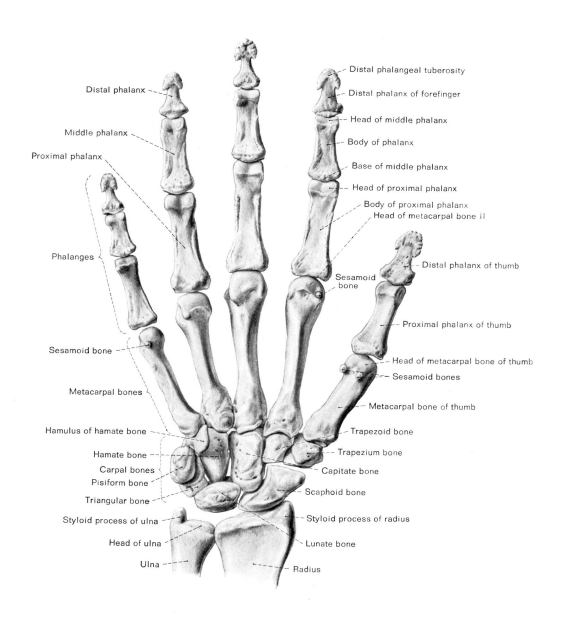

Distal phalanx

Middle phalanx

Proximal phalanx

Phalanges

Sesamoid bone

Metacarpal bones

Hamulus of hamate bone

Hamate bone

Carpal bones

Pisiform bone

Triangular bone

Styloid process of ulna

Head of ulna

Ulna

Distal phalangeal tuberosity

Distal phalanx of forefinger

Head of middle phalanx

Body of phalanx

Base of middle phalanx

Head of proximal phalanx

Body of proximal phalanx

Head of metacarpal bone II

Distal phalanx of thumb

Sesamoid bone

Proximal phalanx of thumb

Head of metacarpal bone of thumb

Sesamoid bones

Metacarpal bone of thumb

Trapezoid bone

Trapezium bone

Capitate bone

Scaphoid bone

Styloid process of radius

Lunate bone

Radius

**Fig. 143.** Skeleton of right hand and wrist with bones in their natural position. Palmar view. Same preparation as in Fig. 142.

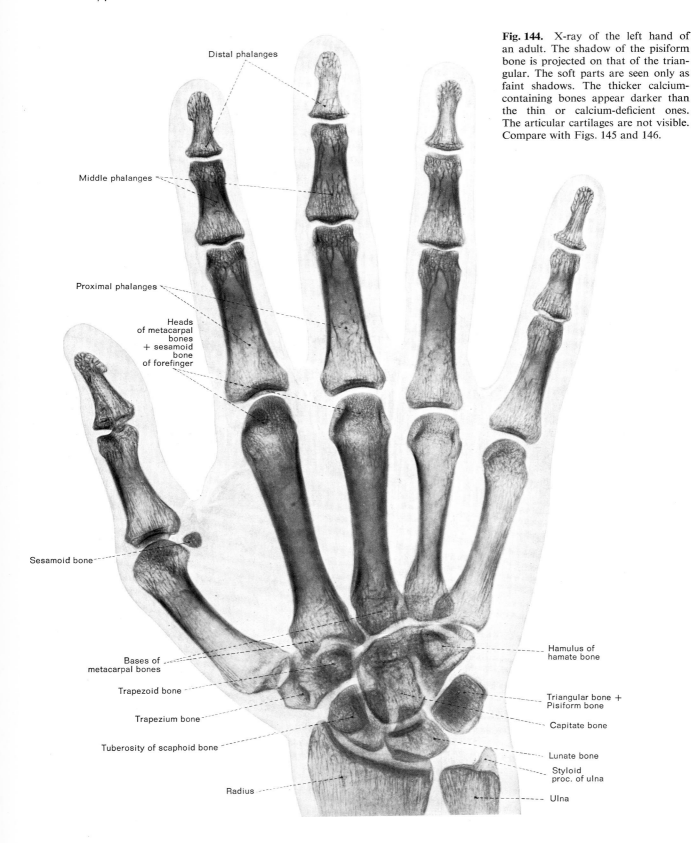

Distal phalanges

Middle phalanges

Proximal phalanges

Heads
of metacarpal
bones
+ sesamoid
bone
of forefinger

Sesamoid bone

Bases of
metacarpal bones

Trapezoid bone

Trapezium bone

Tuberosity of scaphoid bone

Radius

**Fig. 144.** X-ray of the left hand of an adult. The shadow of the pisiform bone is projected on that of the triangular. The soft parts are seen only as faint shadows. The thicker calcium-containing bones appear darker than the thin or calcium-deficient ones. The articular cartilages are not visible. Compare with Figs. 145 and 146.

Hamulus of
hamate bone

Triangular bone +
Pisiform bone

Capitate bone

Lunate bone

Styloid
proc. of ulna

Ulna

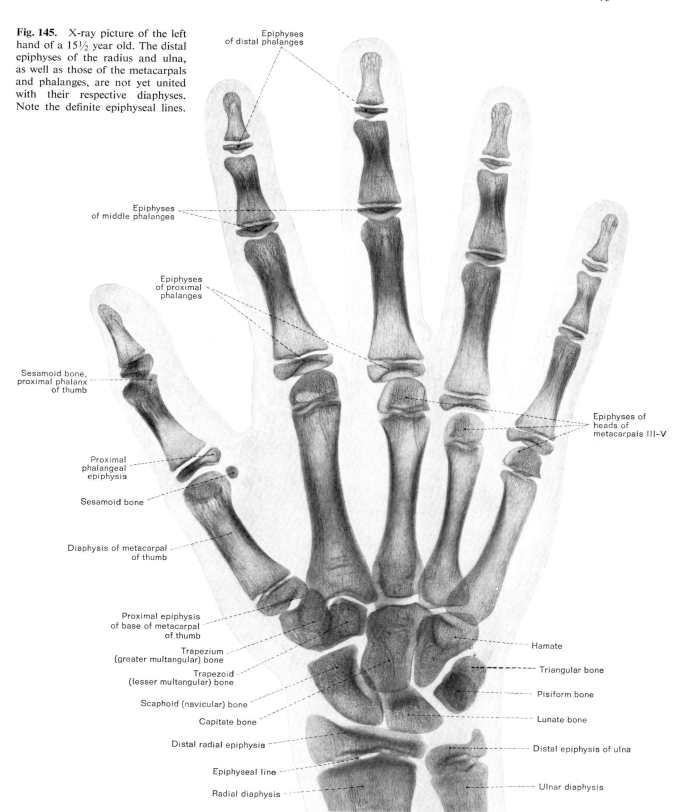

**Fig. 145.** X-ray picture of the left hand of a 15½ year old. The distal epiphyses of the radius and ulna, as well as those of the metacarpals and phalanges, are not yet united with their respective diaphyses. Note the definite epiphyseal lines.

Epiphyses of distal phalanges

Epiphyses of middle phalanges

Epiphyses of proximal phalanges

Sesamoid bone, proximal phalanx of thumb

Proximal phalangeal epiphysis

Sesamoid bone

Diaphysis of metacarpal of thumb

Proximal epiphysis of base of metacarpal of thumb

Trapezium (greater multangular) bone

Trapezoid (lesser multangular) bone

Scaphoid (navicular) bone

Capitate bone

Distal radial epiphysis

Epiphyseal line

Radial diaphysis

Epiphyses of heads of metacarpals III–V

Hamate

Triangular bone

Pisiform bone

Lunate bone

Distal epiphysis of ulna

Ulnar diaphysis

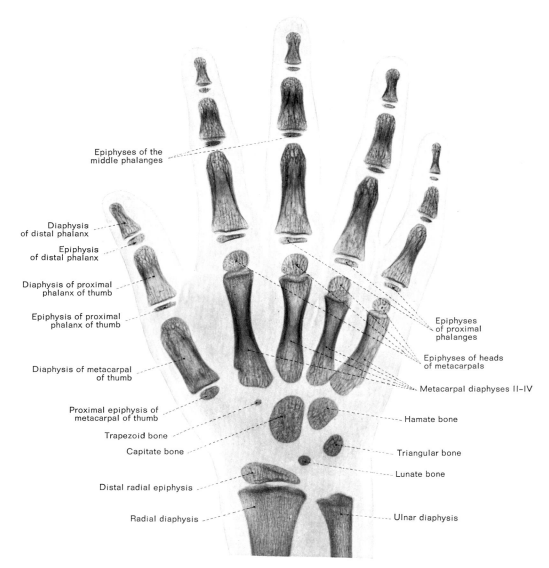

Epiphyses of the
middle phalanges

Diaphysis
of distal phalanx

Epiphysis
of distal phalanx

Diaphysis of proximal
phalanx of thumb

Epiphysis of proximal
phalanx of thumb

Diaphysis of metacarpal
of thumb

Proximal epiphysis of
metacarpal of thumb

Trapezoid bone

Capitate bone

Distal radial epiphysis

Radial diaphysis

Epiphyses
of proximal
phalanges

Epiphyses of heads
of metacarpals

Metacarpal diaphyses II–IV

Hamate bone

Triangular bone

Lunate bone

Ulnar diaphysis

**Fig. 146.**   X-ray picture of the hand of a 5½ year old boy. The phalanges of the fingers have only one proximal epiphysis; the metacarpals II–V have only one distal. From this, one can see the metacarpal of the thumb as the proximal phalanx of the thumb. The center of ossification of the trapezoid and lunate bones are still very small; that of the scaphoid is absent. It is, therefore, possible to determine the age of children through investigation of the ossification. (Compare with Fig. 184.)

# Osteology

## The Pelvic Girdle and Lower Limb

78

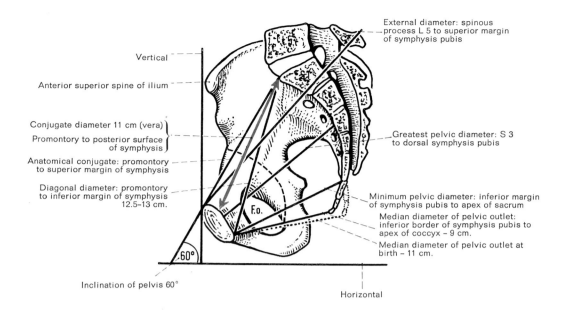

Vertical

Anterior superior spine of ilium

Conjugate diameter 11 cm (vera)
Promontory to posterior surface
of symphysis
Anatomical conjugate: promontory
to superior margin of symphysis

Diagonal diameter: promontory
to inferior margin of symphysis
12.5–13 cm.

F.o.

60°

Inclination of pelvis 60°

External diameter: spinous
process L 5 to superior margin
of symphysis pubis

Greatest pelvic diameter: S 3
to dorsal symphysis pubis

Minimum pelvic diameter: inferior margin
of symphysis pubis to apex of sacrum
Median diameter of pelvic outlet:
inferior border of symphysis pubis to
apex of coccyx – 9 cm.
Median diameter of pelvic outlet at
birth – 11 cm.

Horizontal

**Fig. 147.** Median sagittal section through the pelvis of an adult female, showing important obstetrical diameters and axes. Anatomical conjugate: Diameter from the promontory to the superior margin of the symphysis pubis. Gynecological or true conjugate (vera): Diameter connects the sacrovertebral angle with the middle of the most prominent part of the posterior aspect of the symphysis pubis. The dotted line indicates the pelvic axis.

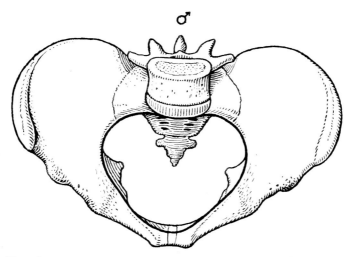

**Fig. 148a.** Male pelvis: Heartshaped pelvic aperture; true pelvis becomes narrower toward the outlet, hence funnel-shaped, subpubic angle.

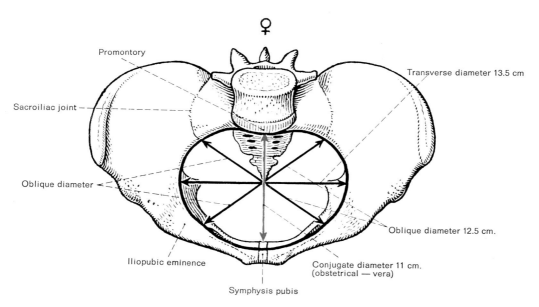

**Fig. 148b.** Female pelvis: Slanting oval of the pelvic aperture; cylindrical true pelvis not narrowed toward outlet, pubic arch.

Note: The sex differences, especially in the shape, size, and diameter of the superior aperture of the pelvic apertures, also as to the sacrum and position of the iliac fossa. The left oblique diameter I (12.5 cm.) from the left iliopubic eminence to the right sacroiliac joint; the right oblique diameter II (12.5 cm) from the right iliopubic eminence to the left sacroiliac joint; conjugate (11 cm) from the promontory to the most prominent part of the posterior aspect of the symphysis of the pubis (red arrow).

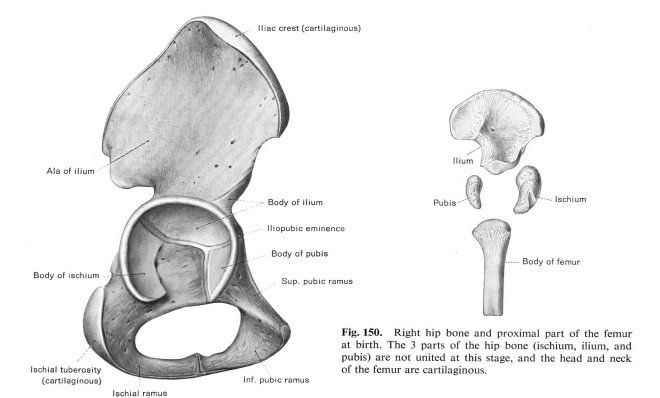

Iliac crest (cartilaginous)

Ala of ilium

Body of ilium

Iliopubic eminence

Body of pubis

Body of ischium

Sup. pubic ramus

Ischial tuberosity
(cartilaginous)

Ischial ramus

Inf. pubic ramus

Ilium

Pubis

Ischium

Body of femur

**Fig. 150.** Right hip bone and proximal part of the femur at birth. The 3 parts of the hip bone (ischium, ilium, and pubis) are not united at this stage, and the head and neck of the femur are cartilaginous.

**Fig. 149.** Hip bone of a child about 5 to 6 years old. Seen from lateral. Ilium, yellow; ischium, green; pubis, blue. The three parts first form a starlike synchondrosis. The separating cartilaginous lines are present only in the young. Later synostosis takes place when they fuse to form the hip bone in the area of the acetabulum.

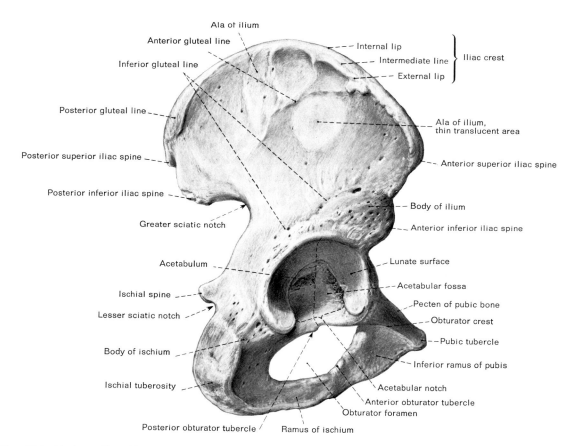

Ala of ilium

Anterior gluteal line

Inferior gluteal line

Posterior gluteal line

Posterior superior iliac spine

Posterior inferior iliac spine

Greater sciatic notch

Acetabulum

Ischial spine

Lesser sciatic notch

Body of ischium

Ischial tuberosity

Posterior obturator tubercle

Ramus of ischium

Obturator foramen

Anterior obturator tubercle

Acetabular notch

Inferior ramus of pubis

Pubic tubercle

Obturator crest

Pecten of pubic bone

Acetabular fossa

Lunate surface

Anterior inferior iliac spine

Body of ilium

Anterior superior iliac spine

Ala of ilium, thin translucent area

Internal lip

Intermediate line } Iliac crest

External lip

**Fig. 151.** Right hip bone. Lateral view.

82

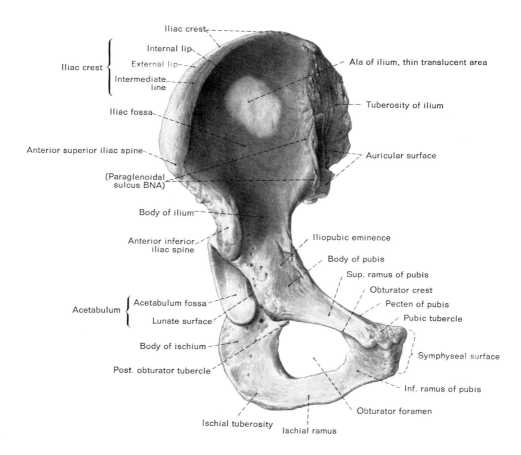

Iliac crest

Internal lip

Iliac crest | External lip

Intermediate line

Iliac fossa

Anterior superior iliac spine

(Paraglenoidal sulcus BNA)

Body of ilium

Anterior inferior iliac spine

Acetabulum { Acetabulum fossa

Lunate surface

Body of ischium

Post. obturator tubercle

Ischial tuberosity

Ischial ramus

Iliac crest

Ala of ilium, thin translucent area

Tuberosity of ilium

Auricular surface

Iliopubic eminence

Body of pubis

Sup. ramus of pubis

Obturator crest

Pecten of pubis

Pubic tubercle

Symphyseal surface

Inf. ramus of pubis

Obturator foramen

**Fig. 152.** Right hip bone. Ventral view.

83

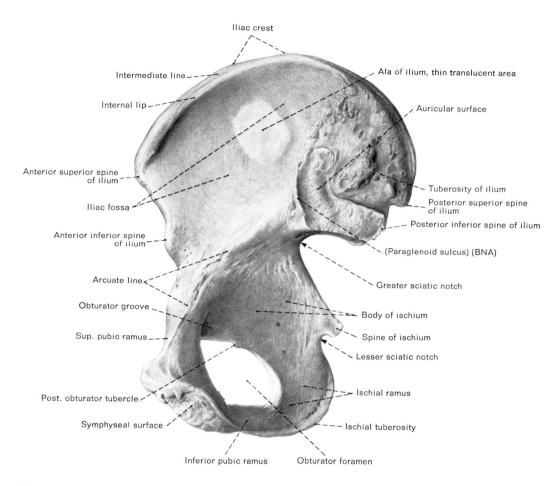

Iliac crest

Intermediate line

Internal lip

Anterior superior spine
of ilium

Iliac fossa

Anterior inferior spine
of ilium

Arcuate line

Obturator groove

Sup. pubic ramus

Post. obturator tubercle

Symphyseal surface

Inferior pubic ramus

Obturator foramen

Ala of ilium, thin translucent area

Auricular surface

Tuberosity of ilium

Posterior superior spine
of ilium

Posterior inferior spine of ilium

(Paraglenoid sulcus) (BNA)

Greater sciatic notch

Body of ischium

Spine of ischium

Lesser sciatic notch

Ischial ramus

Ischial tuberosity

**Fig. 153.** Right hip bone. Medial view.

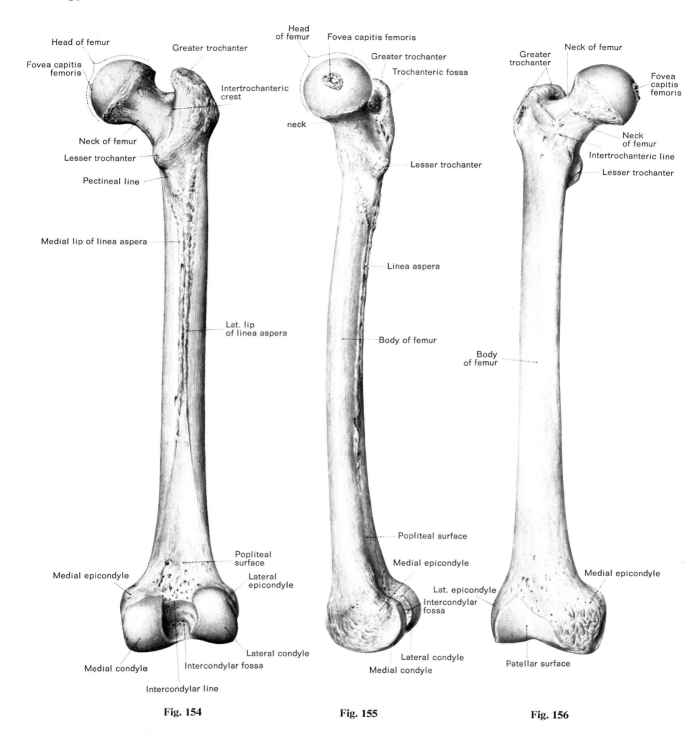

Fig. 154

Fig. 155

Fig. 156

**Figs. 154–156.** Right femur. Fig. 154. Dorsal; Fig. 155. medial; and Fig. 156. ventral views.

85

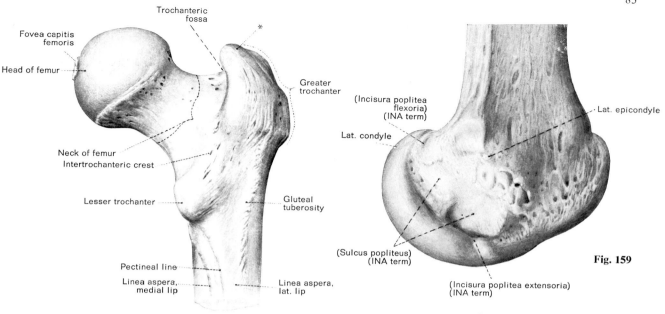

**Fig. 157.** Proximal end of right femur. Dorsal view.
* Tip of greater trochanter

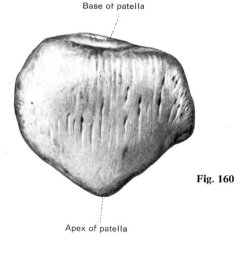

Fig. 159

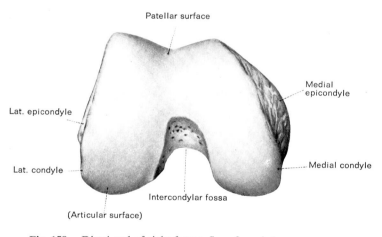

**Fig. 158.** Distal end of right femur. Seen from below.

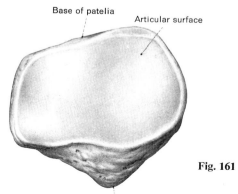

Fig. 160

Fig. 161

**Fig. 159.** Distal end of right femur. Lateral view.
**Fig. 160.** Patella. Ventral view.
**Fig. 161.** Patella. Dorsal view.

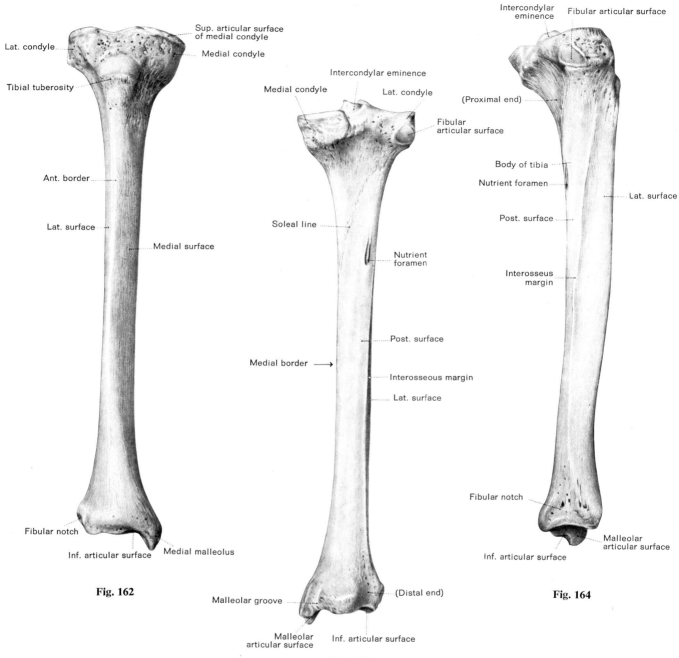

Fig. 162

Lat. condyle
Tibial tuberosity
Ant. border
Lat. surface
Fibular notch
Inf. articular surface
Sup. articular surface of medial condyle
Medial condyle
Medial surface
Medial malleolus

Fig. 163

Medial condyle
Intercondylar eminence
Lat. condyle
Fibular articular surface
Soleal line
Nutrient foramen
Post. surface
Medial border →
Interosseous margin
Lat. surface
Malleolar groove
(Distal end)
Malleolar articular surface
Inf. articular surface

Fig. 164

Intercondylar eminence
Fibular articular surface
(Proximal end)
Body of tibia
Nutrient foramen
Post. surface
Lat. surface
Interosseus margin
Fibular notch
Inf. articular surface
Malleolar articular surface

**Figs. 162–164.** Right tibia. Fig. 162. Ventral; Fig. 163. Dorsal; Fig. 164. Lateral views.

**Figs. 165 and 166.** Right fibula. Fig. 165. Medial; Fig. 166. Lateral views.
**Fig. 167.** Right tibia and fibula. Dorsal view.
**Fig. 168.** Proximal ends of the right tibia and fibula. Proximal view.
**Fig. 169.** Distal ends of right tibia and fibula. Distal view.

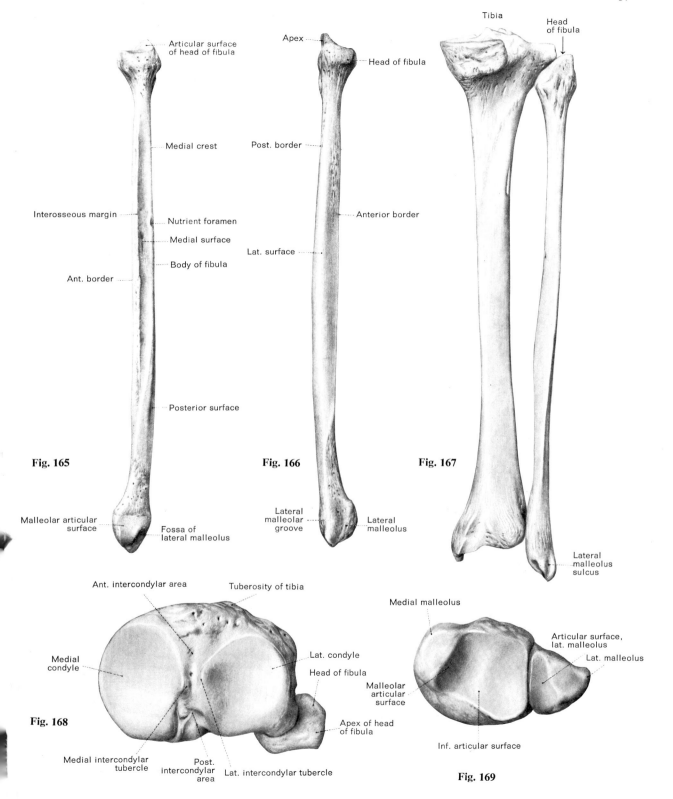

Articular surface of head of fibula

Medial crest

Interosseous margin

Nutrient foramen

Medial surface

Body of fibula

Ant. border

Posterior surface

**Fig. 165**

Malleolar articular surface

Fossa of lateral malleolus

Apex

Head of fibula

Post. border

Anterior border

Lat. surface

**Fig. 166**

Lateral malleolar groove

Lateral malleolus

Tibia

Head of fibula

**Fig. 167**

Lateral malleolus sulcus

Ant. intercondylar area

Tuberosity of tibia

Medial condyle

Lat. condyle

Head of fibula

**Fig. 168**

Medial intercondylar tubercle

Post. intercondylar area

Lat. intercondylar tubercle

Apex of head of fibula

Medial malleolus

Articular surface, lat. malleolus

Lat. malleolus

Malleolar articular surface

Inf. articular surface

**Fig. 169**

88

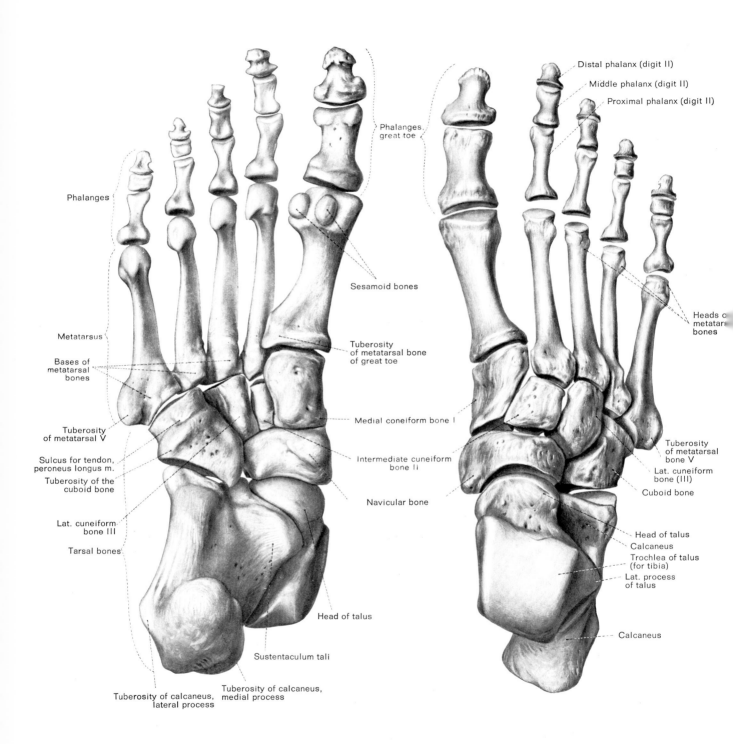

Distal phalanx (digit II)

Middle phalanx (digit II)

Proximal phalanx (digit II)

Phalanges
great toe

Phalanges

Sesamoid bones

Heads of
metatarsal
bones

Metatarsus

Tuberosity
of metatarsal bone
of great toe

Bases of
metatarsal
bones

Tuberosity
of metatarsal V

Medial coneiform bone I

Tuberosity
of metatarsal
bone V

Sulcus for tendon,
peroneus longus m.

Intermediate cuneiform
bone II

Lat. cuneiform
bone (III)

Tuberosity of the
cuboid bone

Navicular bone

Cuboid bone

Lat. cuneiform
bone III

Head of talus

Tarsal bones

Calcaneus

Trochlea of talus
(for tibia)

Lat. process
of talus

Head of talus

Calcaneus

Sustentaculum tali

Tuberosity of calcaneus,
lateral process

Tuberosity of calcaneus,
medial process

**Figs. 170 and 171.** The foot and ankle bones in their natural position. Fig. 170. Plantar view. Fig. 171. Dorsal view.

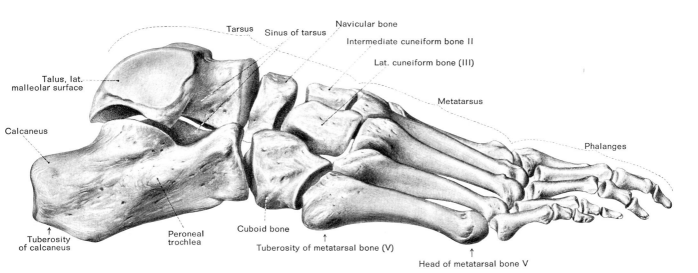

**Fig. 172.** Skeleton of the right foot. Lateral view.

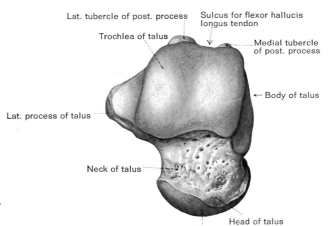

**Fig. 173.** The right talus. Proximal or dorsal view.

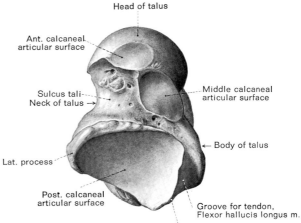

**Fig. 174.** The right talus. Plantar view.

90

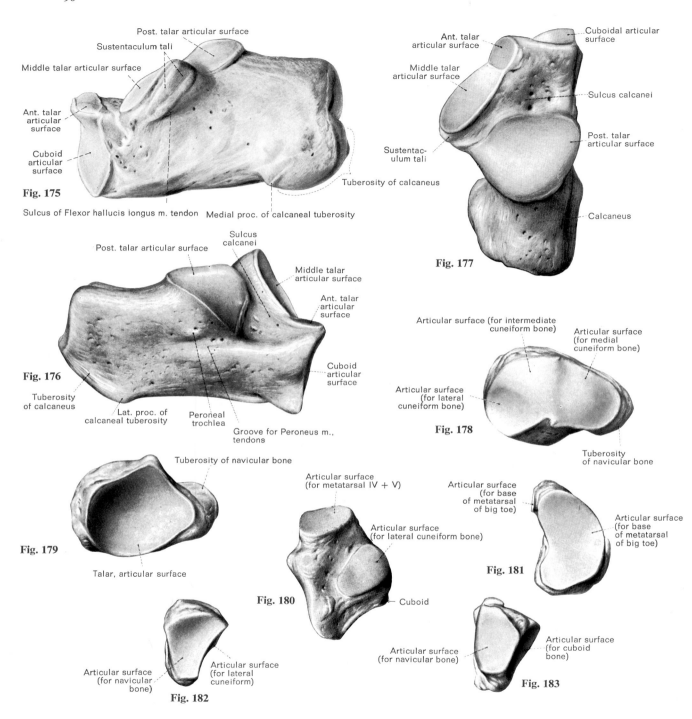

Fig. 175

Post. talar articular surface
Sustentaculum tali
Middle talar articular surface
Ant. talar articular surface
Cuboid articular surface
Sulcus of Flexor hallucis longus m. tendon
Medial proc. of calcaneal tuberosity
Tuberosity of calcaneus

Fig. 177

Ant. talar articular surface
Middle talar articular surface
Sustentaculum tali
Cuboidal articular surface
Sulcus calcanei
Post. talar articular surface
Calcaneus

Fig. 176

Post. talar articular surface
Sulcus calcanei
Middle talar articular surface
Ant. talar articular surface
Cuboid articular surface
Tuberosity of calcaneus
Lat. proc. of calcaneal tuberosity
Peroneal trochlea
Groove for Peroneus m., tendons

Fig. 178

Articular surface (for intermediate cuneiform bone)
Articular surface (for medial cuneiform bone)
Articular surface (for lateral cuneiform bone)
Tuberosity of navicular bone

Fig. 179

Tuberosity of navicular bone
Talar, articular surface

Fig. 180

Articular surface (for metatarsal IV + V)
Articular surface (for lateral cuneiform bone)
Cuboid

Fig. 181

Articular surface (for base of metatarsal of big toe)
Articular surface (for base of metatarsal of big toe)

Fig. 182

Articular surface (for navicular bone)
Articular surface (for lateral cuneiform)

Fig. 183

Articular surface (for navicular bone)
Articular surface (for cuboid bone)

Figs. 175–177.  Right calcaneus. Fig. 175. Medial view. Fig. 176. Lateral view. Fig. 177. Proximal or dorsal view.
Figs. 178 and 179.  Right navicular bone. Fig. 178. Distal view. Fig. 179. Proximal view.
Fig. 180.  Right cuboid. Medial view. (See also Fig. 172.)
Figs. 181–183.  Right cuneiform bones. Fig. 181. Medial cuneiform, distal aspect. Fig. 182. Intermediate cuneiform, proximal aspect. Fig. 183. Lateral cuneiform, proximal aspect.

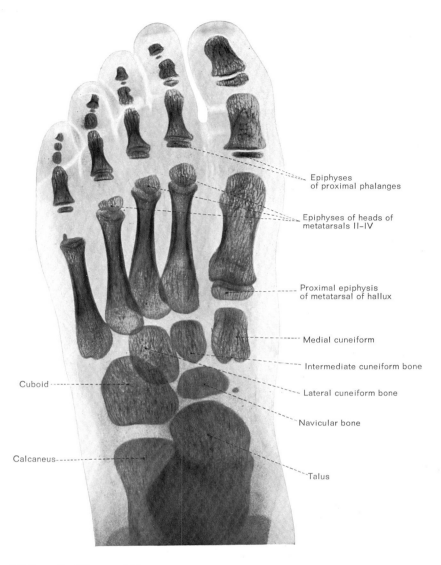

Epiphyses
of proximal phalanges

Epiphyses of heads of
metatarsals II–IV

Proximal epiphysis
of metatarsal of hallux

Medial cuneiform

Intermediate cuneiform bone

Lateral cuneiform bone

Navicular bone

Talus

Cuboid

Calcaneus

**Fig. 184.** X-ray of the left foot of a 5½ year old boy.

Note: The development of the distal-formed epiphyses, the metatarsals II–IV, as well as the proximal epiphyses of the phalanges and that of metatarsal I (compare with Fig. 146). The x-ray picture distinctly shows the epiphyseal "gaps" which make up the cartilaginous epiphyseal juncture, the zone for growth and length.

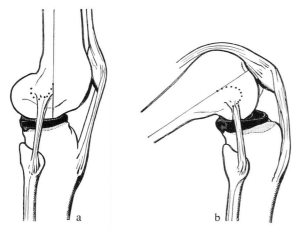

a          b

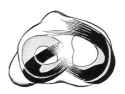

**Fig. 185.** Right knee joint, lateral view. a) Extended. b) Flexed. With stronger flexion, the meniscus, especially the lateral on the cartilaginous plate of the tibia (stippling) will be pushed backward.

**Fig. 186.** View of the head of left superior articular surface of the tibia. Position of meniscus in extension of knee joint, stippled; in flexion, black. Note the greater movement of the lateral meniscus. (Figs. 185 and 186 after H. Virchow from Benninghoff-Goerttler: Lehrbuch der Anatomie des Menschen Vol. I: 10, Urban & Schwarzenberg, Munich–Berlin–Vienna 1968.)

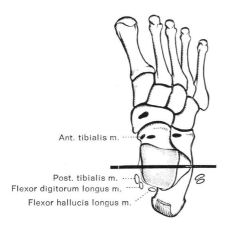

Ant. tibialis m.

Post. tibialis m.
Flexor digitorum longus m.
Flexor hallucis longus m.

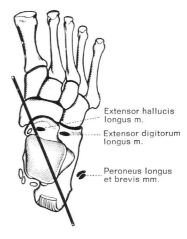

Extensor hallucis longus m.

Extensor digitorum longus m.

Peroneus longus et brevis mm.

**Fig. 187.** Axis of the upper ankle joint, the talocrural articulation, with the tendons of the muscles for this joint. Tendons of the extensors, black; tendons of the flexors, white. Compare with Fig. 188.

**Fig. 188.** Axis of the lower ankle joint, the talocalcaneo-navicular and subtalar articulations, with the tendons of the muscles for these joints. Tendons of the pronators, black; tendons of the supinators, white). Compare with Fig. 187. (Figs. 187 and 188 after S. Mollier from Benninghoff-Goerttler: Lehrbuch der Anatomie des Menschen, Vol. I: 10, pub. by Urban & Schwarzenberg, Munich–Berlin–Vienna, 1968.)

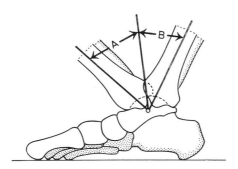

A     B

◀ **Fig. 189.** Flexion and extension in the upper ankle joint, the talocrural articulation, when the foot is solidly planted and the leg below the knee is moved back and forth. (From S. Mollier: Plastische Anatomie, 2. pub. by Bergmann, Munich, 1938.)

# Syndesmology

*Joints and Ligaments of the Vertebral Column, Thorax, Skull*

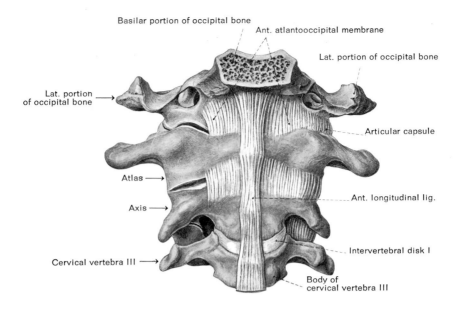

Basilar portion of occipital bone

Ant. atlantooccipital membrane

Lat. portion of occipital bone

Lat. portion of occipital bone

Articular capsule

Atlas

Axis

Ant. longitudinal lig.

Intervertebral disk I

Cervical vertebra III

Body of cervical vertebra III

**Fig. 190.** Part of the occipital bone, the first three vertebrae, the anterior atlantooccipital membrane, and the cranial end of the anterior longitudinal ligament. Articular capsules are removed on the right. Ventral view.

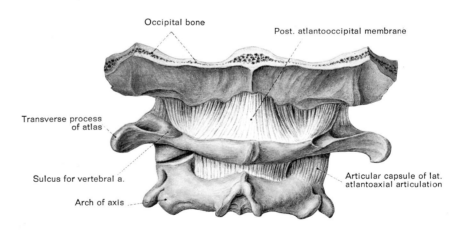

Occipital bone

Post. atlantooccipital membrane

Transverse process of atlas

Sulcus for vertebral a.

Arch of axis

Articular capsule of lat. atlantoaxial articulation

**Fig. 191.** Part of the occipital bone, atlas, and axis with their ligaments, and the posterior atlantooccipital membrane. The articular capsule of the lateral atlantoaxial articulation removed on left. Dorsal view.

Note: The atlantooccipital, lateral atlantoaxial, and median atlantoaxial articulations form a functional unit with the effect of a ball and socket joint. Dissection of the articular portions demonstrates the safeguard against dislocation.

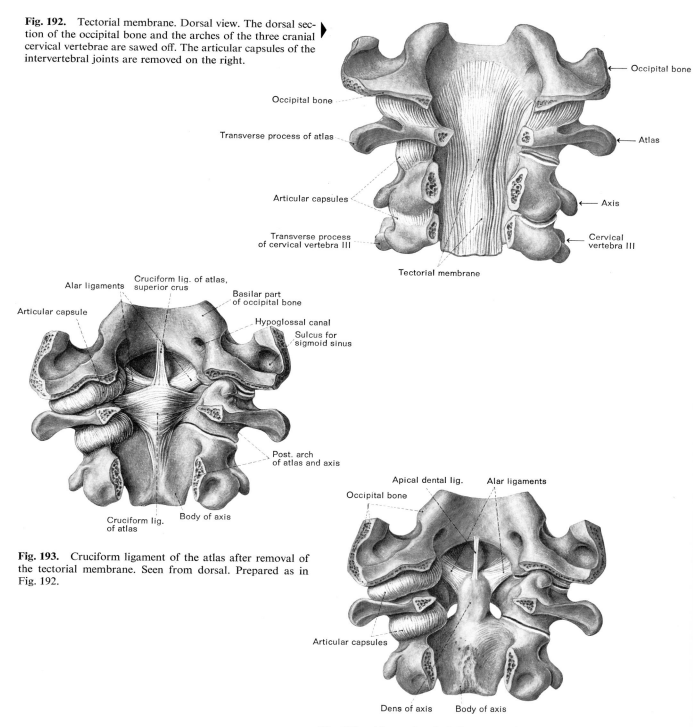

**Fig. 192.** Tectorial membrane. Dorsal view. The dorsal section of the occipital bone and the arches of the three cranial cervical vertebrae are sawed off. The articular capsules of the intervertebral joints are removed on the right.

Occipital bone

Transverse process of atlas

Articular capsules

Transverse process of cervical vertebra III

Tectorial membrane

Occipital bone

Atlas

Axis

Cervical vertebra III

Alar ligaments

Cruciform lig. of atlas, superior crus

Articular capsule

Basilar part of occipital bone

Hypoglossal canal

Sulcus for sigmoid sinus

Post. arch of atlas and axis

Cruciform lig. of atlas

Body of axis

**Fig. 193.** Cruciform ligament of the atlas after removal of the tectorial membrane. Seen from dorsal. Prepared as in Fig. 192.

Apical dental lig.

Alar ligaments

Occipital bone

Articular capsules

Dens of axis

Body of axis

**Fig. 194.** Alar and apical ligaments after removal of the cruciform ligament of the atlas. Seen from dorsal. Prepared as in Fig. 192.

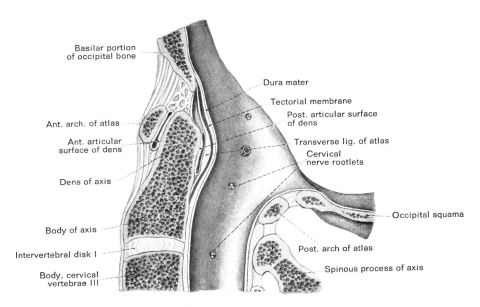

Basilar portion
of occipital bone

Dura mater

Tectorial membrane

Post. articular surface
of dens

Ant. arch. of atlas

Ant. articular
surface of dens

Transverse lig. of atlas

Cervical
nerve rootlets

Dens of axis

Occipital squama

Body of axis

Intervertebral disk I

Post. arch of atlas

Spinous process of axis

Body, cervical
vertebrae III

**Fig. 195.**　Atlantoaxial articulation. Median longitudinal section.

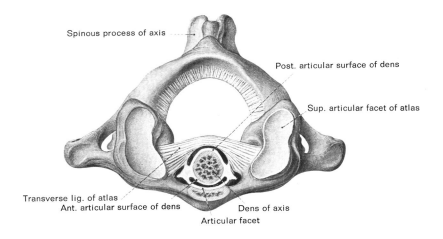

Spinous process of axis

Post. articular surface of dens

Sup. articular facet of atlas

Transverse lig. of atlas
Ant. articular surface of dens

Dens of axis

Articular facet

**Fig. 196.**　Median atlantoaxial articulation. The atlas is removed from the atlantooccipital articulation. The dens of the axis and the ventral arch of the atlas are sawed through horizontally. Cranial view.

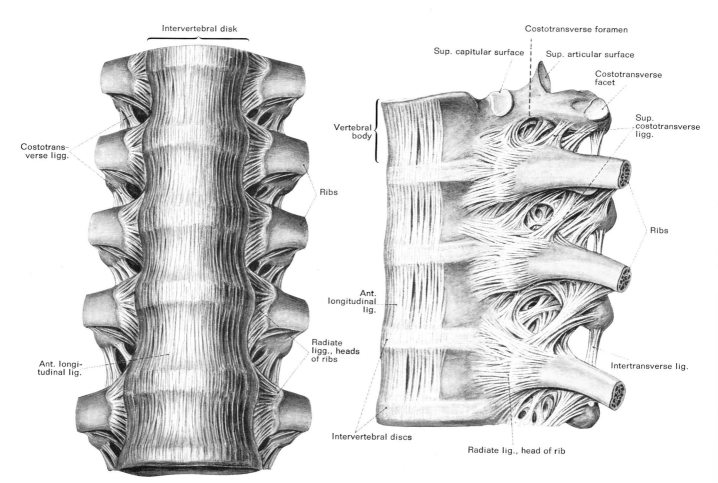

Fig. 197. Preparation of the anterior longitudinal ligament of the caudal section of the thoracic vertebral column with the costovertebral articulations. Ventral view.

Fig. 198. Preparation of the middle and caudal thoracic vertebrae and ribs. The most cranial rib was disarticulated and removed. Left lateral view.

Note: The heads of the ribs articulate with the (12) vertebrae and the (10) intervertebral disks forming the costovertebral articulations. These are gliding joints between the heads of the ribs and the demifacet of two adjacent vertebrae. Only the 11th and 12th thoracic vertebrae have a whole costal facet on the upper lateral surface of the vertebrae.

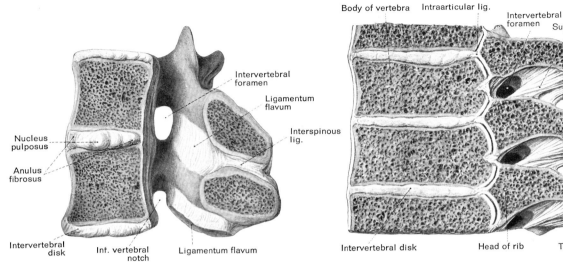

Nucleus
pulposus

Anulus
fibrosus

Intervertebral
disk

Inf. vertebral
notch

Ligamentum flavum

Intervertebral
foramen

Ligamentum
flavum

Interspinous
lig.

Body of vertebra    Intraarticular lig.

Intervertebral
foramen    Sup. costotransverse lig.

Lat. costotransverse lig.

Intervertebral disk

Head of rib

Tubercle of rib

**Fig. 199.** Two thoracic vertebrae with their ligaments (ligamenta flava). Cut through the median sagittal plane.

**Fig. 200.** Sawcut through the vertebral bodies, the costovertebral articulations and the vertebral ends of the ribs. The cut is at the 45° angle to the median plane. The interarticular crest is closely bound up with the intervertebral disk through the intraarticular ligament. The rib belongs to the body of the vertebra below.

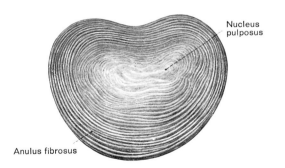

Nucleus
pulposus

Anulus fibrosus

**Fig. 201.** Articulating surface view of an isolated intervertebral disk. Lumbar vertebra.

99

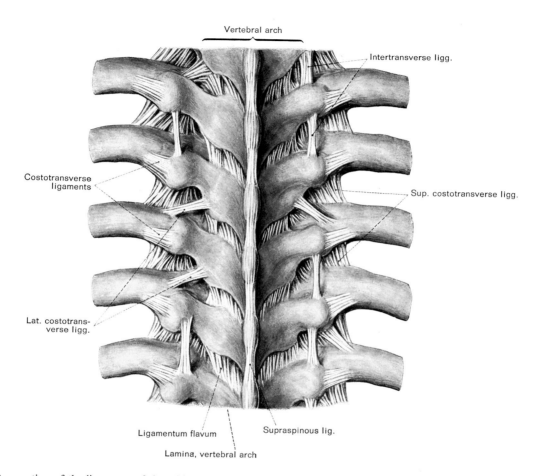

Vertebral arch

Intertransverse ligg.

Costotransverse
ligaments

Sup. costotransverse ligg.

Lat. costotrans-
verse ligg.

Ligamentum flavum

Supraspinous lig.

Lamina, vertebral arch

**Fig. 202.** Preparation of the ligaments of the middle and caudal thoracic vertebrae and ribs. Articulations of the vertebrae. Dorsal view.

100

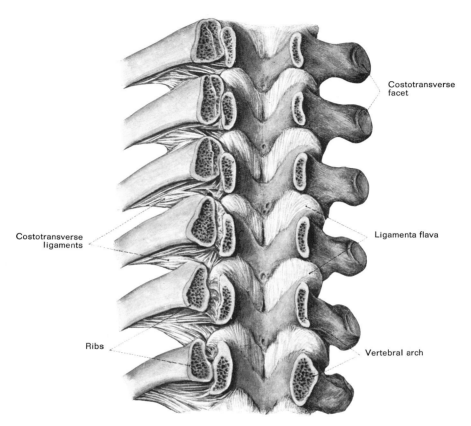

Costotransverse
facet

Costotransverse
ligaments

Ligamenta flava

Ribs

Vertebral arch

**Fig. 203.** Ligamenta flava of the thoracic vertebrae. (Seen from inside the vertebral canal.) The vertebral bodies are sawed off to display the lamina. The ribs on the left are disarticulate and removed; on the right, they are in their natural position.

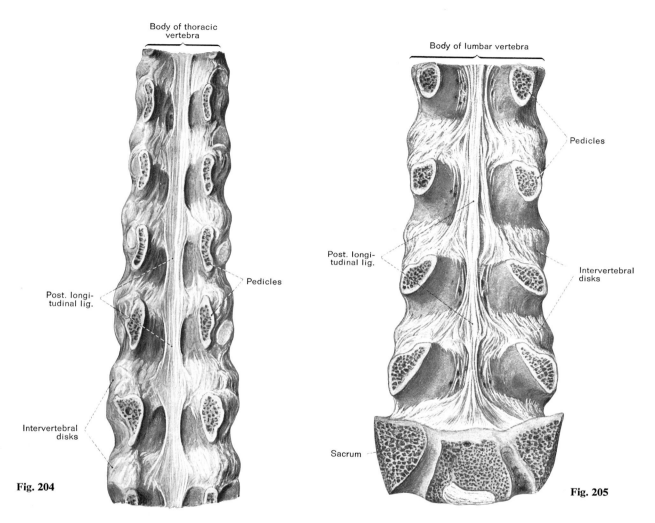

Body of thoracic vertebra

Body of lumbar vertebra

Pedicles

Post. longi-
tudinal lig.

Intervertebral
disks

Pedicles

Post. longi-
tudinal lig.

Intervertebral
disks

Sacrum

**Fig. 204**

**Fig. 205**

**Figs. 204 and 205.** Posterior longitudinal ligament and intervertebral disk. Vertebral canal opened by removing the vertebral arches from the dorsal side. Fig. 204. Caudal region of the thoracic vertebrae. Fig. 205. Region of the lumbar portion of the spine and the sacrum.

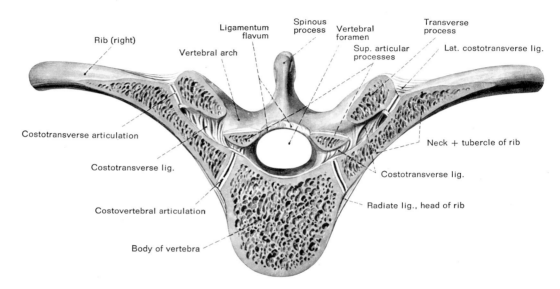

**Fig. 206.** Horizontal section through a thoracic vertebra, with the costovertebral articulations.

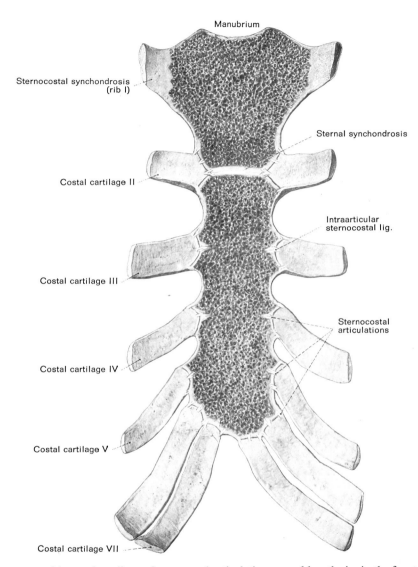

Manubrium

Sternocostal synchondrosis
(rib I)

Sternal synchondrosis

Costal cartilage II

Intraarticular
sternocostal lig.

Costal cartilage III

Sternocostal
articulations

Costal cartilage IV

Costal cartilage V

Costal cartilage VII

**Fig. 207.** The sternum with costal cartilages. Sternocostal articulations sawed lengthwise in the frontal plane.

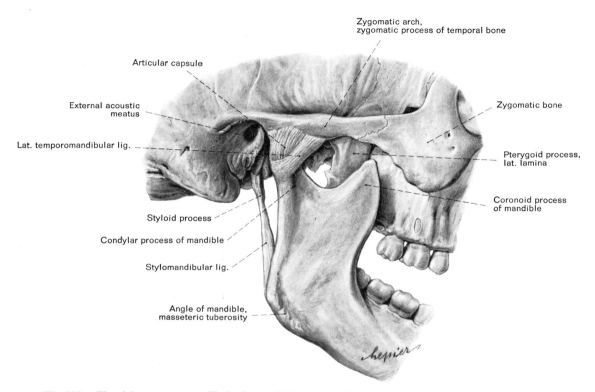

**Fig. 208.** The right temporomandibular joint with ligaments. Lateral view.

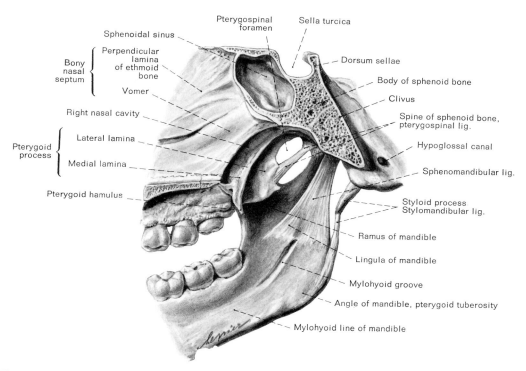

Pterygospinal foramen

Sella turcica

Sphenoidal sinus

Bony nasal septum { Perpendicular lamina of ethmoid bone

Dorsum sellae

Body of sphenoid bone

Vomer

Clivus

Right nasal cavity

Spine of sphenoid bone, pterygospinal lig.

Pterygoid process { Lateral lamina

Hypoglossal canal

Medial lamina

Sphenomandibular lig.

Pterygoid hamulus

Styloid process
Stylomandibular lig.

Ramus of mandible

Lingula of mandible

Mylohyoid groove

Angle of mandible, pterygoid tuberosity

Mylohyoid line of mandible

**Fig. 209.** The right temporomandibular joint with ligaments. Medial view.

# Syndesmology

---

*Joints and Ligaments of the Shoulder Girdle and Upper Limb*

---

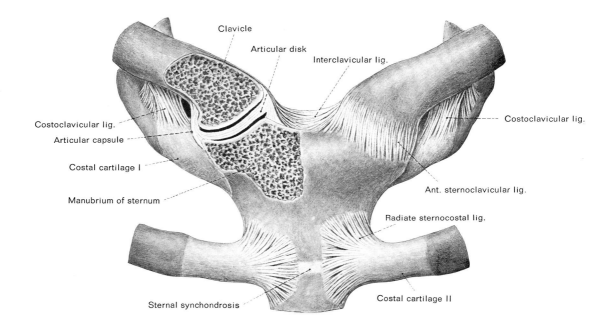

Clavicle

Articular disk

Interclavicular lig.

Costoclavicular lig.

Costoclavicular lig.

Articular capsule

Costal cartilage I

Ant. sternoclavicular lig.

Manubrium of sternum

Radiate sternocostal lig.

Sternal synchondrosis

Costal cartilage II

**Fig. 210.** Both sternoclavicular joints (and the articulations of the cranial ribs with the sternum). Ventral view. The right sternoclavicular joint was opened by a frontal sawcut.

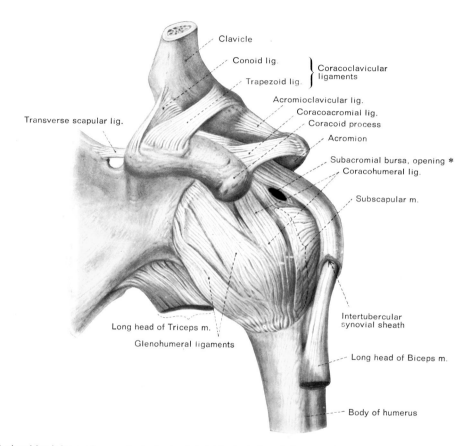

Clavicle

Conoid lig.

Trapezoid lig.

Coracoclavicular ligaments

Acromioclavicular lig.
Coracoacromial lig.
Coracoid process
Acromion

Transverse scapular lig.

Subacromial bursa, opening *
Coracohumeral lig.

Subscapular m.

Intertubercular synovial sheath

Long head of Triceps m.

Glenohumeral ligaments

Long head of Biceps m.

Body of humerus

**Fig. 211.** Left shoulder joint and acromioclavicular joint. Ventral view. * Communication point with the subacromial bursa.

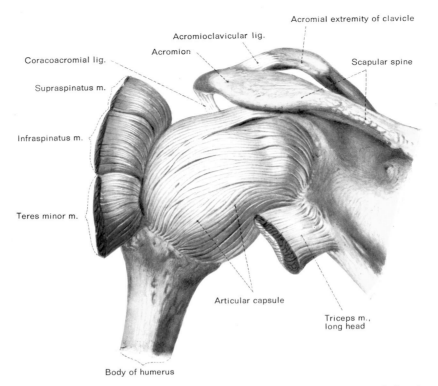

Coracoacromial lig.

Acromion

Acromioclavicular lig.

Acromial extremity of clavicle

Scapular spine

Supraspinatus m.

Infraspinatus m.

Teres minor m.

Articular capsule

Triceps m., long head

Body of humerus

**Fig. 212.** Left shoulder joint. Dorsal view. The muscle attachments of the Supraspinatus, Infraspinatus, Teres minor, and the long head of the Triceps muscles show the relationship to the joint capsule.

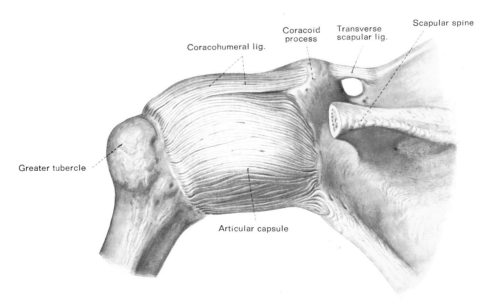

Coracohumeral lig.

Coracoid process

Transverse scapular lig.

Scapular spine

Greater tubercle

Articular capsule

**Fig. 213.** Left shoulder joint without muscle attachments. Dorsocranial view. The acromium is cut off with a saw.

111

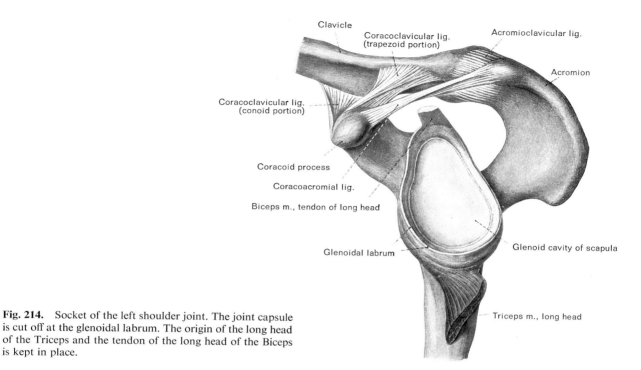

Clavicle
Coracoclavicular lig.
(trapezoid portion)
Acromioclavicular lig.
Acromion
Coracoclavicular lig.
(conoid portion)
Coracoid process
Coracoacromial lig.
Biceps m., tendon of long head
Glenoidal labrum
Glenoid cavity of scapula
Triceps m., long head

**Fig. 214.** Socket of the left shoulder joint. The joint capsule is cut off at the glenoidal labrum. The origin of the long head of the Triceps and the tendon of the long head of the Biceps is kept in place.

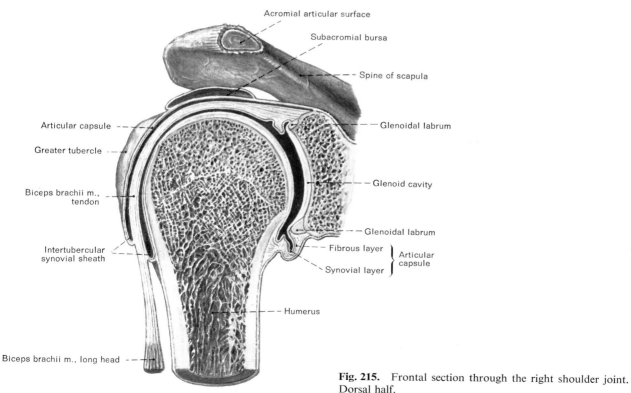

Acromial articular surface
Subacromial bursa
Spine of scapula
Articular capsule
Greater tubercle
Glenoidal labrum
Glenoid cavity
Biceps brachii m., tendon
Glenoidal labrum
Fibrous layer
Synovial layer
Articular capsule
Intertubercular synovial sheath
Humerus
Biceps brachii m., long head

**Fig. 215.** Frontal section through the right shoulder joint. Dorsal half.

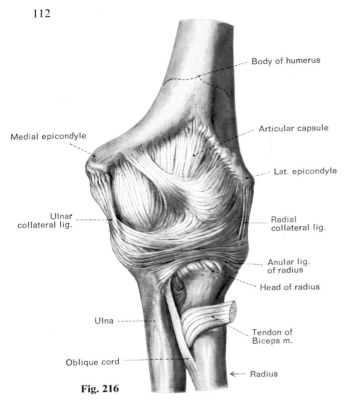

Body of humerus

Articular capsule

Lat. epicondyle

Medial epicondyle

Radial
collateral lig.

Ulnar
collateral lig.

Anular lig.
of radius

Head of radius

Ulna

Tendon of
Biceps m.

Oblique cord

Radius

**Fig. 216**

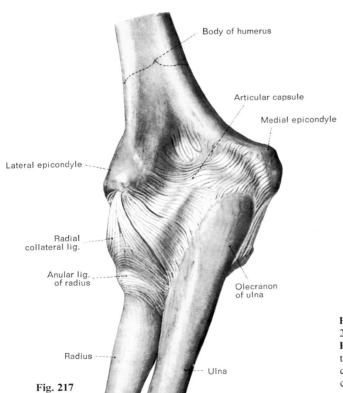

Body of humerus

Articular capsule

Medial epicondyle

Lateral epicondyle

Radial
collateral lig.

Anular lig.
of radius

Olecranon
of ulna

Radius

Ulna

**Fig. 217**

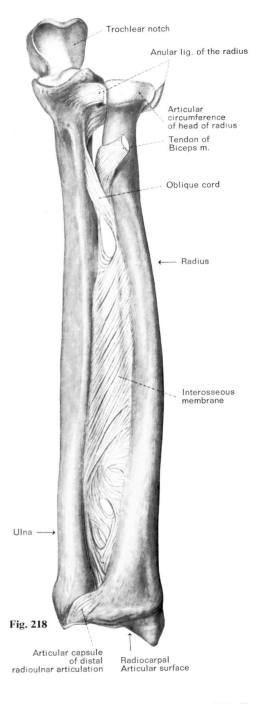

Trochlear notch

Anular lig. of the radius

Articular
circumference
of head of radius

Tendon of
Biceps m.

Oblique cord

Radius

Interosseous
membrane

Ulna

**Fig. 218**

Articular capsule
of distal
radioulnar articulation

Radiocarpal
Articular surface

**Figs. 216 and 217.** Left elbow joint (articulatio cubiti). Fig.
216. Palmar view. Fig. 217. Dorsoradial view.
**Fig. 218.** Both left forearm bones, the radius and ulna, and
the interosseus membrane. The elbow joint was opened, the
capsule removed; the anular ligament of the radius has been
cut to expose the cylindrical head of the radius.

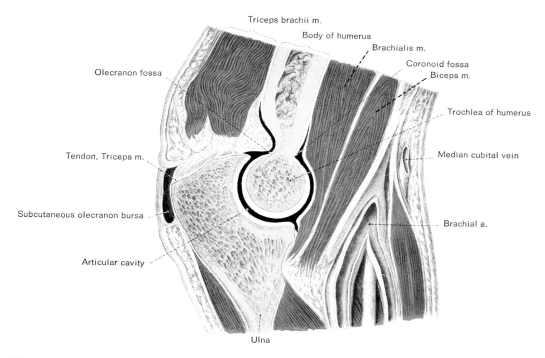

**Fig. 219.** Sagittal section (frozen) of the left elbow joint, humeroulnar articulation.

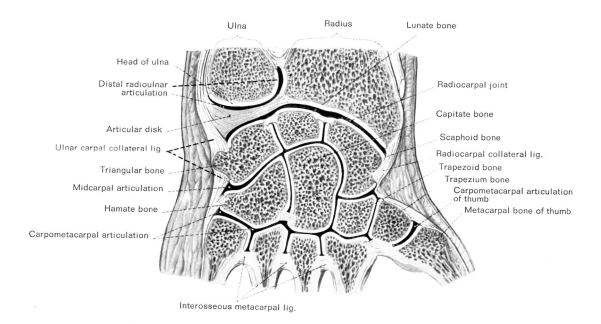

**Fig. 220.** Section through the wrist joint, cut parallel to the dorsal surface of the hand.

114

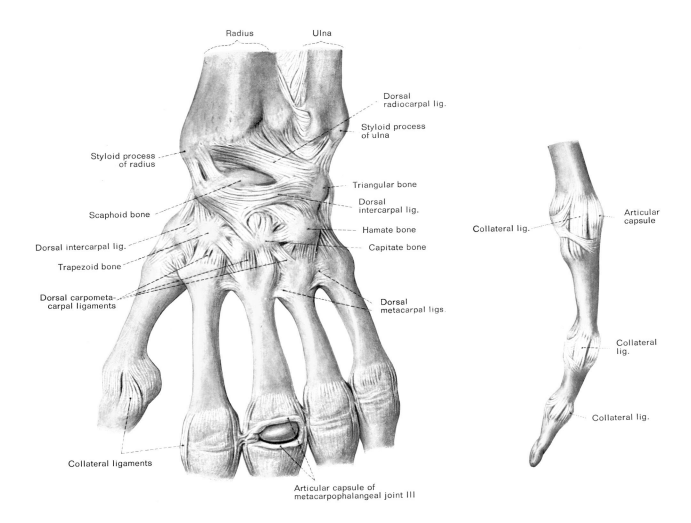

Radius

Ulna

Dorsal
radiocarpal lig.

Styloid process
of ulna

Styloid process
of radius

Triangular bone

Dorsal
intercarpal lig.

Scaphoid bone

Hamate bone

Dorsal intercarpal lig.

Capitate bone

Trapezoid bone

Dorsal carpometa-
carpal ligaments

Dorsal
metacarpal ligs.

Collateral ligaments

Articular capsule of
metacarpophalangeal joint III

Collateral lig.

Articular
capsule

Collateral
lig.

Collateral lig.

**Fig. 221.** Articulations and ligaments of the hand and wrist. **Fig. 222.** Articulations of the middle finger. Lateral view.
Dorsal view.

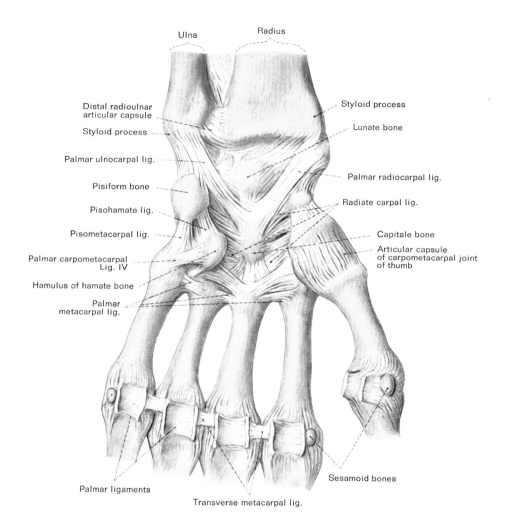

Ulna

Radius

Distal radioulnar
articular capsule

Styloid process

Styloid process

Lunate bone

Palmar ulnocarpal lig.

Palmar radiocarpal lig.

Pisiform bone

Radiate carpal lig.

Pisohamate lig.

Pisometacarpal lig.

Capitale bone

Articular capsule
of carpometacarpal joint
of thumb

Palmar carpometacarpal
Lig. IV

Hamulus of hamate bone

Palmar
metacarpal lig.

Sesamoid bones

Palmar ligaments

Transverse metacarpal lig.

**Fig. 223.** Articulations and ligaments of the hand and wrist. Palmar view. The flexor retinaculum (ligamentum carpi transversum) was removed. The sesamoid bones of the thumb, index and little finger were exposed.

# Syndesmology

*Joints and Ligaments of the Pelvic Girdle and Lower Limb*

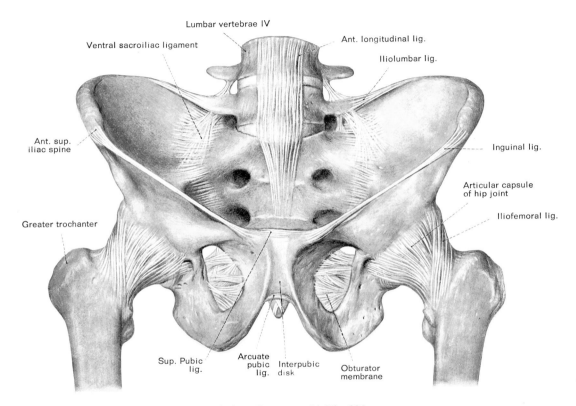

Lumbar vertebrae IV

Ventral sacroiliac ligament

Ant. longitudinal lig.

Iliolumbar lig.

Ant. sup.
iliac spine

Inguinal lig.

Articular capsule
of hip joint

Iliofemoral lig.

Greater trochanter

Sup. Pubic
lig.

Arcuate
pubic
lig.

Interpubic
disk

Obturator
membrane

**Fig. 224.** Male pelvis with its ligaments. Ventral view. Compare with Fig. 225.

Note: 1. The differences between the male and female pelves are primarily related to an enlarged pelvic outlet in the female to facilitate the function of childbearing.

### The Chief Differences between Male and Female Pelves:

(1) The **subpubic angle** or arch is wider and more rounded in the female pelvis than in the male.
(2) The **ischial tuberosities** are more widely separated and everted in the female pelvis than in the male.
(3) The **symphysis pubis** is more shallow in the female. The distance between the arcuate ligament and the superior pubic ligament is greater in the male pelvis.
(4) The **ilia** have more flare in the female pelvis. This results in a shallow, wide, pelvis major in the female; and a narrower, deeper pelvis major in the male.
(5) The **sacrum** is broader and less curved in the female.
(6) The **obturator foramen** is smaller and somewhat triangular in shape in the female.

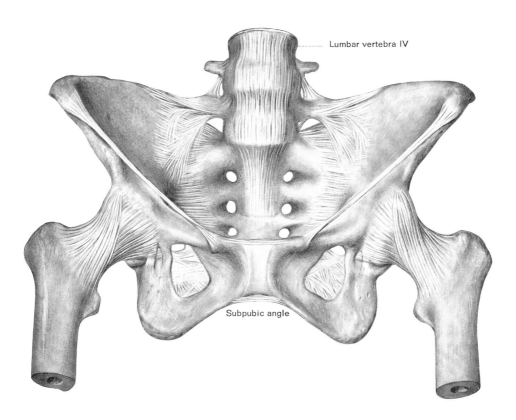

Lumbar vertebra IV

Subpubic angle

**Fig. 225.** Female pelvis with its ligaments. Ventral view.

### The Chief Differences between Male and Female Pelves: (Continued)

(7) The **cavity of the true pelvis (pelvis minor)** is wider and more shallow in the female than in the male.

(8) The outline of the **superior aperture of the pelvis minor** is more nearly circular in the female. This is, in in part, related to the protrusion of the **promontory** into the male pelvis minor to give it more of a heart shape.

(9) The **inferior outlet of the pelvis minor** is larger in the female.

(10) The **sciatic notches** are wider and more shallow in the female pelvis and the **ischial spines** do not protrude so far into the pelvis minor. The interspinous distance is, therefore, greater in the female.

(11) The **coccyx is more movable** and able to accommodate for increased size of the birth canal near the termination of pregnancy (Fig. 147).

(12) The **bones of the female pelvis are more delicate** and lighter in weight than those of the male pelvis.

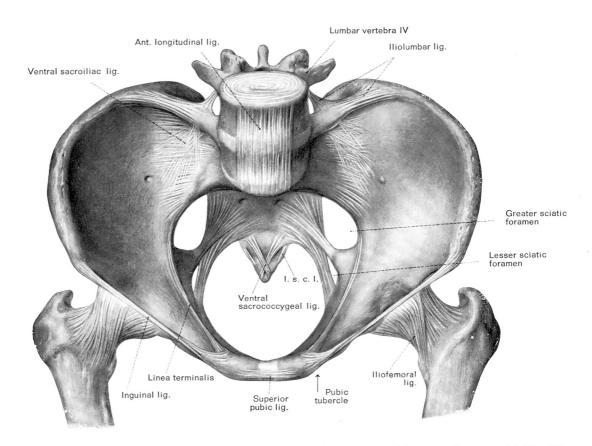

**Fig. 226.** Male pelvis with its ligaments. Cranial view. l. s. c. l. = lateral sacrococcygeal ligament. Compare with Fig. 227.

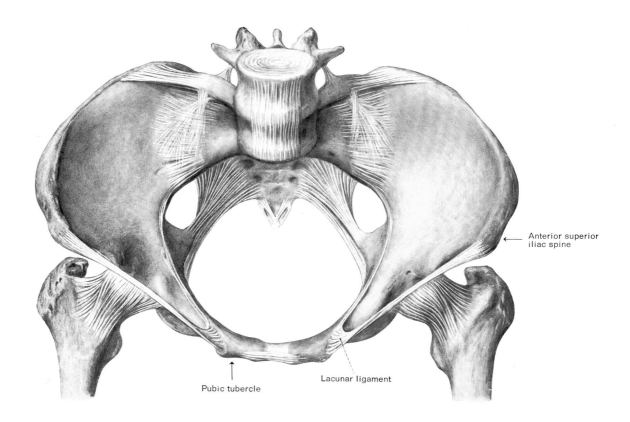

Anterior superior
iliac spine

Pubic tubercle

Lacunar ligament

**Fig. 227.** Female pelvis with its ligaments. Cranial view. Compare with Fig. 226.

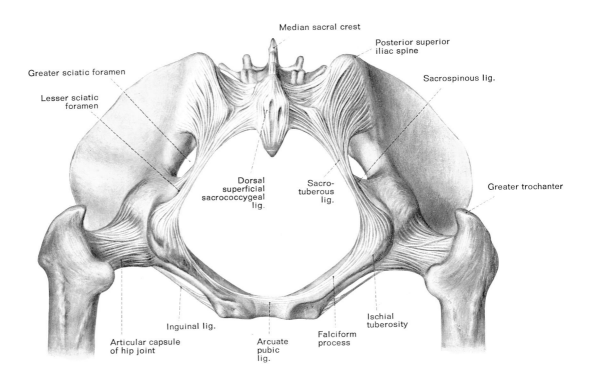

**Fig. 228.** Female pelvis with its ligaments. Caudal view.

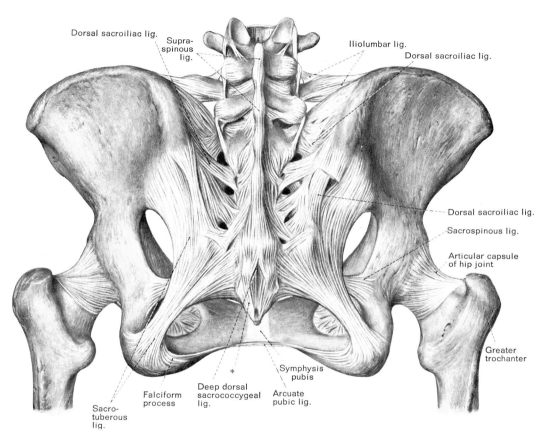

Dorsal sacroiliac lig.

Supra-spinous lig.

Iliolumbar lig.

Dorsal sacroiliac lig.

Dorsal sacroiliac lig.

Sacrospinous lig.

Articular capsule of hip joint

Greater trochanter

Symphysis pubis

Arcuate pubic lig.

Deep dorsal sacrococcygeal lig.

Falciform process

Sacro-tuberous lig.

*

**Fig. 229.** Female pelvis with its ligaments. Dorsal view. On the right, a superficial layer of the dorsal sacroiliac ligament has been removed. * Superficial dorsal sacrococcygeal ligament.

124

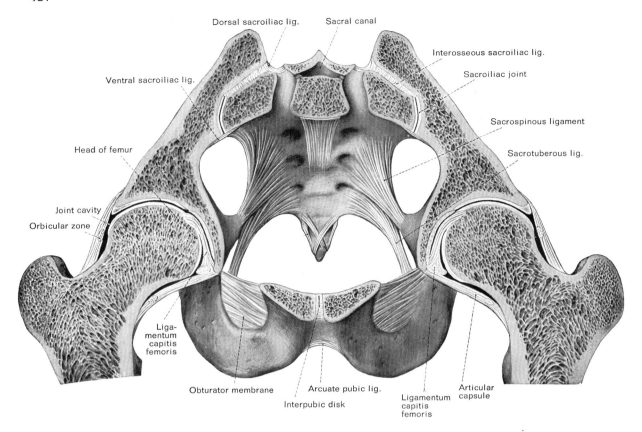

Dorsal sacroiliac lig.

Sacral canal

Interosseous sacroiliac lig.

Ventral sacroiliac lig.

Sacroiliac joint

Sacrospinous ligament

Sacrotuberous lig.

Head of femur

Joint cavity

Orbicular zone

Liga-
mentum
capitis
femoris

Obturator membrane

Interpubic disk

Arcuate pubic lig.

Ligamentum
capitis
femoris

Articular
capsule

**Fig. 230.** Frontal section of the pelvis and both hip joints, somewhat perpendicular to the pelvic axis. The preparation shows, in addition to the hip joints, the symphysis pubis with its articular space, the sacroiliac articulations, the pelvic view of the sacrospinous and sacrotuberous ligaments.

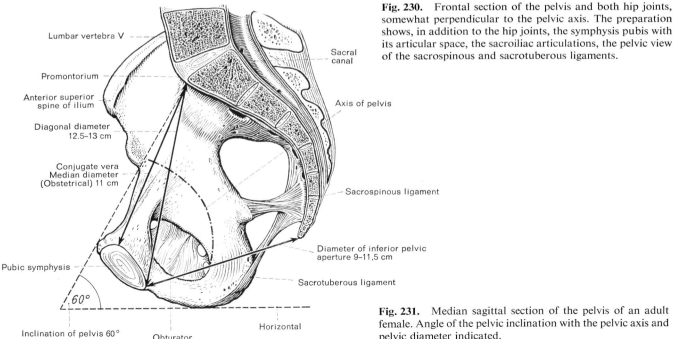

Lumbar vertebra V

Promontorium

Anterior superior
spine of ilium

Diagonal diameter
12.5–13 cm

Conjugate vera
Median diameter
(Obstetrical) 11 cm

Pubic symphysis

Sacral
canal

Axis of pelvis

Sacrospinous ligament

Diameter of inferior pelvic
aperture 9–11,5 cm

Sacrotuberous ligament

60°

Inclination of pelvis 60°

Obturator
membrane

Horizontal

**Fig. 231.** Median sagittal section of the pelvis of an adult female. Angle of the pelvic inclination with the pelvic axis and pelvic diameter indicated.

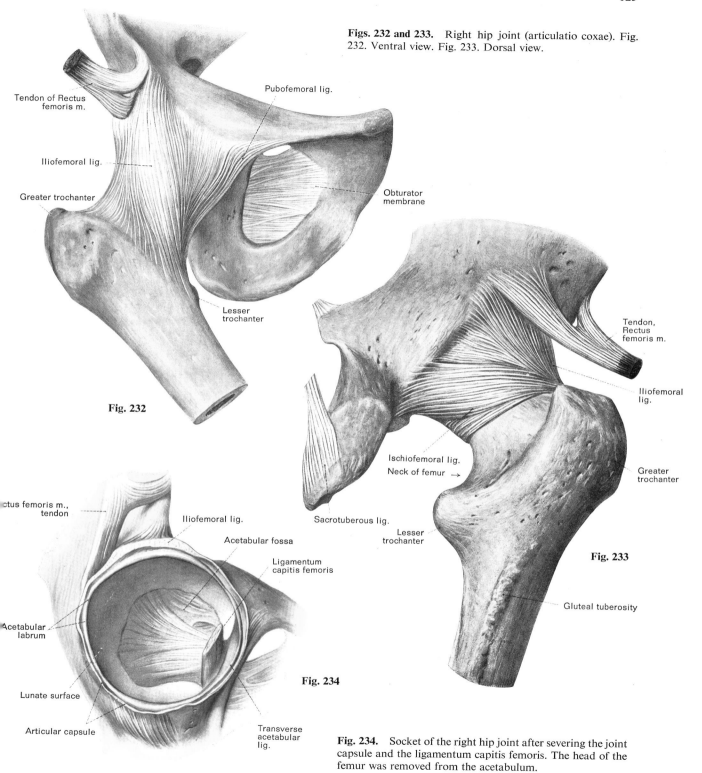

**Figs. 232 and 233.** Right hip joint (articulatio coxae). Fig. 232. Ventral view. Fig. 233. Dorsal view.

Tendon of Rectus femoris m.

Iliofemoral lig.

Greater trochanter

Pubofemoral lig.

Obturator membrane

Lesser trochanter

**Fig. 232**

Tendon, Rectus femoris m.

Iliofemoral lig.

Ischiofemoral lig.

Neck of femur →

Greater trochanter

Sacrotuberous lig.

Lesser trochanter

**Fig. 233**

Gluteal tuberosity

ctus femoris m., tendon

Iliofemoral lig.

Acetabular fossa

Ligamentum capitis femoris

Acetabular labrum

Lunate surface

Articular capsule

Transverse acetabular lig.

**Fig. 234**

**Fig. 234.** Socket of the right hip joint after severing the joint capsule and the ligamentum capitis femoris. The head of the femur was removed from the acetabulum.

126

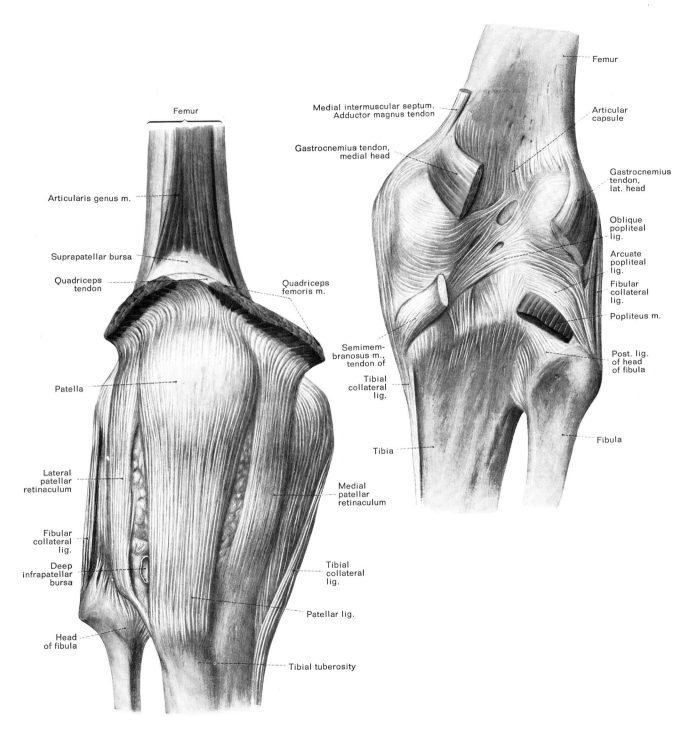

Femur

Articularis genus m.

Suprapatellar bursa

Quadriceps tendon

Patella

Lateral patellar retinaculum

Fibular collateral lig.

Deep infrapatellar bursa

Head of fibula

Quadriceps femoris m.

Medial patellar retinaculum

Tibial collateral lig.

Patellar lig.

Tibial tuberosity

Medial intermuscular septum, Adductor magnus tendon

Gastrocnemius tendon, medial head

Semimem- branosus m., tendon of

Tibial collateral lig.

Tibia

Femur

Articular capsule

Gastrocnemius tendon, lat. head

Oblique popliteal lig.

Arcuate popliteal lig.

Fibular collateral lig.

Popliteus m.

Post. lig. of head of fibula

Fibula

**Fig. 235.** Extended right knee joint (articulatio genus). Anterior view.

**Fig. 236.** Extended right knee joint. Posterior view.

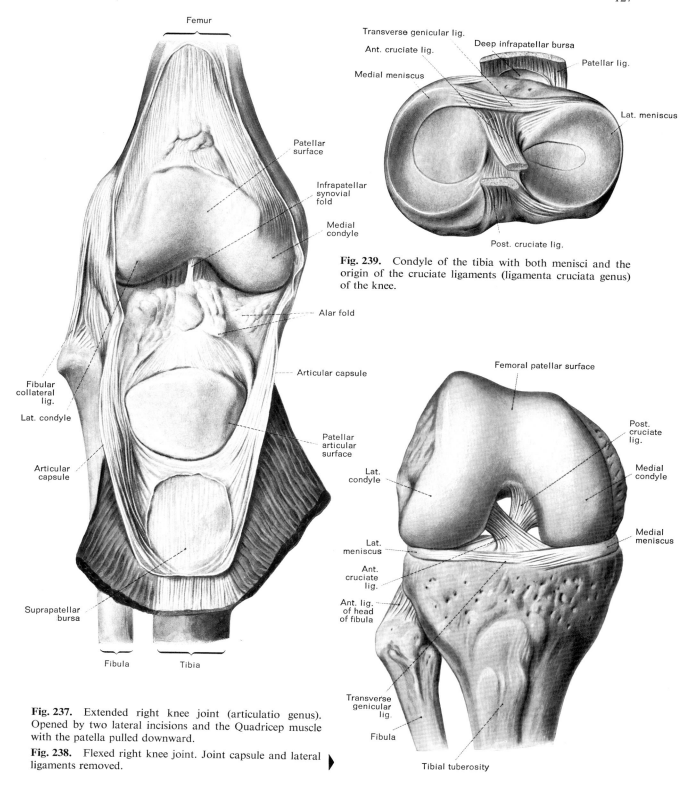

**Fig. 239.** Condyle of the tibia with both menisci and the origin of the cruciate ligaments (ligamenta cruciata genus) of the knee.

**Fig. 237.** Extended right knee joint (articulatio genus). Opened by two lateral incisions and the Quadricep muscle with the patella pulled downward.

**Fig. 238.** Flexed right knee joint. Joint capsule and lateral ligaments removed.

Labels in Fig. 237:
Femur — Patellar surface — Infrapatellar synovial fold — Medial condyle — Alar fold — Articular capsule — Patellar articular surface — Fibular collateral lig. — Lat. condyle — Articular capsule — Suprapatellar bursa — Fibula — Tibia

Labels in Fig. 239:
Transverse genicular lig. — Ant. cruciate lig. — Medial meniscus — Deep infrapatellar bursa — Patellar lig. — Lat. meniscus — Post. cruciate lig.

Labels in Fig. 238:
Femoral patellar surface — Post. cruciate lig. — Medial condyle — Medial meniscus — Lat. condyle — Lat. meniscus — Ant. cruciate lig. — Ant. lig. of head of fibula — Transverse genicular lig. — Fibula — Tibial tuberosity

128

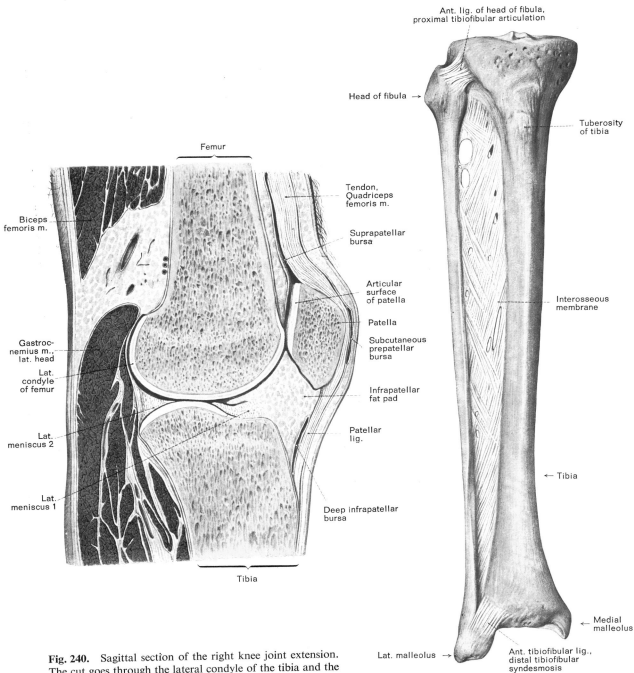

Femur

Biceps
femoris m.

Gastroc-
nemius m.,
lat. head

Lat.
condyle
of femur

Lat.
meniscus 2

Lat.
meniscus 1

Tibia

Tendon,
Quadriceps
femoris m.

Suprapatellar
bursa

Articular
surface
of patella

Patella

Subcutaneous
prepatellar
bursa

Infrapatellar
fat pad

Patellar
lig.

Deep infrapatellar
bursa

Ant. lig. of head of fibula,
proximal tibiofibular articulation

Head of fibula →

Tuberosity
of tibia

Interosseous
membrane

← Tibia

Medial
malleolus

Lat. malleolus →

Ant. tibiofibular lig.,
distal tibiofibular
syndesmosis

**Fig. 240.** Sagittal section of the right knee joint extension. The cut goes through the lateral condyle of the tibia and the lateral meniscus. The latter was cut in two places: anterior and posterior. The congruity of the articular surfaces covered with cartilage are made possible by means of menisci, the plica alares and the fat bodies of the joint. The articular cavity is enlarged through the communication with the labyrinthine bursa.

**Fig. 241.** The right tibiofibular articulation with their ligaments. Anterior view.

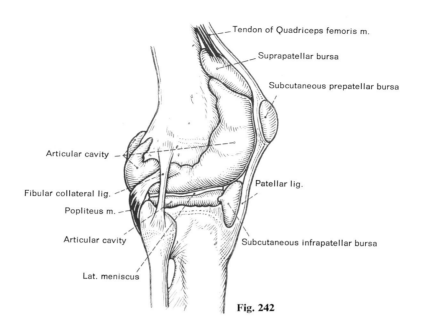

Tendon of Quadriceps femoris m.

Suprapatellar bursa

Subcutaneous prepatellar bursa

Articular cavity

Fibular collateral lig.

Popliteus m.

Articular cavity

Patellar lig.

Subcutaneous infrapatellar bursa

Lat. meniscus

**Fig. 242**

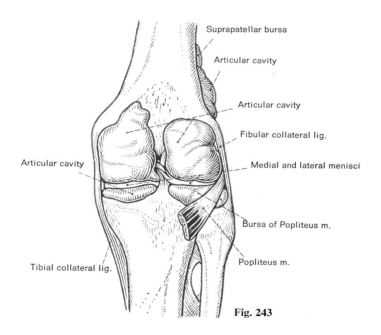

Suprapatellar bursa

Articular cavity

Articular cavity

Fibular collateral lig.

Articular cavity

Medial and lateral menisci

Bursa of Popliteus m.

Tibial collateral lig.

Popliteus m.

**Fig. 243**

**Figs. 242 and 243.** Joint effusion of the right knee joint (articulatio genus). Fig. 242. Seen from lateral. Fig. 243. Seen from dorsal.

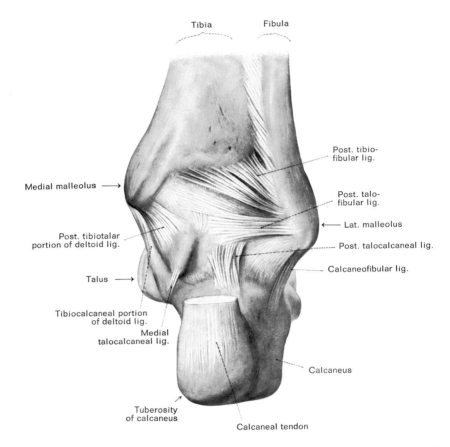

Tibia

Fibula

Medial malleolus ⟶

Post. tibio-
fibular lig.

Post. talo-
fibular lig.

⟵ Lat. malleolus

Post. talocalcaneal lig.

Post. tibiotalar
portion of deltoid lig.

Calcaneofibular lig.

Talus ⟶

Tibiocalcaneal portion
of deltoid lig.

Medial
talocalcaneal lig.

Calcaneus

Tuberosity
of calcaneus

Calcaneal tendon

**Fig. 244.**   The distal tibiofibular syndesmosis and ankle joint (articulatio talocruralis). Only a stump of the calcaneal tendon remains. Dorsal view.

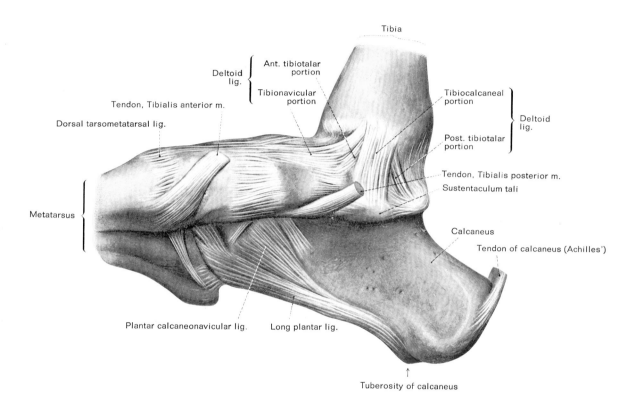

**Fig. 245.** Ligaments between the foot and the leg (ligamenta tarsi). Medial view.

132

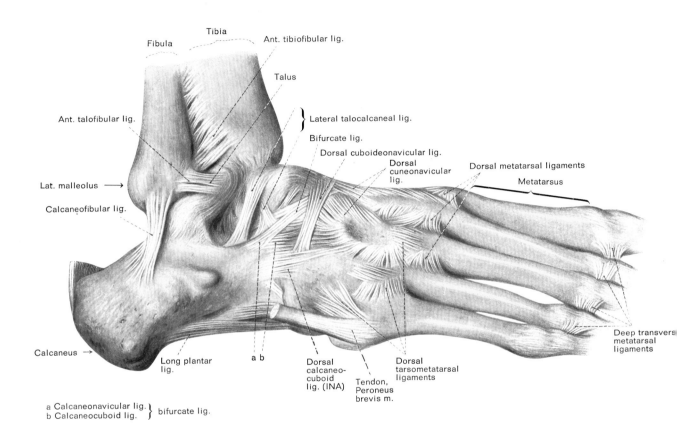

Tibia

Fibula

Ant. tibiofibular lig.

Talus

Lateral talocalcaneal lig.

Ant. talofibular lig.

Bifurcate lig.

Dorsal cuboideonavicular lig.

Dorsal cuneonavicular lig.

Dorsal metatarsal ligaments

Metatarsus

Lat. malleolus $\longrightarrow$

Calcaneofibular lig.

Deep transverse metatarsal ligaments

Calcaneus $\rightarrow$

Long plantar lig.

a b

Dorsal calcaneo-cuboid lig. (INA)

Tendon, Peroneus brevis m.

Dorsal tarsometatarsal ligaments

a Calcaneonavicular lig.
b Calcaneocuboid lig. } bifurcate lig.

**Fig. 246.** Ligaments of the foot (ligamenta pedis). Dorsolateral view.

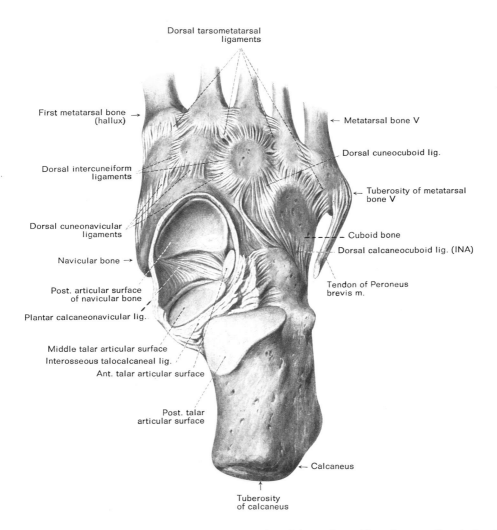

Dorsal tarsometatarsal
ligaments

First metatarsal bone →
(hallux)

← Metatarsal bone V

Dorsal cuneocuboid lig.

Dorsal intercuneiform
ligaments

← Tuberosity of metatarsal
bone V

Dorsal cuneonavicular
ligaments

Navicular bone →

Cuboid bone

Dorsal calcaneocuboid lig. (INA)

Post. articular surface
of navicular bone

Plantar calcaneonavicular lig.

Tendon of Peroneus
brevis m.

Middle talar articular surface
Interosseous talocalcaneal lig.
Ant. talar articular surface

Post. talar
articular surface

← Calcaneus

Tuberosity
of calcaneus

**Fig. 247.** Talocalcaneonavicular articulation, lower ankle joint. Viewed from above. The talus was disarticulated and removed to display its articulations, especially the navicular socket for its head.

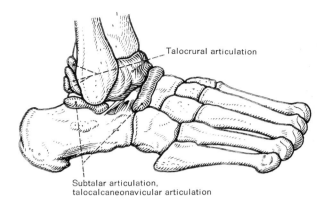

**Fig. 248.** Joint effusion of the upper and lower ankle joints on the right foot, (articulatio talocruralis, articulatio subtalaris, articulatio talocalcaneonavicularis). Lateral view (after Benninghoff, Goerttler, Lehrbuch der Anatomie des Menschen, Vol. I).

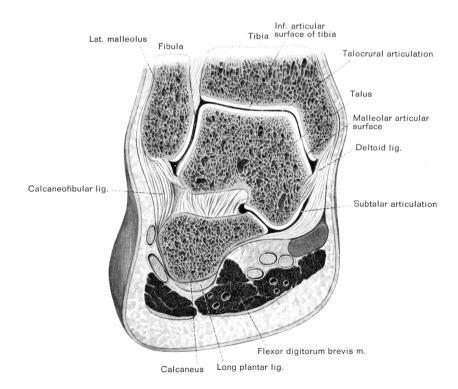

**Fig. 249.** Frontal frozen section through the upper ankle joint (articulatio talocruralis) and the dorsal compartment of the lower ankle joint (articulatio subtalaris).

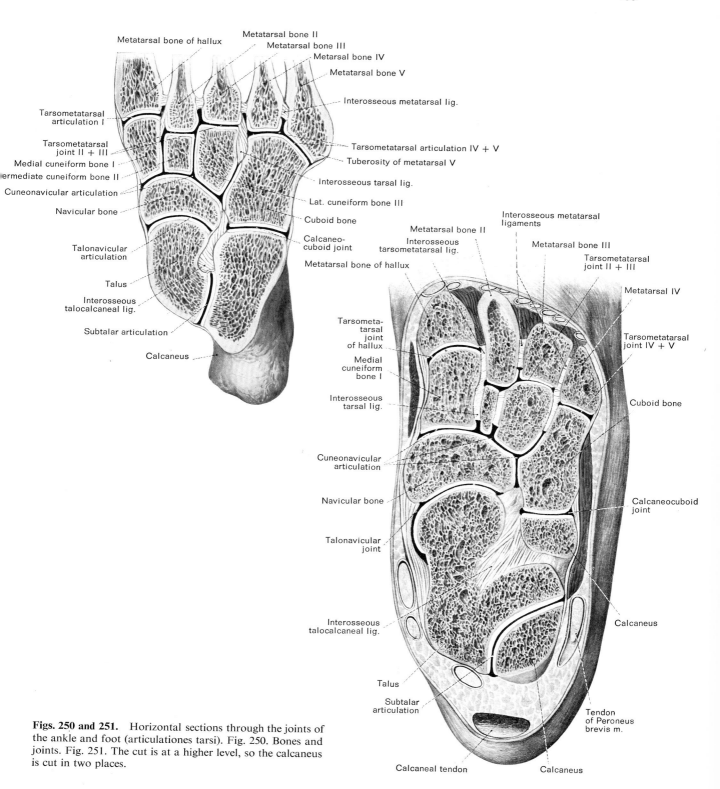

Metatarsal bone of hallux
Metatarsal bone II
Metatarsal bone III
Metarsal bone IV
Metatarsal bone V
Interosseous metatarsal lig.
Tarsometatarsal articulation I
Tarsometatarsal joint II + III
Medial cuneiform bone I
ermediate cuneiform bone II
Cuneonavicular articulation
Navicular bone
Tarsometatarsal articulation IV + V
Tuberosity of metatarsal V
Interosseous tarsal lig.
Lat. cuneiform bone III
Cuboid bone
Calcaneo-cuboid joint
Talonavicular articulation
Talus
Interosseous talocalcaneal lig.
Subtalar articulation
Calcaneus

Interosseous metatarsal ligaments
Metatarsal bone II
Interosseous tarsometatarsal lig.
Metatarsal bone III
Tarsometatarsal joint II + III
Metatarsal bone of hallux
Metatarsal IV
Tarsometatarsal joint IV + V
Tarsometa-tarsal joint of hallux
Medial cuneiform bone I
Interosseous tarsal lig.
Cuboid bone
Cuneonavicular articulation
Navicular bone
Calcaneocuboid joint
Talonavicular joint
Interosseous talocalcaneal lig.
Calcaneus
Talus
Subtalar articulation
Tendon of Peroneus brevis m.
Calcaneal tendon
Calcaneus

**Figs. 250 and 251.** Horizontal sections through the joints of the ankle and foot (articulationes tarsi). Fig. 250. Bones and joints. Fig. 251. The cut is at a higher level, so the calcaneus is cut in two places.

136

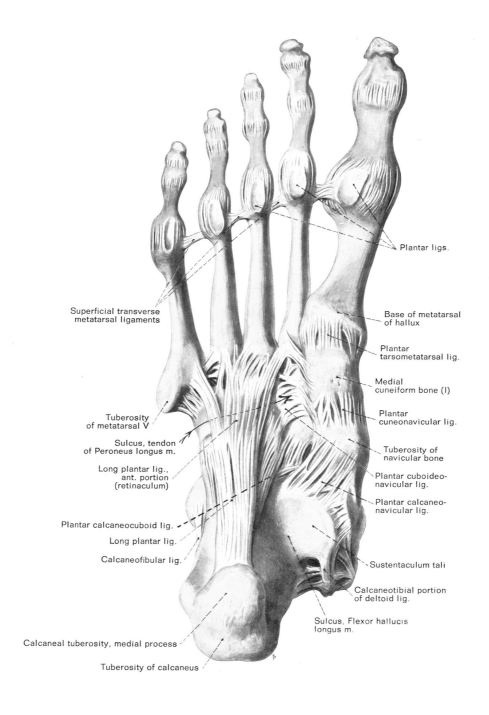

Plantar ligs.

Superficial transverse
metatarsal ligaments

Base of metatarsal
of hallux

Plantar
tarsometatarsal lig.

Medial
cuneiform bone (I)

Plantar
cuneonavicular lig.

Tuberosity
of metatarsal V

Sulcus, tendon
of Peroneus longus m.

Tuberosity of
navicular bone

Plantar cuboideo-
navicular lig.

Long plantar lig.,
ant. portion
(retinaculum)

Plantar calcaneo-
navicular lig.

Plantar calcaneocuboid lig.

Long plantar lig.

Calcaneofibular lig.

Sustentaculum tali

Calcaneotibial portion
of deltoid lig.

Sulcus, Flexor hallucis
longus m.

Calcaneal tuberosity, medial process

Tuberosity of calcaneus

**Fig. 252.** Ligaments of the plantar surface of the foot. Superficial layers.

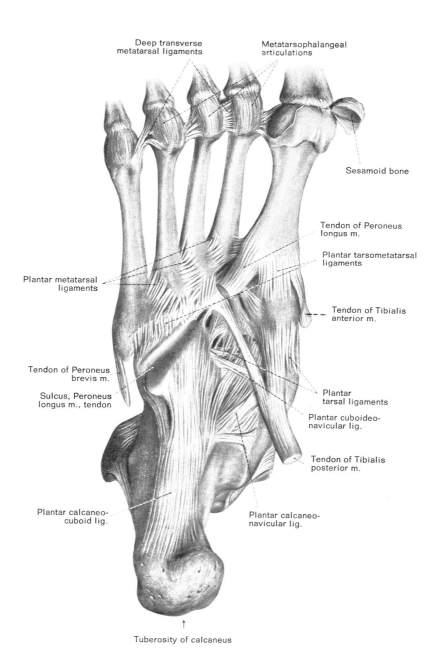

**Fig. 253.** Ligaments of the plantar surface of the foot. Deep layers. The metatarsal joint of the great toe was opened, exposing a sesamoid bone.

# Myology

---

*Muscles of the Neck, Trunk, and Pelvis*

---

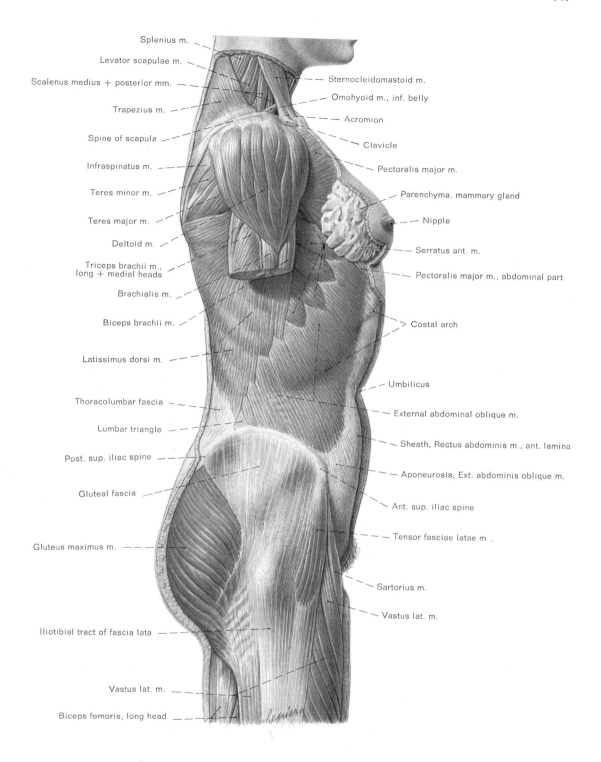

Splenius m.

Levator scapulae m.

Scalenus medius + posterior mm.

Trapezius m.

Spine of scapula

Infraspinatus m.

Teres minor m.

Teres major m.

Deltoid m.

Triceps brachii m., long + medial heads

Brachialis m.

Biceps brachii m.

Latissimus dorsi m.

Thoracolumbar fascia

Lumbar triangle

Post. sup. iliac spine

Gluteal fascia

Gluteus maximus m.

Iliotibial tract of fascia lata

Vastus lat. m.

Biceps femoris, long head

Sternocleidomastoid m.

Omohyoid m., inf. belly

Acromion

Clavicle

Pectoralis major m.

Parenchyma, mammary gland

Nipple

Serratus ant. m.

Pectoralis major m., abdominal part

Costal arch

Umbilicus

External abdominal oblique m.

Sheath, Rectus abdominis m., ant. lamina

Aponeurosis, Ext. abdominis oblique m.

Ant. sup. iliac spine

Tensor fasciae latae m .

Sartorius m.

Vastus lat. m.

**Fig. 254.**  Musculature of the neck, trunk, and thigh of an adult female. Mammary gland dissected.

142

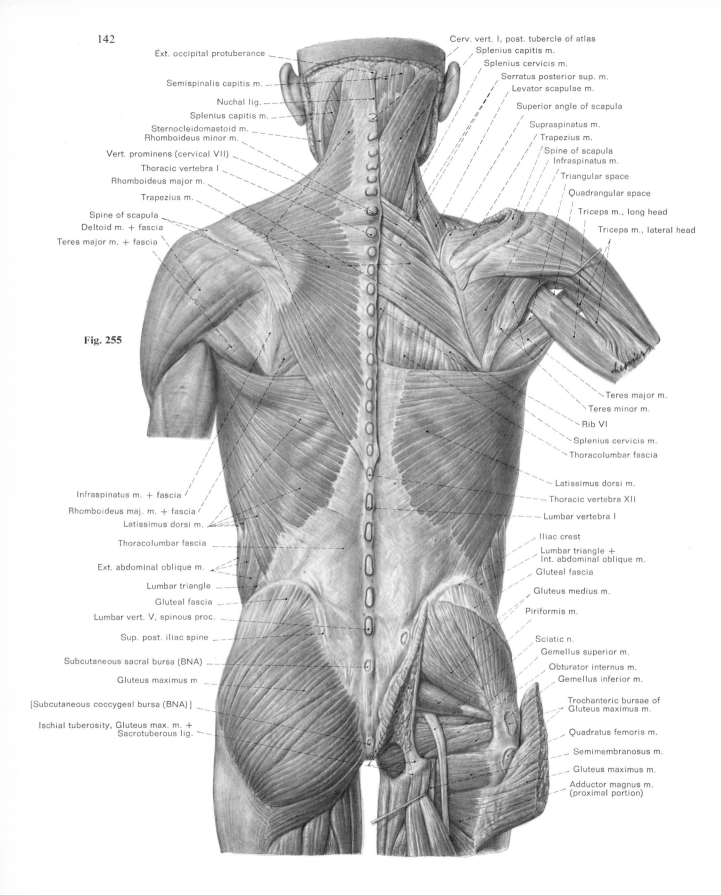

Ext. occipital protuberance

Semispinalis capitis m.

Nuchal lig.

Splenius capitis m.

Sternocleidomastoid m.
Rhomboideus minor m.

Vert. prominens (cervical VII)

Thoracic vertebra I

Rhomboideus major m.

Trapezius m.

Spine of scapula
Deltoid m. + fascia
Teres major m. + fascia

Fig. 255

Infraspinatus m. + fascia

Rhomboideus maj. m. + fascia

Latissimus dorsi m.

Thoracolumbar fascia

Ext. abdominal oblique m.

Lumbar triangle

Gluteal fascia

Lumbar vert. V, spinous proc.

Sup. post. iliac spine

Subcutaneous sacral bursa (BNA)

Gluteus maximus m

[Subcutaneous coccygeal bursa (BNA)]

Ischial tuberosity, Gluteus max. m. +
Sacrotuberous lig.

Cerv. vert. I, post. tubercle of atlas
Splenius capitis m.
Splenius cervicis m.
Serratus posterior sup. m.
Levator scapulae m.
Superior angle of scapula
Supraspinatus m.
Trapezius m.
Spine of scapula
Infraspinatus m.
Triangular space
Quadrangular space
Triceps m., long head
Triceps m., lateral head

Teres major m.
Teres minor m.
Rib VI
Splenius cervicis m.
Thoracolumbar fascia

Latissimus dorsi m.
Thoracic vertebra XII
Lumbar vertebra I
Iliac crest
Lumbar triangle +
Int. abdominal oblique m.
Gluteal fascia
Gluteus medius m.
Piriformis m.
Sciatic n.
Gemellus superior m.
Obturator internus m.
Gemellus inferior m.
Trochanteric bursae of
Gluteus maximus m.
Quadratus femoris m.
Semimembranosus m.
Gluteus maximus m.
Adductor magnus m.
(proximal portion)

## Muscles of the Back – First Layer (Fig. 255)

| Name | Origin | Insertion |
|---|---|---|
| **1. Trapezius muscle** <br> A flat triangular muscle (see Fig. 254); tendinous tissue in region where the cervical and the thoracic spinous processes meet | Medial third of superior nuchal line; external occipital protuberance; cervical spinous processes via the nuchal ligament; spines of thoracic vertebrae and their supraspinous ligaments | Lateral third of clavicle (Fig. 275); acromion; spine of scapula |

*Nerve:* Spinal accessory nerve plus C 3, 4

*Action:* Cranial fibers elevate the scapula, the caudal depress it; the middle fibers pull the scapula dorsally, suspend the shoulder girdle, help rotate the scapula. Normal tension helps maintain the square shoulder. When the accessory is cut, the shoulder droops.

| | | |
|---|---|---|
| **2. Latissimus dorsi muscle** <br> A large triangular muscle | By way of the thoracolumbar fascia (aponeurosis), from the 6 caudal thoracic, all lumbar spines, sacrum, and external lip of iliac crest. Muscular slips from 3 or 4 caudal ribs and inferior angle of scapula | By a flat tendon to floor of intertubercular sulcus of humerus, ventral to Teres major insertion; Latissimus dorsi bursa between tendons |

*Nerve:* Thoracodorsal nerve of the brachial plexus (C 6, 7, 8)

*Action:* Extends and adducts the humerus and rotates it medially. Draws the arm and shoulder downward and backward

| | | |
|---|---|---|
| **3. Rhomboideus major muscle** | Spines of the 2nd to 5th thoracic vertebrae | Medial border of scapula, caudal to the spine of the scapula |
| **4. Rhomboideus minor muscle** | Spines of 7th cervical and 1st thoracic vertebra; the nuchal ligament | Medial border of scapula, cranial to the spine of the scapula |

*Nerve:* For both: Dorsal scapular nerve from the brachial plexus (C 4, 5)

*Action:* Draws the scapula upward and medially. Holds scapula to trunk along with the Serratus anterior muscle.

| | | |
|---|---|---|
| **5. Levator scapulae muscle** <br> Borders the Scalenus posterior muscle ventrally | The posterior tubercles of the transverse processes of the upper 4 cervical vertebrae | Superior angle of the scapula (and the immediate adjacent region) to the base of the spine of the scapula |

*Nerve:* Cervical plexus and the dorsal scapular nerve (C 3, 4)

*Action:* Pulls the scapula upward and medially (along with the Trapezius muscle). If the scapula is fixed, it pulls the neck laterally

**Fig. 255.** Shoulder, neck, back, and gluteal muscles. *Left:* Superficial layers. *Right:* Deeper layers.

144

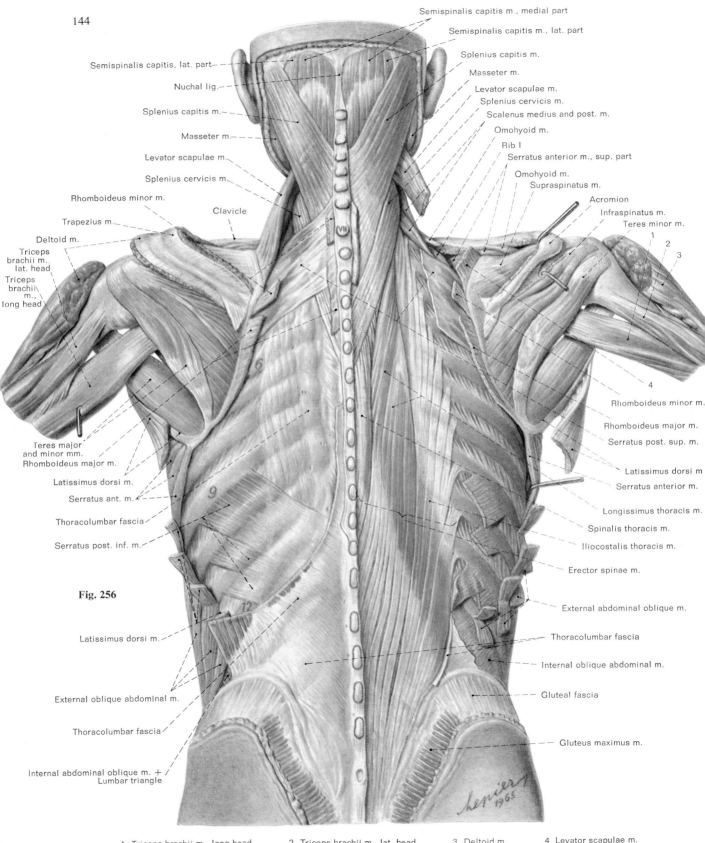

Semispinalis capitis m., medial part
Semispinalis capitis m., lat. part
Splenius capitis m.
Masseter m.
Levator scapulae m.
Splenius cervicis m.
Scalenus medius and post. m.
Omohyoid m.
Rib I
Serratus anterior m., sup. part
Omohyoid m.
Supraspinatus m.
Acromion
Infraspinatus m.
Teres minor m.
1
2
3
4
Rhomboideus minor m.
Rhomboideus major m.
Serratus post. sup. m.
Latissimus dorsi m
Serratus anterior m.
Longissimus thoracis m.
Spinalis thoracis m.
Iliocostalis thoracis m.
Erector spinae m.
External abdominal oblique m.
Thoracolumbar fascia
Internal oblique abdominal m.
Gluteal fascia
Gluteus maximus m.

Semispinalis capitis, lat. part
Nuchal lig.
Splenius capitis m.
Masseter m.
Levator scapulae m.
Splenius cervicis m.
Rhomboideus minor m.
Trapezius m.
Deltoid m.
Clavicle
Triceps brachii m., lat. head
Triceps brachii m., long head
Teres major and minor mm.
Rhomboideus major m.
Latissimus dorsi m.
Serratus ant. m.
Thoracolumbar fascia
Serratus post. inf. m.

Fig. 256

Latissimus dorsi m.

External oblique abdominal m.

Thoracolumbar fascia

Internal abdominal oblique m. +
Lumbar triangle

1  Triceps brachii m., long head        2  Triceps brachii m., lat. head        3  Deltoid m.        4  Levator scapulae m.

## Muscles of the Back – Respiratory Muscles  (Fig. 256)

| Name | *Origin* | *Insertion* |
|---|---|---|
| **1. Serratus posterior superior muscle** A thin, quadrilateral muscle | Nuchal ligament, spinous processes of 7th cervical and the first 2 or 3 thoracic vertebrae | Ribs 2–5, lateral to their angles |
| **2. Serratus posterior inferior muscle** (more broad than above) | By way of thoracolumbar fascia from last 2 thoracic and upper 2 lumbar spinous processes | Inferior borders of last 4 ribs, lateral to their angels |

*Nerve:*   For both: Intercostal nerves (superior T 1–4; inferior T 9–12)

*Action:*   Serratus posterior superior muscle elevates first 4 ribs, assists in inspiration. Serratus posterior inferior muscle pulls last 4 ribs caudally, helps in expiration

## Deep Muscles of the Back – The True Back Muscles: Splenius capitis and cervicis muscles (Figs. 256, 257)

The two muscles are close together at their origin (from the spinous processes). Gradually, as they approach their individual insertions, they become separated into two specific muscles.

| | | |
|---|---|---|
| **1. Splenius capitis muscle** The splenius muscles get their innervations from the true back muscles | Nuchal ligament, spinous processes of 3rd (4th) to 7th cervical and first 3 thoracic vertebrae | Lateral third of the superior nuchal line (and the mastoid process of the temporal bone) |

*Nerve:*   Dorsal rami of nerves C 2–5, lateral branches

*Action:*   Muscles of both sides, acting together, extend the head and neck; one side acting alone, rotates the head to the same side

| | | |
|---|---|---|
| **2. Splenius cervicis muscle** | Spines of 3rd (or 4th) to 6th thoracic vertebrae | Posterior tubercles of the transverse processes of the first 3 cervical vertebrae |

*Nerve:*   Dorsal rami of nerves C 2–5, lateral branches (same as Splenius capitis)

*Action:*   Muscles of both sides acting together extend the neck and head. Muscles of one side rotates the upper cervical vertebrae and, by its action on the atlas, rotates the head to the same side

**Fig. 256.**   Shoulder, neck, and back musculature. Deeper layers of long back muscles.

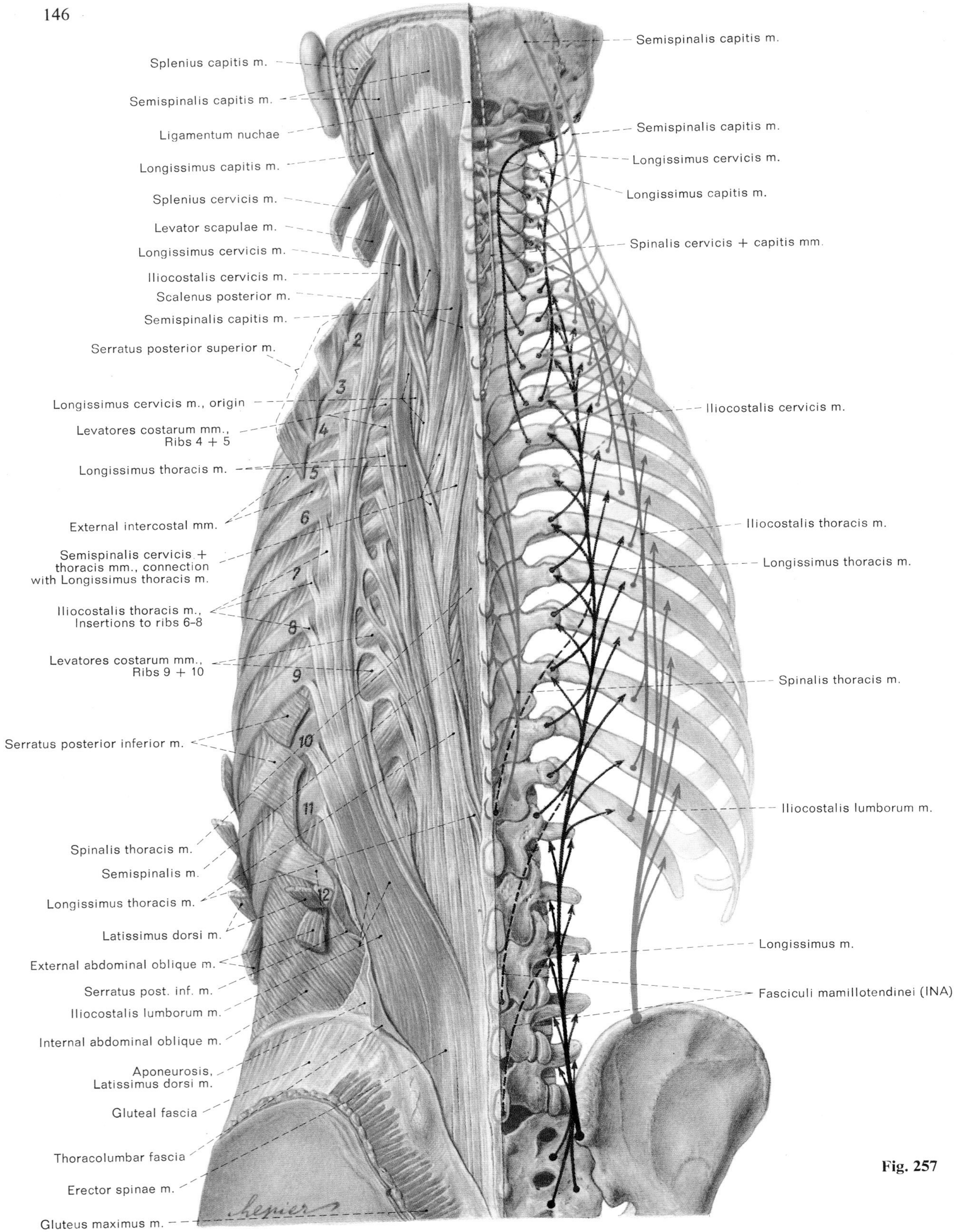

146

Splenius capitis m.

Semispinalis capitis m.

Ligamentum nuchae

Longissimus capitis m.

Splenius cervicis m.

Levator scapulae m.

Longissimus cervicis m.

Iliocostalis cervicis m.

Scalenus posterior m.

Semispinalis capitis m.

Serratus posterior superior m.

Longissimus cervicis m., origin

Levatores costarum mm.,
Ribs 4 + 5

Longissimus thoracis m.

External intercostal mm.

Semispinalis cervicis +
thoracis mm., connection
with Longissimus thoracis m.

Iliocostalis thoracis m.,
Insertions to ribs 6–8

Levatores costarum mm.,
Ribs 9 + 10

Serratus posterior inferior m.

Spinalis thoracis m.

Semispinalis m.

Longissimus thoracis m.

Latissimus dorsi m.

External abdominal oblique m.

Serratus post. inf. m.

Iliocostalis lumborum m.

Internal abdominal oblique m.

Aponeurosis,
Latissimus dorsi m.

Gluteal fascia

Thoracolumbar fascia

Erector spinae m.

Gluteus maximus m.

Semispinalis capitis m.

Semispinalis capitis m.

Longissimus cervicis m.

Longissimus capitis m.

Spinalis cervicis + capitis mm.

Iliocostalis cervicis m.

Iliocostalis thoracis m.

Longissimus thoracis m.

Spinalis thoracis m.

Iliocostalis lumborum m.

Longissimus m.

Fasciculi mamillotendinei (INA)

Fig. 257

# The Erector Spinae Muscles (Sacrospinalis) (Fig. 257)

| Name | Origin | Insertion |
|---|---|---|
| **1. Iliocostalis muscle** (lateral column): Ilium to ribs to ribs (red lines) | | |
| *a–c continuous without sharp delineations*   a) *Lumbar section:* Iliocostalis lumborum muscle | As the Erector spinae muscle joins with the Longissimus muscle from the external lip of the iliac crest | The angles of ribs 5 to 12 Cranial: tendinous Caudal: fleshy |
| b) *Dorsal section:* Iliocostalis thoracic muscle | Individual slips from the 12th to the 7th ribs | By thin tendons on angles of the upper 6 ribs and to the transverse process of the 7th cervical vertebra |
| c) *Cervical section:* Iliocostalis cervicis m. | Cranial and middle ribs (2nd to 6th) | Transverse processes of the 4th to the 7th cervical vertebrae |
| **2. Longissimus muscle** (intermediate column, the longest) Sacrum to transverse process to transverse process (black lines) | | |
| a) *Longissimus thoracis m.* blends with Longissimus cervicis and then with the Spinalis muscle | As the Erector spinae muscle joins with the Iliocostalis muscle from the sacrum and transverse processes of lumbar vertebrae (tendinous) with some slips from transverse processes of thoracic vertebrae | *Cranial:* rounded tendons *Caudal:* fleshy *Medial:* Accessory processes of upper lumbar vertebrae; transverse processes of thoracic vertebrae *Lateral:* Slips to costal processes of lumbar vertebrae and all ribs between the angles and tubercles |
| b) *Longissimus cervicis m.* | Transverse processes of upper 4 or 5 thoracic vertebrae | Transverse processes of 2nd to 6th cervical vertebrae (tendinous) |
| c) *Longissimus capitis m.* | Transverse processes of the upper thoracic vertebrae and the transverse and articular processes of middle and lower cervical vertebrae | Dorsal margin of the mastoid process of the temporal bone |
| **3. Spinalis muscles** (medial column): Spinous process to spinous process (blue lines) | | |
| *Spinalis thoracis muscle* (continuation of Sacrospinalis muscle) | Spinous processes of the caudal thoracic vertebrae (blending with the Longissimus muscle) | Spinous processes of 3rd to 9th thoracic vertebrae |
| *Spinalis cervicis muscle* (inconstant) | Lower 2 cervical and first 2 thoracic spinous processes | Spinous processes of axis and 2nd and 3rd cervical vertebrae |
| *Spinalis capitis muscle* (Rarely a separate muscle, usually fused with the Semispinalis capitis muscle) | Spinous processes of the lower cervical and upper thoracic vertebrae | With Semispinalis capitis muscle between the superior and inferior nuchal line on the occipital bone |

*Nerve:*   Dorsal rami of all spinal nerves (cervical, thoracic, and lumbar)

*Action:*   Muscles of both sides, acting together, extend the vertebral column and assist in maintaining erect posture. Muscles of one side, acting alone, bend vertebral column to the side

**Fig. 257.** Neck and long back muscles. Left: Deeper layers. Right: Diagram of origins, course, and insertion of the back muscles. Outline of spinous processes of: lumbar vertebrae, bright blue; the thoracic vertebrae, red; the cervical vertebrae green. The longissimus muscle column, black.

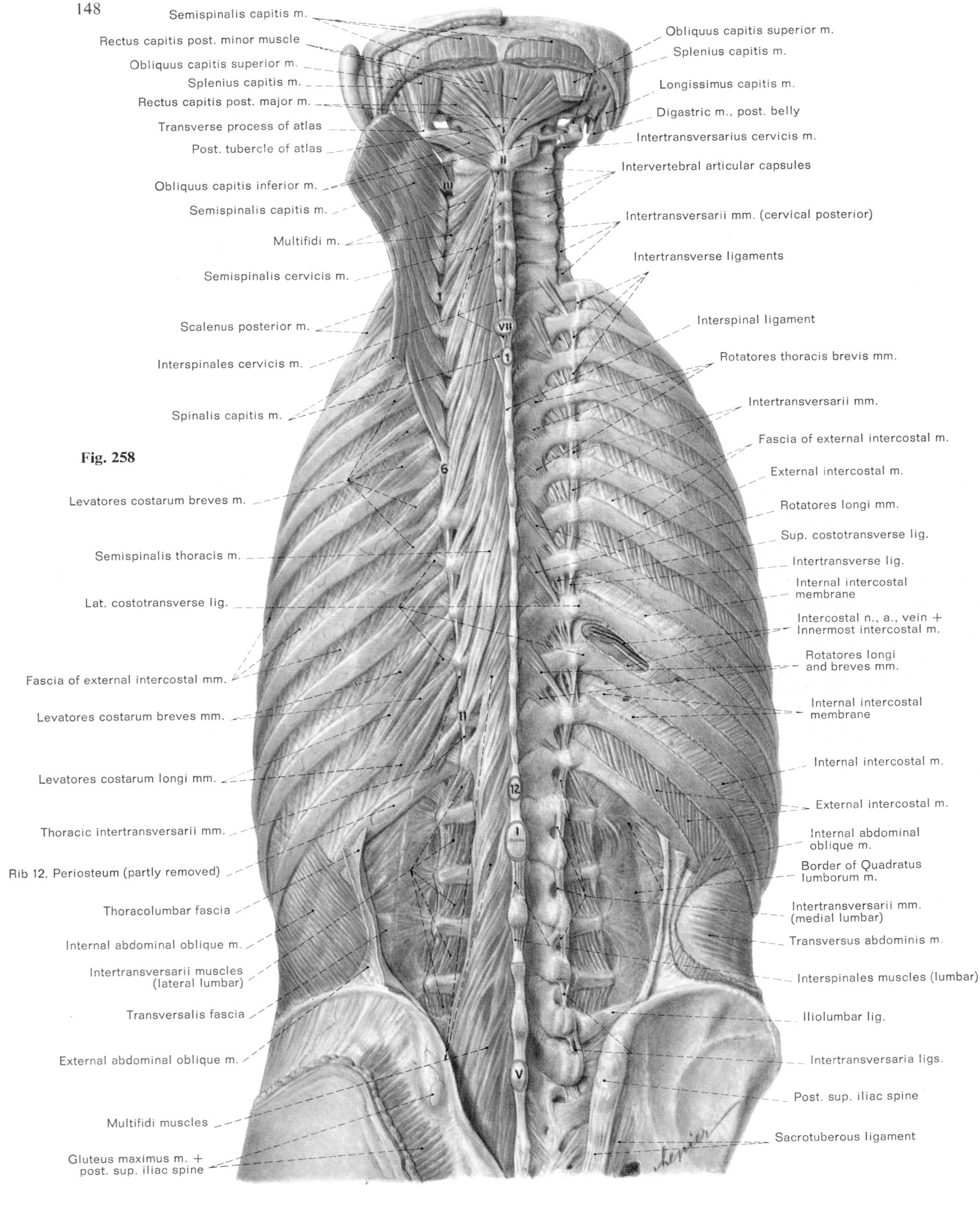

148

Semispinalis capitis m.

Rectus capitis post. minor muscle

Obliquus capitis superior m.

Splenius capitis m.

Rectus capitis post. major m.

Transverse process of atlas

Post. tubercle of atlas

Obliquus capitis inferior m.

Semispinalis capitis m.

Multifidi m.

Semispinalis cervicis m.

Scalenus posterior m.

Interspinales cervicis m.

Spinalis capitis m.

**Fig. 258**

Levatores costarum breves m.

Semispinalis thoracis m.

Lat. costotransverse lig.

Fascia of external intercostal mm.

Levatores costarum breves mm.

Levatores costarum longi mm.

Thoracic intertransversarii mm.

Rib 12, Periosteum (partly removed)

Thoracolumbar fascia

Internal abdominal oblique m.

Intertransversarii muscles (lateral lumbar)

Transversalis fascia

External abdominal oblique m.

Multifidi muscles

Gluteus maximus m. + post. sup. iliac spine

Obliquus capitis superior m.

Splenius capitis m.

Longissimus capitis m.

Digastric m., post. belly

Intertransversarius cervicis m.

Intervertebral articular capsules

Intertransversarii mm. (cervical posterior)

Intertransverse ligaments

Interspinal ligament

Rotatores thoracis brevis mm.

Intertransversarii mm.

Fascia of external intercostal m.

External intercostal m.

Rotatores longi mm.

Sup. costotransverse lig.

Intertransverse lig.

Internal intercostal membrane

Intercostal n., a., vein + Innermost intercostal m.

Rotatores longi and breves mm.

Internal intercostal membrane

Internal intercostal m.

External intercostal m.

Internal abdominal oblique m.

Border of Quadratus lumborum m.

Intertransversarii mm. (medial lumbar)

Transversus abdominis m.

Interspinales muscles (lumbar)

Iliolumbar lig.

Intertransversaria ligs.

Post. sup. iliac spine

Sacrotuberous ligament

## Deep Layer of Back Muscles, Transversospinal Muscles  (Figs. 256-258, 260)

| Name | Origin | Insertion |
|------|--------|-----------|
| **1. Semispinalis thoracis muscle**<br>**Semispinalis cervicis muscle**<br>(without separate boundaries) | Pass obliquely upward and medially from the transverse process to the spinous processes, hence the name transversospinal. Absent in the lumbar vertebrae | |
| | Transverse processes of all thoracic vertebrae | Spinous processes 4 to 6 segments higher than their origin, including the spine of the axis |
| **Semispinalis capitis m.**<br>(transversooccipital, largest muscle in back of neck with 1 or 2 conspicuous tendinous intersections. Fig. 257) | Transverse processes of 3 cervical and 5 or 6 thoracic vertebrae | Between the superior and inferior nuchal line |

*Nerve:*  Dorsal rami of the cervical and thoracic nerves

*Action:*  Extend vertebral column (especially the cervical vertebrae) and head, bending the head backwards. Unilateral innervation draws the muscle of the head toward the opposing side. Together, with the Sternocleidomastoid m., supports the head

| Name | Origin | Insertion |
|------|--------|-----------|
| **2. Multifidi muscles**<br>(spans 2 or 3 vertebrae) | Dorsal surface of the sacrum; transverse processes of lumbar, thoracic, and lower cervical vertebrae | Spinous process of lumbar, thoracic, and cervical vertebrae up to the axis |
| **3. Rotatores cervicis muscles**<br>The short rotator muscles link adjacent vertebrae; the long ones skip one vertebra<br>**Rotatores thoracis muscles**<br>**Rotatores lumborum muscles** | Transverse process of the cervical vertebrae<br><br>Transverse process of thoracic vertebrae<br>Transverse process of the lumbar vertebrae | Roots of the spinous processes of the adjacent or the second vertebra above |

*Nerve:*  Dorsal rami of the spinal nerves: cervical, thoracic, and (lumbar) nerves

*Action:*  Also of the transversospinal group. When acting bilaterally, they all extend the vertebral column. When acting individually and unilaterally, they bend the vertebral column to the side and rotate the vertebrae

**◀ Fig. 258.**   Deep neck and back musculature. Transversopinal group.

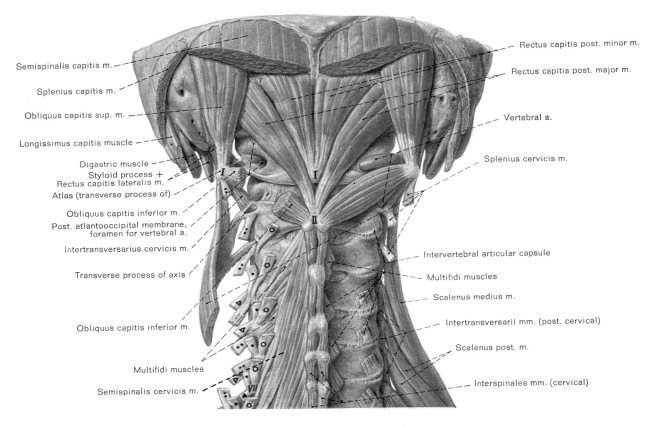

Semispinalis capitis m.

Splenius capitis m.

Obliquus capitis sup. m.

Longissimus capitis muscle

Digastric muscle

Styloid process +
Rectus capitis lateralis m.

Atlas (transverse process of)

Obliquus capitis inferior m.

Post. atlantooccipital membrane,
foramen for vertebral a.

Intertransversarius cervicis m.

Transverse process of axis

Obliquus capitis inferior m.

Multifidi muscles

Semispinalis cervicis m.

Rectus capitis post. minor m.

Rectus capitis post. major m.

Vertebral a.

Splenius cervicis m.

Intervertebral articular capsule

Multifidi muscles

Scalenus medius m.

Intertransversarii mm. (post. cervical)

Scalenus post. m.

Interspinales mm. (cervical)

**Fig. 259.** Middle and deep layers of the neck musculature. The suboccipital triangle.

Note: The vertebral artery (Fig. 259) is deep in the suboccipital triangle, bounded by the Obliquus capitis superior and inferior muscles and the Rectus capitis posterior major muscle. After passing through the transverse foramen of the atlas, the vertebral artery runs directly medial in its groove in the atlas, and passes through the posterior atlantooccipital membrane and the dura, through the large occipital foramen to supply part of the brain.

## Short Suboccipital Muscles (Transversospinal muscles) (Figs. 258, 259)

| Name | Origin | Insertion |
|---|---|---|
| 1. Rectus capitis posterior major muscle | Spinous process of the axis (II) | Inferior nuchal line (of occipital bone) |
| 2. Rectus capitis posterior minor muscle | Posterior tubercle of atlas (I) | Medial part of the inferior nuchal line of the occipital bone |
| 3. Rectus capitis lateralis muscle (Fig. 281) | Transverse process of the atlas | Jugular process of the occipital bone |
| 4. Obliquus capitis superior muscle | Transverse process of the atlas | Occipital bone, above the inferior nuchal line |
| 5. Obliquus capitis inferior muscle | Spinous process of the axis (II) | Transverse process of the atlas |

*Nerve:* Suboccipital nerve (dorsal ramus of the first cervical nerve)

*Action:* Extend and rotate head. The Rectus capitis posterior major and Obliquus capitis inferior muscles turn the head to the same side; the Rectus capitis lateralis bends the head laterally (unilateral innervation)

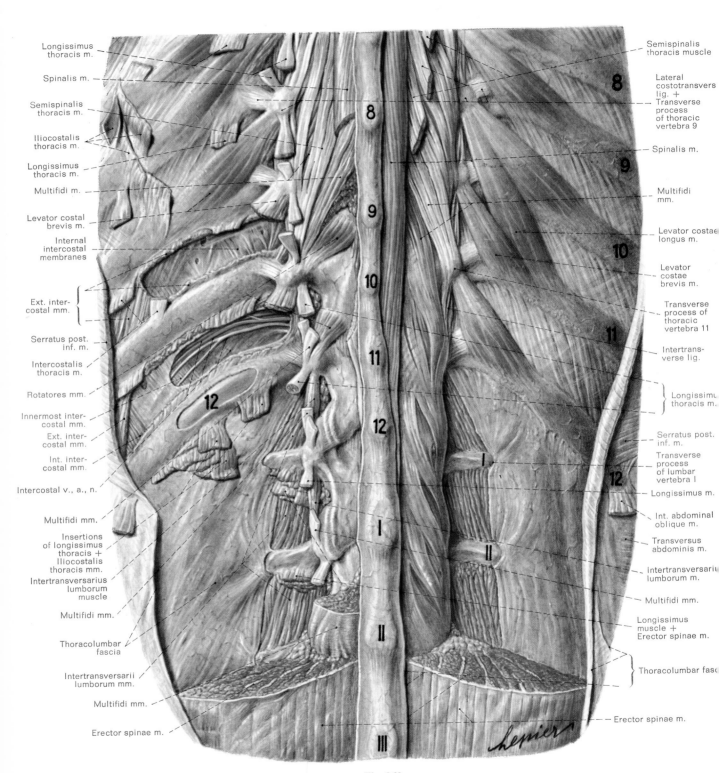

Longissimus thoracis m.
Spinalis m.
Semispinalis thoracis m.
Iliocostalis thoracis m.
Longissimus thoracis m.
Multifidi m.
Levator costal brevis m.
Internal intercostal membranes
Ext. intercostal mm.
Serratus post. inf. m.
Intercostalis thoracis m.
Rotatores mm.
Innermost intercostal mm.
Ext. intercostal mm.
Int. intercostal mm.
Intercostal v., a., n.
Multifidi mm.
Insertions of longissimus thoracis + Iliocostalis thoracis mm.
Intertransversarius lumborum muscle
Multifidi mm.
Thoracolumbar fascia
Intertransversarii lumborum mm.
Multifidi mm.
Erector spinae m.

Semispinalis thoracis muscle
Lateral costotransverse lig. + Transverse process of thoracic vertebra 9
Spinalis m.
Multifidi mm.
Levator costae longus m.
Levator costae brevis m.
Transverse process of thoracic vertebra 11
Intertransverse lig.
Longissimus thoracis m.
Serratus post. inf. m.
Transverse process of lumbar vertebra I
Longissimus m.
Int. abdominal oblique m.
Transversus abdominis m.
Intertransversarii lumborum m.
Multifidi mm.
Longissimus muscle + Erector spinae m.
Thoracolumbar fascia
Erector spinae m.

Fig. 260

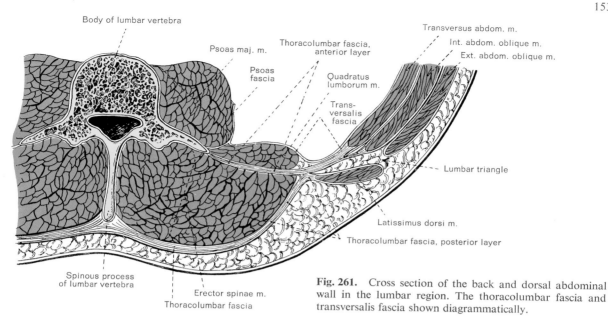

Body of lumbar vertebra

Psoas maj. m.

Thoracolumbar fascia,
anterior layer

Psoas
fascia

Quadratus
lumborum m.

Transversus abdom. m.

Int. abdom. oblique m.

Ext. abdom. oblique m.

Trans-
versalis
fascia

Lumbar triangle

Latissimus dorsi m.

Thoracolumbar fascia, posterior layer

Spinous process
of lumbar vertebra

Erector spinae m.

Thoracolumbar fascia

**Fig. 261.** Cross section of the back and dorsal abdominal wall in the lumbar region. The thoracolumbar fascia and transversalis fascia shown diagrammatically.

Note: Thoracolumbar fascia (lumbodorsal aponeurosis): A tendonous sheath from the Transversus abdominis, the Latissimus dorsi, and the Serratus posterior inferior muscles. It is fastened on the spinous processes with the posterior layer, on the transverse processes of the lumbar vertebrae with the anterior layers, and is between the 12th rib and crista iliaca.

Lumbar triangle (trigonum lumbale) is a small triangular interval of the back bordered by the External oblique abdominal muscle and by the Latissimus dorsi and the iliac crest (Figs. 255, 261). Occasionally it is the site of a hernia.

Transversalis fascia: The inner surface of the peritoneal musculature is separated from the peritoneum by the fascia transversalis. Among other things, it strengthens the dorsal wall of the inguinal canal. The principal outpouching of the transversalis fascia is the internal spermatic fascia (tunica vaginalis communis) which invests the inner part of the spermatic cord and testis.

Intercostal vessels, intercostal nerve (ramus ventralis of a thoracic nerve): In the middle part of Fig. 260, the intercostal vessels and the intercostal nerve are displayed through a window in the intercostal muscles. They run lateral to the costal sulcus: the posterior intercostal vein is above; the posterior intercostal artery, in the middle; and the intercostal nerve, below.

**Fig. 260.** Deep back muscles: Rotatores, Multifidi, and Levator costae. The spinous processes of the vertebral column were designated in the thoracic region with Arabic numerals 8–12; in the lumbar region with Roman numerals I–III. The first two transverse processes of the lumbar vertebrae are also labeled I and II. The ribs 8–12 on the right are shown with Arabic numerals.

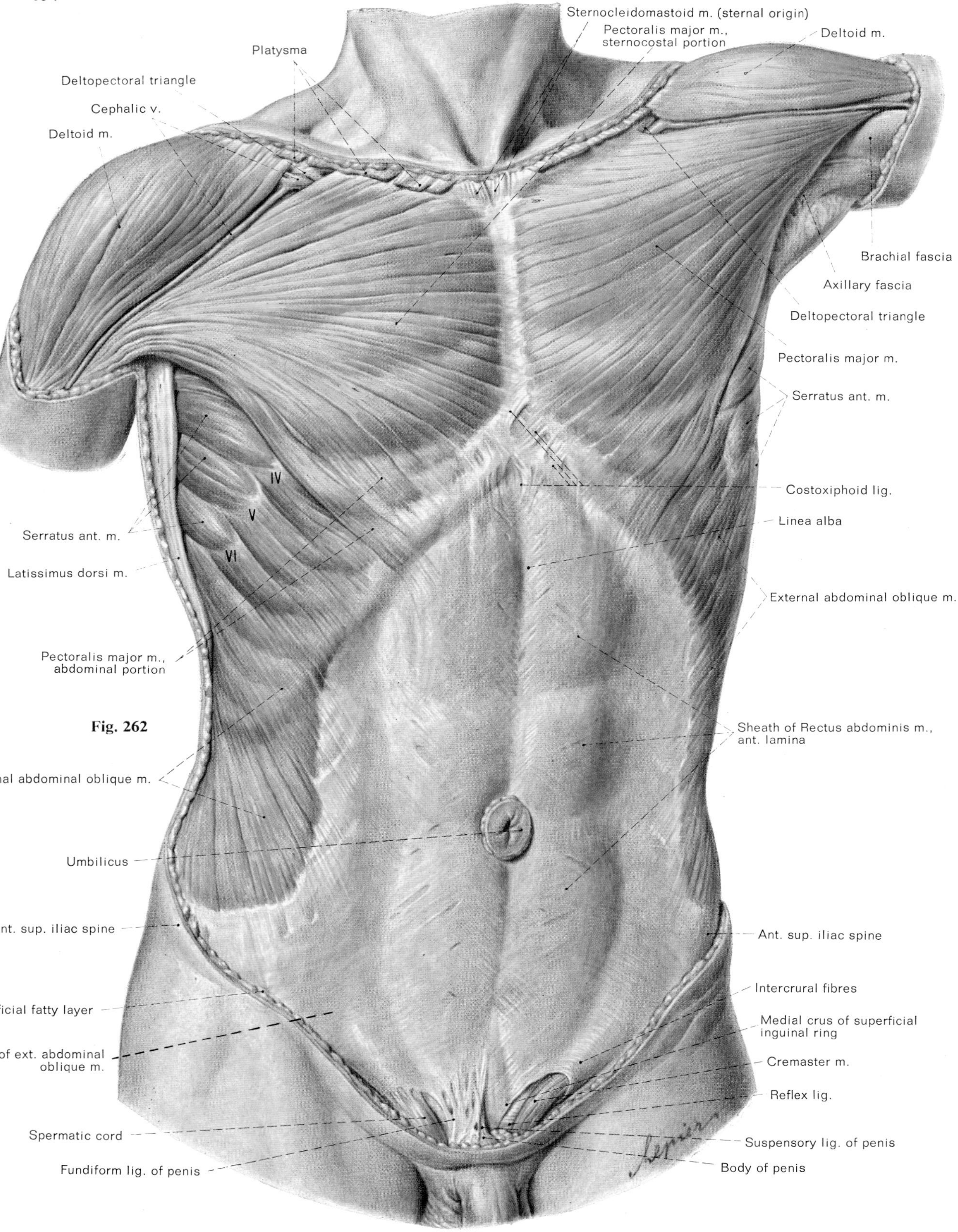

154

Sternocleidomastoid m. (sternal origin)

Pectoralis major m., sternocostal portion

Deltoid m.

Platysma

Deltopectoral triangle

Cephalic v.

Deltoid m.

Brachial fascia

Axillary fascia

Deltopectoral triangle

Pectoralis major m.

Serratus ant. m.

IV

V

VI

Serratus ant. m.

Latissimus dorsi m.

Costoxiphoid lig.

Linea alba

External abdominal oblique m.

Pectoralis major m., abdominal portion

Fig. 262

Sheath of Rectus abdominis m., ant. lamina

External abdominal oblique m.

Umbilicus

Ant. sup. iliac spine

Ant. sup. iliac spine

Superficial fatty layer

Intercrural fibres

Medial crus of superficial inguinal ring

Aponeurosis of ext. abdominal oblique m.

Cremaster m.

Reflex lig.

Spermatic cord

Suspensory lig. of penis

Fundiform lig. of penis

Body of penis

### Thoracic and Abdominal Muscles (Figs. 262, 269)

| Name | Origin | Insertion |
|---|---|---|
| **1. Pectoralis major muscle** Strong, predominantly fleshy; tendinous only at insertion | *Clavicular portion:* Sternal half of clavicle *Sternocostal portion:* Ventral surface of sternum and costal cartilages 2 to 6 *Abdominal portion:* A slip from the aponeurosis of the External abdominal oblique muscle | All fibers converge toward a flat tendon (5 cm broad) which is inserted into the crest of the greater tubercle of the humerus |

*Nerve:* Lateral and medial pectoral nerves from the brachial plexus (C 5 – T 1)

*Action:* Flexes, adducts, and rotates the arm medially. Powerful adduction (lowering the raised arm). In many cases, works with other muscles (Latissimus dorsi and Trapezius muscles)

| | | |
|---|---|---|
| **2. Pectoralis minor muscle** (Weak and moderately flat) | Ribs 2 to 5 near the cartilage-bone junction | Coracoid process of the scapula (medial border) |

*Nerve:* Medial pectoral nerve (C 8 – T 1)

*Action:* Depresses the shoulder, raises ribs in forced inspiration; seldom functions alone, but with the Serratus anterior and Trapezius muscles, etc.

| | | |
|---|---|---|
| **3. Subclavius muscle** | Short, thick tendon on 1st rib at junction of cartilage and bone | Acromial end of clavicle |

*Nerve:* Subclavius nerve from the brachial plexus

*Action:* Adequate for such a small muscle; assists in drawing the shoulder forward and downward

| | | |
|---|---|---|
| **4. Serratus anterior muscle** | With fleshy digitations from first 9 ribs, consisting of 3 parts. The middle is the weakest; the caudal, the strongest | |
| (Superior part) | Ribs 1 and 2, somewhat converging | Superior angle of the scapula |
| (Middle part) | Ribs 2–4, diverging | Medial margin of scapula |
| (Inferior part) | Ribs 5–9, strongly converging | Inferior angle of scapula |

*Nerve:* Long thoracic nerve from the brachial plexus (C 5, 6, 7)

*Action:* Holds scapula closely to the body, draws scapula forward as in a pushing action. Assists in flexion and abduction of the arm

**Fig. 262.** Pectoral and abdominal musculature. Ventral view of superficial layer. Ribs: IV–VI.

156

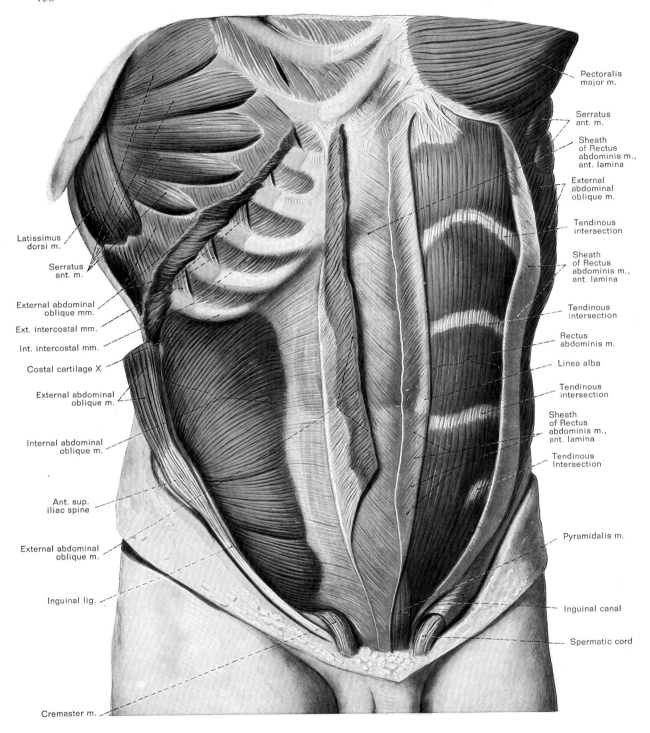

Pectoralis major m.

Serratus ant. m.

Sheath of Rectus abdominis m., ant. lamina

External abdominal oblique m.

Tendinous intersection

Sheath of Rectus abdominis m., ant. lamina

Tendinous intersection

Rectus abdominis m.

Linea alba

Tendinous intersection

Sheath of Rectus abdominis m., ant. lamina

Tendinous Intersection

Pyramidalis m.

Inguinal canal

Spermatic cord

Latissimus dorsi m.

Serratus ant. m.

External abdominal oblique mm.

Ext. intercostal mm.

Int. intercostal mm.

Costal cartilage X

External abdominal oblique m.

Internal abdominal oblique m.

Ant. sup. iliac spine

External abdominal oblique m.

Inguinal lig.

Cremaster m.

**Fig. 263.** Abdominal musculature, second layer (from ventral and right). *Left:* The outer layer of rectus sheath has been opened along its midline, to display the Rectus abdominis and Pyramidalis muscles. *Right:* The external abdominal oblique muscle has been transected and 3 flaps reflected to display the Internal abdominal oblique muscle.

## Muscles of the Abdomen, Superficial Layers (Figs. 262, 263)

| Name | Origin | Insertion |
|---|---|---|
| **1. External abdominal oblique muscle**<br>Course of the fibers from lateral-cranial toward the medial-caudal | Fleshy digitations from lower 8 ribs. The dorsal border is free | On external lip of iliac crest, on the inguinal ligament and outer layer of the rectus sheath |

*Nerve:* Intercostal nerves, branches of lumbar plexus (iliohypogastric and ilioinguinal nerves)

*Action:* Maintains abdominal pressure to keep viscera in position; forces viscera up to elevate diaphragm during expiration; increases abdominal pressure to initiate and aid the rectum in evacuation of its contents; both sides flex vertebral column; one side bends it laterally and rotates it

| Name | Origin | Insertion |
|---|---|---|
| **2. Internal abdominal oblique muscle**<br>Course of fibers at right angles to the External oblique | Intermediate lip of iliac crest; thoraco-lumbar fascia; lateral two-thirds of inguinal ligament | Fleshy digitations to lower 3 ribs (9–12), the linea alba, aponeurosis helps in formation of rectus sheath (see Fig. 263) |

*Nerve:* Same as above

*Action:* Same as for External, but rotates toward the same side, supports the External of the opposing side, bends the body laterally

| Name | Origin | Insertion |
|---|---|---|
| **3. Cremaster muscle** | Caudal fibers of the Internal oblique m. (often from Transverse abdominal muscle) | Goes with the spermatic cord to the testis |

*Nerve:* Genital branch of the genitofemoral nerve

*Action:* Supports and elevates the testis

| Name | Origin | Insertion |
|---|---|---|
| **4. Transversus abdominus muscle** | 1. *Costal:* Deep surfaces of costal cartilages of lower 6 ribs<br>2. *Vertebral:* The thoracolumbar fascia from the transverse processes of the lumbar vertebrae<br>3. *Pelvic:* Internal lip of iliac crest, lateral third of inguinal ligament | Aponeurosis helps form rectus sheath; attaches to xiphoid process and linea alba; helps form falx inguinalis which attaches to superior border of the pubis and pectineal line |

*Nerve:* Intercostal nerves, branches of lumbar plexus (iliohypogastric, ilioinguinal, genitofemoral nerves)

*Action:* Contraction and expansion of abdominal wall, and maintains abdominal pressure to keep viscera in position

158

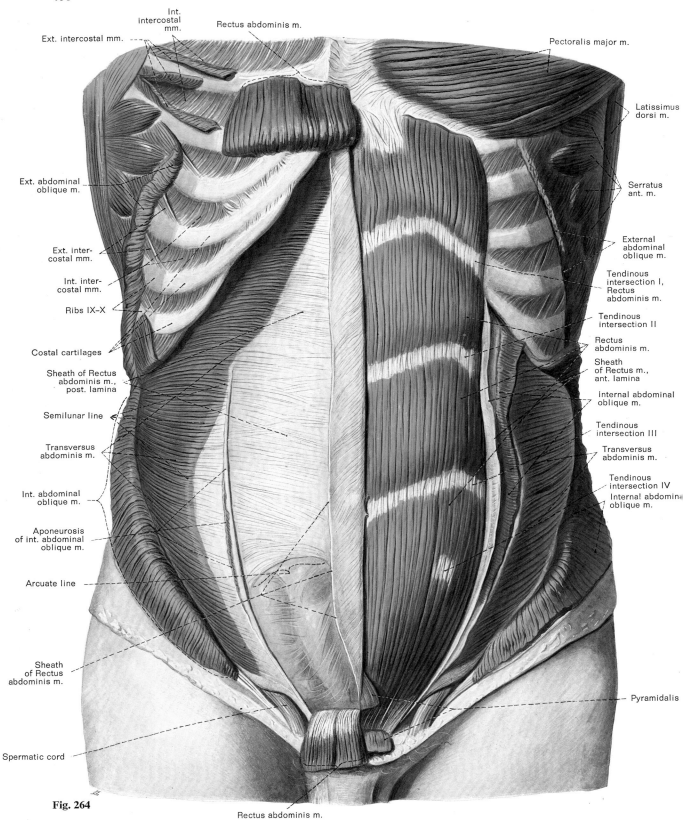

Ext. intercostal mm.

Int. intercostal mm.

Rectus abdominis m.

Pectoralis major m.

Latissimus dorsi m.

Ext. abdominal oblique m.

Serratus ant. m.

External abdominal oblique m.

Ext. intercostal mm.

Tendinous intersection I, Rectus abdominis m.

Int. intercostal mm.

Tendinous intersection II

Ribs IX–X

Rectus abdominis m.

Costal cartilages

Sheath of Rectus m., ant. lamina

Sheath of Rectus abdominis m., post. lamina

Internal abdominal oblique m.

Semilunar line

Tendinous intersection III

Transversus abdominis m.

Transversus abdominis m.

Tendinous intersection IV

Int. abdominal oblique m.

Internal abdominal oblique m.

Aponeurosis of int. abdominal oblique m.

Arcuate line

Sheath of Rectus abdominis m.

Pyramidalis

Spermatic cord

**Fig. 264**

Rectus abdominis m.

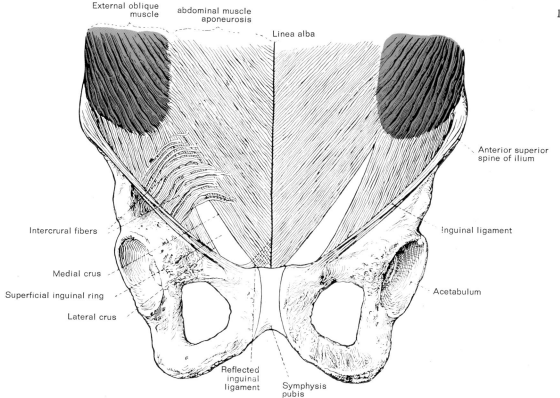

External oblique
muscle

abdominal muscle
aponeurosis

Linea alba

Anterior superior
spine of ilium

Intercrural fibers

Inguinal ligament

Medial crus

Superficial inguinal ring

Lateral crus

Acetabulum

Reflected
inguinal
ligament

Symphysis
pubis

**Fig. 265.** A diagrammatic view of the aponeurosis of the External abdominal oblique muscles, including the intercrural fibers that form the superficial inguinal ring.

### Straight Muscles of the Abdomen (Figs. 263-264)

| Name | Origin | Insertion |
|---|---|---|
| **1. Rectus abdominis muscle** Contains 3 or 4 tendinous inter-sections | 5th to 7th cartilage, xiphoid process | Cranial border of the pubis between the pubic tubercle and the symphysis |

*Nerves:* Middle and caudal intercostal nerves (T 7 – T 12) (rarely upper lumbar nerves)

*Action:* Flexes the vertebral column; pulls the sternum toward the pubis (antagonist of long back muscles); tenses anterior abdominal wall; and assists in compressing the abdominal contents

| | | |
|---|---|---|
| **2. Pyramidalis muscle** (inconstant) | Ventral surface of pubis and anterior pubic ligament | Linea alba cranial to symphysis |

*Nerve:* Branch of 12th thoracic nerve

*Action:* Tenses the linea alba. The size of the triangular muscle varies

**Fig. 264.** Deep layers of the muscles of the abdomen. *Left:* The Rectus abdominis muscle exposed, Pyramidalis muscle is cut to show the rectus tendon; in addition, the Internal abdominal oblique muscle is cut. *Right:* The Rectus abdominis and Internal oblique muscles were resected to display all the Transversus abdominis muscle and the dorsal layer of the rectus sheath with the linea arcuata and linea semilunaris.

160

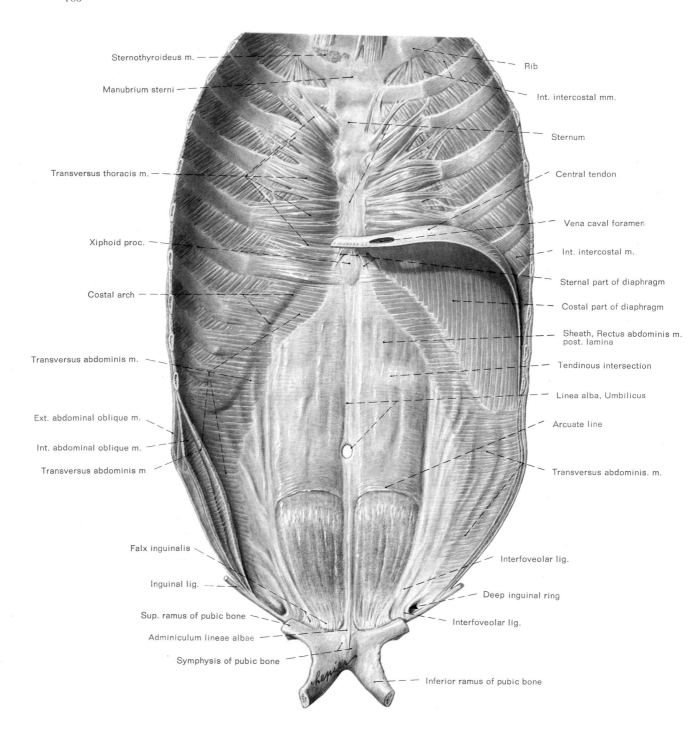

Sternothyroideus m. —

Manubrium sterni —

Transversus thoracis m. —

Xiphoid proc. —

Costal arch —

Transversus abdominis m. —

Ext. abdominal oblique m. —

Int. abdominal oblique m. —

Transversus abdominis m.

Falx inguinalis —

Inguinal lig. —

Sup. ramus of pubic bone —

Adminiculum lineae albae —

Symphysis of pubic bone —

— Rib

— Int. intercostal mm.

— Sternum

— Central tendon

— Vena caval foramen

— Int. intercostal m.

— Sternal part of diaphragm

— Costal part of diaphragm

— Sheath, Rectus abdominis m. post. lamina

— Tendinous intersection

— Linea alba, Umbilicus

— Arcuate line

— Transversus abdominis. m.

— Interfoveolar lig.

— Deep inguinal ring

— Interfoveolar lig.

— Inferior ramus of pubic bone

**Fig. 266.** Inner view of the ventral thoracic and abdominal musculature.

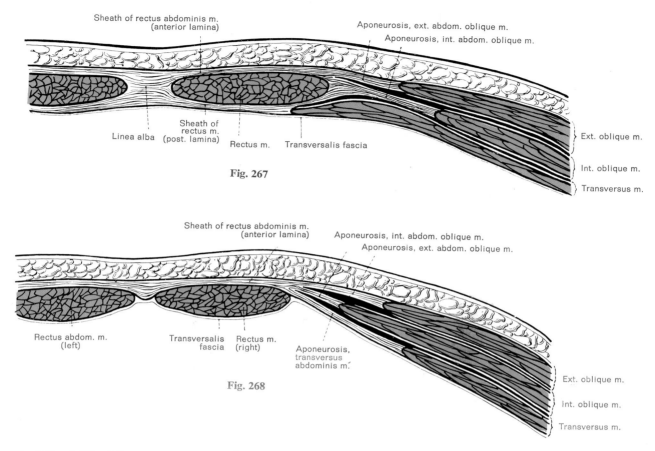

Figs. 267 and 268. Diagrams of cross sections of the ventral abdominal wall. Formation and relationship of the rectus sheath and the aponeurotic tendons of the flat abdominal muscles. Fig. 267. Cranial to the umbilicus. Fig. 268. In the middle between the umbilicus and the symphysis pubis.

Note: The rectus sheath above the linea arcuata is made up of the aponeurosis of 3 wide abdominal muscles: the External oblique and half of the Internal oblique form the ventral layer; the other half of the Internal oblique and the Transversus abdominis form the dorsal layer. Below the linea arcuata, all 3 aponeuroses pass ventral to the rectus muscle; the dorsal wall of the sheath is formed here by only the fascia transversalis.

162

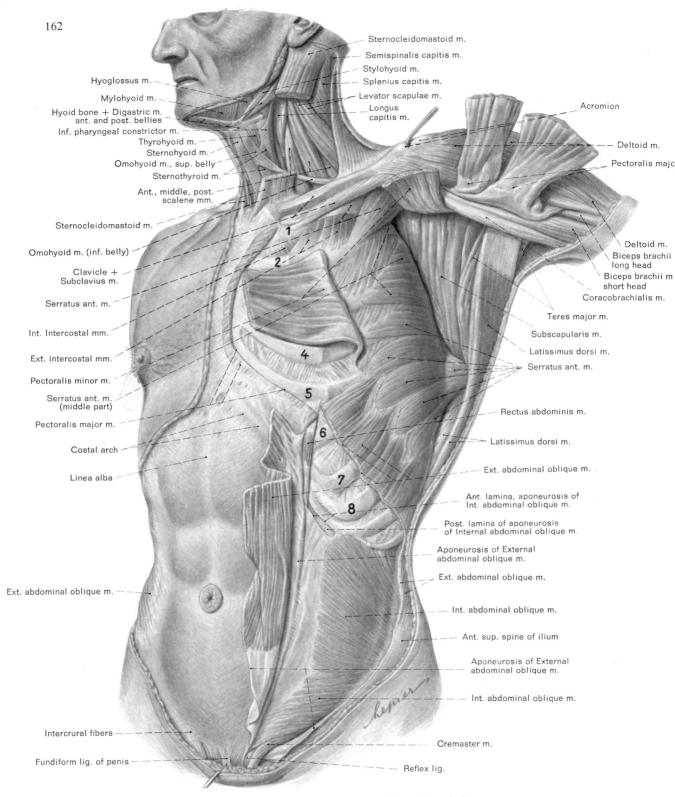

Sternocleidomastoid m.
Semispinalis capitis m.
Stylohyoid m.
Splenius capitis m.
Levator scapulae m.
Longus capitis m.

Hyoglossus m.
Mylohyoid m.
Hyoid bone + Digastric m. ant. and post. bellies
Inf. pharyngeal constrictor m.
Thyrohyoid m.
Sternohyoid m.
Omohyoid m., sup. belly
Sternothyroid m.
Ant., middle, post. scalene mm.

Sternocleidomastoid m.
Omohyoid m. (inf. belly)
Clavicle + Subclavius m.
Serratus ant. m.
Int. Intercostal mm.
Ext. intercostal mm.
Pectoralis minor m.
Serratus ant. m. (middle part)
Pectoralis major m.
Costal arch
Linea alba

Ext. abdominal oblique m.

Intercrural fibers
Fundiform lig. of penis

Acromion

Deltoid m.
Pectoralis majo[r]

Deltoid m.
Biceps brachii long head
Biceps brachii [m] short head
Coracobrachialis m.
Teres major m.
Subscapularis m.
Latissimus dorsi m.
Serratus ant. m.

Rectus abdominis m.
Latissimus dorsi m.
Ext. abdominal oblique m.
Ant. lamina, aponeurosis of Int. abdominal oblique m.
Post. lamina of aponeurosis of Internal abdominal oblique m.
Aponeurosis of External abdominal oblique m.
Ext. abdominal oblique m.
Int. abdominal oblique m.
Ant. sup. spine of ilium
Aponeurosis of External abdominal oblique m.
Int. abdominal oblique m.

Cremaster m.
Reflex lig.

**Fig. 269.** Deep layers of neck, thoracic, and abdominal musculature. Ventrolateral view.

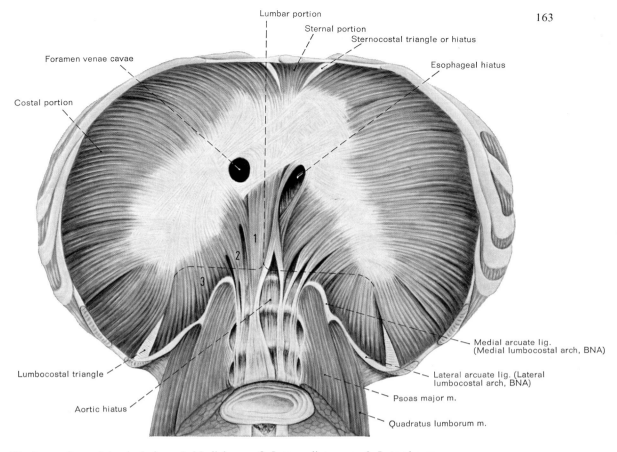

Lumbar portion

Sternal portion

Sternocostal triangle or hiatus

Esophageal hiatus

Foramen venae cavae

Costal portion

Medial arcuate lig. (Medial lumbocostal arch, BNA)

Lateral arcuate lig. (Lateral lumbocostal arch, BNA)

Psoas major m.

Quadratus lumborum m.

Lumbocostal triangle

Aortic hiatus

**Fig. 270.** Diaphragm from abdominal view: 1. Medial crus. 2. Intermediate crus. 3. Lateral crus.

## Diaphragm (Figs. 266, 270)

| Name | Origin | | Insertion |
|------|--------|--|-----------|
| **Sternal portion** | Inner surface of xiphoid process | | In the central tendon: *vena caval foramen* <br> In the lumbar portion: the *esophageal hiatus* |
| **Costal portion** | Inner surface of 6 caudal ribs (cartilages) | | |
| **Lumbar portion** | *Medial crus + intermediate crus* (tendinous) | Ventral surface of lumbar vertebrae 2–4 (tendon), between the component of both sides: *hiatus aortica* | |
| | *Lateral crus* | Transverse process of lumbar vertebra 1 (2); medial and lateral lumbar costal arches | |

*Nerve:* Phrenic nerve from the cervical plexus C 4 (3–5)

*Action:* Respiratory muscle (diaphragmatic breathing) produces inspiration, sustains abdominal muscular pressure

164

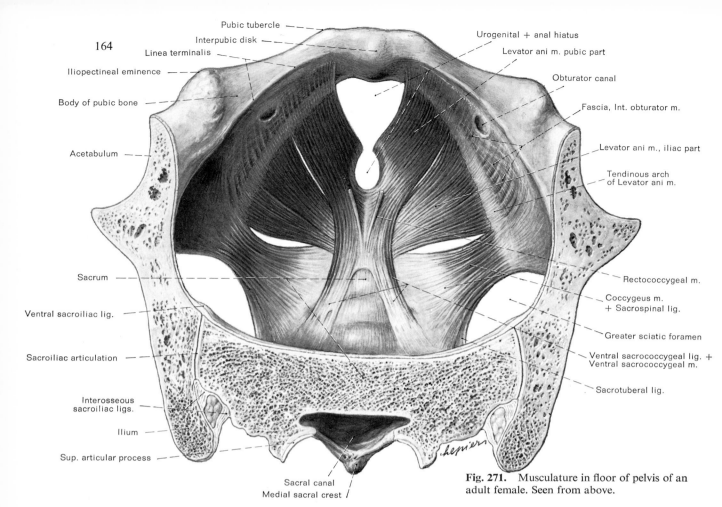

Pubic tubercle
Interpubic disk
Linea terminalis
Iliopectineal eminence
Body of pubic bone
Acetabulum
Sacrum
Ventral sacroiliac lig.
Sacroiliac articulation
Interosseous sacroiliac ligs.
Ilium
Sup. articular process
Sacral canal
Medial sacral crest

Urogenital + anal hiatus
Levator ani m. pubic part
Obturator canal
Fascia, Int. obturator m.
Levator ani m., iliac part
Tendinous arch of Levator ani m.
Rectococcygeal m.
Coccygeus m. + Sacrospinal lig.
Greater sciatic foramen
Ventral sacrococcygeal lig. + Ventral sacrococcygeal m.
Sacrotuberal lig.

**Fig. 271.** Musculature in floor of pelvis of an adult female. Seen from above.

| Name | Origin | Insertion |
|---|---|---|
| **Quadratus lumborum muscle** 4-sided muscle in dorsal wall of abdomen (Fig. 273) | Internal lip of crest of ilium; iliolumbar ligament | 12th rib, (medial border); transverse processes of upper 4 lumbar vertebrae |

*Nerve:* Branches of 12th thoracic and upper 3 lumbar nerves (T 12; L 1–4)

*Action:* Depresses and fixes last rib (expiration); abducts or bends trunk to same side, when acting unilaterally

### Muscles of the Pelvic Floor (Figs. 271, 272)

**I. Pelvic diaphragm**

| | | |
|---|---|---|
| **1. Levator ani muscle,** funnel-shaped, made up of several muscle parts: Pubococcygeus, Puborectalis, Iliococcygeus, Levator prostatae mm. | Tendinous arch of Levator ani muscle (spans the Obturator internus muscle from the symphysis to the ischial spine) | Sacrum, coccyx, and External sphincter muscle |

*Nerve:* Pudendal plexus, sacral nerves (S 3–5)

*Action:* Supports and slightly raises the pelvic floor

| | | |
|---|---|---|
| **2. Coccygeus muscle** | Ischial spine | Sacrum and coccyx |

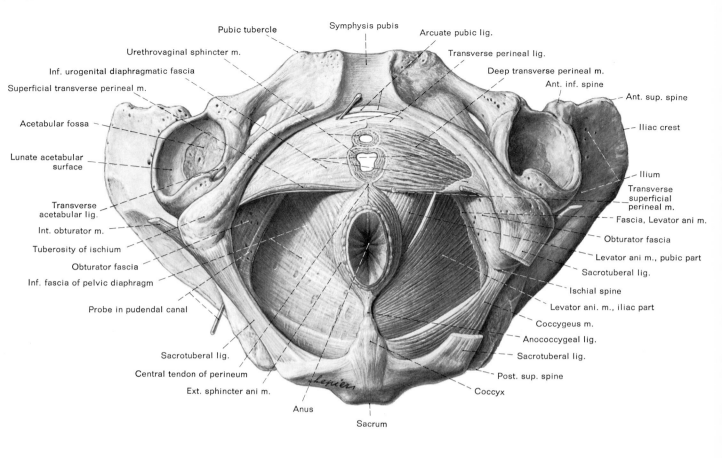

**Fig. 272.** Musculature in floor of pelvis of an adult female. Perineal view. Sound in pudendal canal.

## Muscles of the Pelvic Floor (continued)

**II. External sphincter ani muscle**
(subcutaneous, superficial, and deep portions)

**III. Urogenital diaphragm**

1. **Transversus perinei profundus muscle:** Stretches between the ischial rami, completed by the transverse ligament of the perineum and the arcuate ligament of the pubis. The male urethra or the urethra and vagina pass through this.

2. **Transversus perinei superficialis muscle** (variable)
Perineal branches of the pudendal nerve (S 2–4)

**Central tendon of perineum:** A knotty-like tendinous tissue for all muscles of the pelvic floor. It is interlaced anteriorly with the Sphincter ani externus muscle, with the dorsal border of the Transversus perinei profundus muscle, involving in addition, the Levator ani and the Bulbospongiosus muscles.

165

166

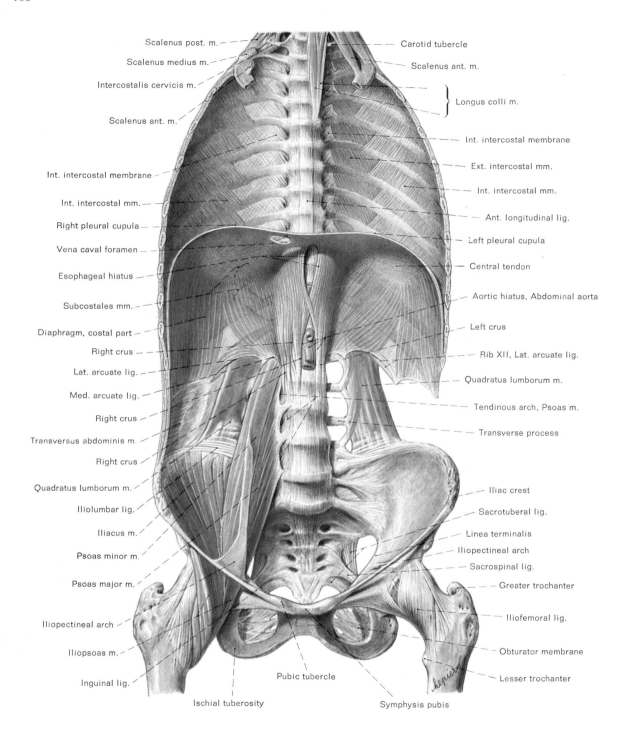

**Fig. 273.** The thoracic cavity, the diaphragm, the dorsal psoas musculature, and the pelvis. Ventral view.

# Myology

## Muscles of the Head and Neck

168

**Fig. 274.** Platysma. The skin and subcutaneous fatty tissue were removed from the lower jaw region of the right side of the neck and upper thorax.

**Fig. 275.** Head, neck, and upper thorax, showing triangles of the neck. The facial muscles for expression and part of the muscles of mastication, cervical muscles, the Deltoid, Pectoralis major, carotid triangle, and brachial plexus. The lower part of the parotid gland is pulled back with a hook.

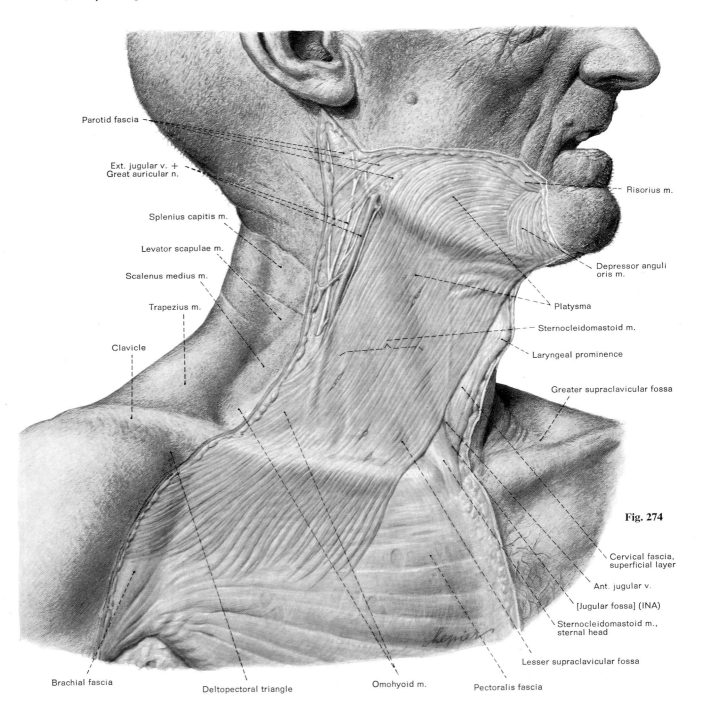

Parotid fascia

Ext. jugular v. + Great auricular n.

Splenius capitis m.

Levator scapulae m.

Scalenus medius m.

Trapezius m.

Clavicle

Brachial fascia

Deltopectoral triangle

Omohyoid m.

Pectoralis fascia

Risorius m.

Depressor anguli oris m.

Platysma

Sternocleidomastoid m.

Laryngeal prominence

Greater supraclavicular fossa

Fig. 274

Cervical fascia, superficial layer

Ant. jugular v.

[Jugular fossa] (INA)

Sternocleidomastoid m., sternal head

Lesser supraclavicular fossa

Accessory parotid gland + parotid duct

Zygomaticus major m.

Epicranius m. + Tempor oparietal m.

Orbicularis oculi m.

Buccinator m.

Zygomaticus minor m.

Medial palpebral lig.

Levator labii superioris m.

Ant. auricular m.

Post. auricular m.

Occipitofrontalis m., occipital belly

Levator labii superioris alaeque nasi m.

Nasalis m., transverse part

Nasalis m., alar part

Levator anguli oris m.

Orbicularis oris m.

Parotid gland, superficial portion

Depressor anguli oris m.

Semispinalis capitis m.

Submandibular gland

Buccal fat pad + Masseter m.

Hyoglossus m.

Digastric m., post. belly

Stylohyoid m.

Internal jugular v.

Splenius capitis m.

Sternocleidomastoid m.

Mentalis m.

Depressor labii inferioris m.

Levator scapulae m.

Mylohyoid m.

Scalenus medius m.

Digastric m., ant. belly

Hyoid bone

Thyrohyoid m.,

Laryngeal prominence

Trapezius m.

Acromion

Inf. pharyngeal constrictor m.

Common carotid a.

Deltoid m.

Fig. 275

Omohyoid m., sup. belly

Thyroid gland

Sternothyroid m.

Sternohyoid m.

Sternothyroid m.

Deltoid m.

Cephalic v.

Omohyoid m., Inf. belly

Clavicle

Pectoralis major m.

Scalenus ant. m.

Jugular v. (bulb)

Brachial plexus

Interclavicular lig.

## The Suprahyoid Muscles*  (Figs. 276, 277, 279, 289)

| Name | Origin | Insertion |
|---|---|---|
| **1. Digastric muscle** Divided into 2 bellies by a tendon. These are fastened through a short tendon to the margin of the hyoid bone | Mastoid notch of temporal bone (posterior belly) | Digastric fossa of mandible (anterior belly) |

*Nerve:*  Anterior belly: mylohyoid nerve. Posterior belly: facial nerve

*Action:*  Opens jaws (depresses lower jaw); elevates (fixes) the hyoid bone

| Name | Origin | Insertion |
|---|---|---|
| **2. Stylohyoid muscle** Passes on either side of tendon of the Digastric muscle | Styloid process of temporal bone | Lateral margin of the body of the hyoid bone near the greater cornu |

*Nerve:*  Facial nerve

*Action:*  Fixes hyoid bone; it pulls the hyoid bone backward and upward during deglutition

| Name | Origin | Insertion |
|---|---|---|
| **3. Mylohyoid muscle** The muscles of both sides in midline are united by a raphe | Mylohyoid line of the mandible. The muscles form a fleshy plate across the mandibular arch | Mylohyoid raphe and cranial margin of body of hyoid bone |

*Nerve:*  Mylohyoid nerve from mandibular division of trigeminal nerve

*Action:*  Elevates oral floor and tongue during deglutition; depresses mandible, or elevates hyoid bone

| Name | Origin | Insertion |
|---|---|---|
| **4. Geniohyoid Muscle** It borders directly on the tongue muscles, especially the Genioglossus | Inferior mental spine of the mandible, short tendon | Ventral margin of body of hyoid bone |
| | Muscles on both sides lie close together, a thin connective tissue-like septum separates them in the midline | |

*Nerve:*  Hypoglossal nerve

*Action:*  Supports the action of Mylohyoid muscle (elevates the tongue); elevates and fixes hyoid bone; depresses mandible

---

* In contrast to the Infrahyoid muscles, the Suprahyoid muscles belong to the muscles of the head, since they connect only bones of the head. The Digastric muscle is not a true Hyoid muscle, since it is only indirectly connected with the hyoid bone.

| Name | Origin | Insertion |
|---|---|---|

**1. Sternocleidomastoid muscle** (Fig. 275)

| | | |
|---|---|---|
| Sternal head: | Ventral surface of the manubrium sterni | Lateral surface of mastoid processe; superior nuchal line of occipital bone |
| Clavicular head: | Cranial surface of medial third of clavicle | |

*Nerve:* Spinal accessory nerve; fibers from second cervical nerve

*Action:* Various: Both sides together, hold head, move chin upward and pull back of head down. One side alone, turns chin upward and to opposite side. The understanding of this muscle clarifies the anatomy of the neck

### Infrahyoid Muscles (Figs. 275, 279, 280)

| | | |
|---|---|---|
| **1. Sternohyoid muscle** (thin, narrow muscle) | Inner surface of manubrium sterni and sternoclavicular joint | Body of hyoid bone |
| **2. Sternothyroid muscle** (shorter, wider muscle) | 1st costal cartilage; dorsal surface of manubrium sterni, caudal to Sternohyoid muscle | Outer surface of thyroid cartilage (opposite the origin of Thyrohyoid muscle) |
| **3. Thyrohyoid muscle** (small quadrilateral muscle) | Outer surface of the thyroid cartilage | Inferior border of greater cornu of hyoid bone |
| **4. Omohyoid muscle** (two fleshy bellies united in middle by a single tendon) | Superior margin of scapula between superior angle and scapular notch (inferior belly) | Caudal border of lateral section of body of hyoid bone (sup. belly) |

*Nerve:* Ansa cervicalis

*Action:* Fixes hyoid bone firmly; with Suprahyoid muscles, assist in movements of tongue, hyoid bone, and larynx in swallowing and phonation. With the Thyrohyoid m. (and hyoid bone fixed) elevates larynx in act of swallowing and production of high notes. The Sternothyroid m. does the opposite in drawing down the larynx to produce low notes. Muscles assist in respiration (pull sternum cranially in inspiration)

### Auricular Muscles (Fig. 275)

| | | |
|---|---|---|
| **Anterior auricular muscle** | Temporal fascia, superficial lamina | Base of cartilaginous external ear |
| **Posterior auricular muscle** | Tendon of insertion of Sternocleidomastoid muscle | |

*Nerve:* Facial nerve

*Action:* Moves the external ear (pinna)

172

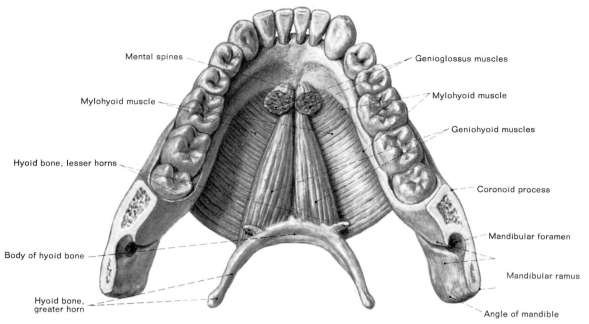

**Fig. 276.** Mylohyoid and Geniohyoid muscles, seen from occlusal surface (1/1). Hyoid bone with greater and lesser cornua, Mylohyoid and Geniohyoid muscles. Genioglossus muscle stumps of origin were preserved.

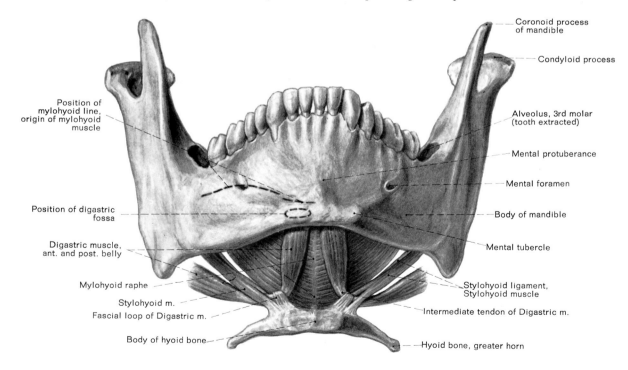

**Fig. 277.** Mandible, hyoid bone, muscles of the hyoid bone, seen from in front and below. The origin of the Mylohyoid muscle and the digastric fossa on the inner surface of the mandible are indicated by interrupted lines.

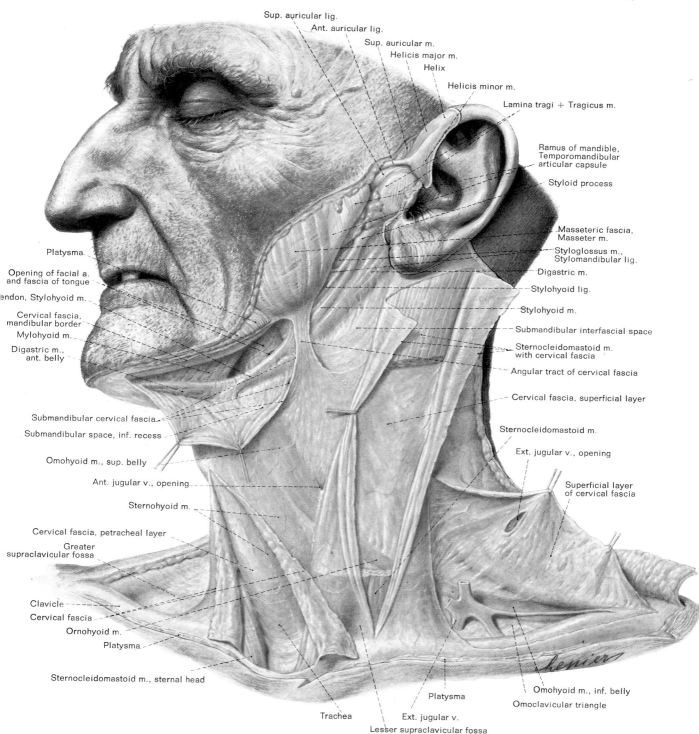

Sup. auricular lig.

Ant. auricular lig.

Sup. auricular m.

Helicis major m.

Helix

Helicis minor m.

Lamina tragi + Tragicus m.

Ramus of mandible, Temporomandibular articular capsule

Styloid process

Masseteric fascia, Masseter m.

Styloglossus m., Stylomandibular lig.

Digastric m.

Stylohyoid lig.

Stylohyoid m.

Submandibular interfascial space

Sternocleidomastoid m. with cervical fascia

Angular tract of cervical fascia

Cervical fascia, superficial layer

Sternocleidomastoid m.

Ext. jugular v., opening

Superficial layer of cervical fascia

Platysma

Opening of facial a. and fascia of tongue

endon, Stylohyoid m.

Cervical fascia, mandibular border

Mylohyoid m.

Digastric m., ant. belly

Submandibular cervical fascia

Submandibular space, inf. recess

Omohyoid m., sup. belly

Ant. jugular v., opening

Sternohyoid m.

Cervical fascia, petracheal layer

Greater supraclavicular fossa

Clavicle

Cervical fascia

Ornohyoid m.

Platysma

Sternocleidomastoid m., sternal head

Trachea

Ext. jugular v.

Lesser supraclavicular fossa

Platysma

Omohyoid m., inf. belly

Omoclavicular triangle

**Fig. 278.** The cervical fascia and the exposed areas after the removal of a greater portion of the musculature of the neck and submandibular region, including the vessels and nerves. Ventrolateral view.

174

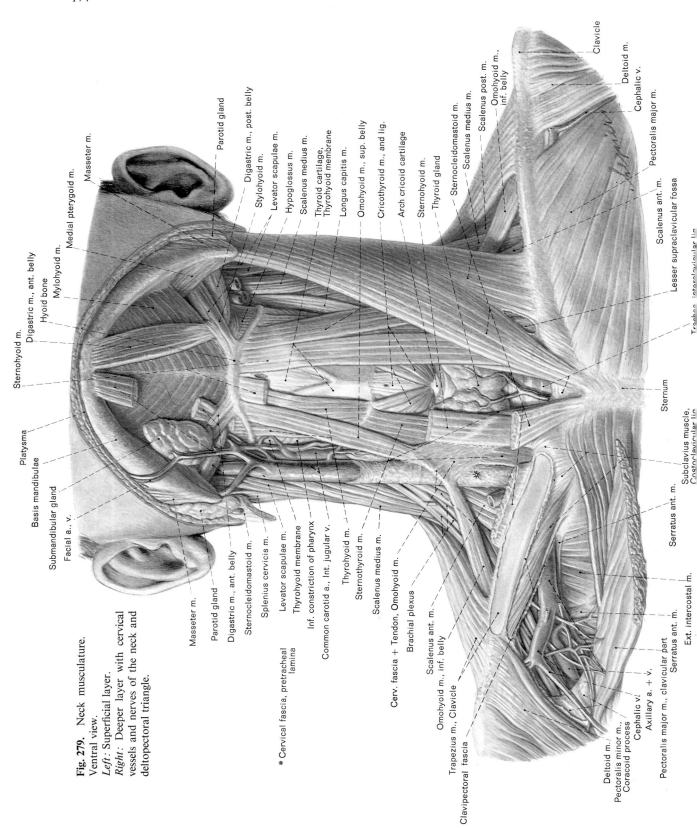

**Fig. 279.** Neck musculature. Ventral view.
*Left:* Superficial layer.
*Right:* Deeper layer with cervical vessels and nerves of the neck and deltopectoral triangle.

Sternohyoid m.

Platysma

Basis mandibulae

Submandibular gland

Facial a. + v.

Masseter m.

Parotid gland

Digastric m., ant. belly

Sternocleidomastoid m.

Splenius cervicis m.

Levator scapulae m.

Thyrohyoid membrane

Inf. constriction of pharynx

Common carotid a., Int. jugular v.

Thyrohyoid m.

Sternothyroid m.

Scalenus medius m.

*Cerv. fascia, pretracheal lamina

Cerv. fascia + Tendon, Omohyoid m.

Scalenus ant. m.

Omohyoid m., inf. belly

Trapezius m., Clavicle

Clavipectoral fascia

Deltoid m.

Pectoralis minor m., Coracoid process

Cephalic v.

Axillary a. + v.

Pectoralis major m., clavicular part

Masseter m.

Medial pterygoid m.

Mylohyoid m.

Hyoid bone

Digastric m., ant. belly

Parotid gland

Digastric m., post. belly

Stylohyoid m.

Levator scapulae m.

Hypoglossus m.

Scalenus medius m.

Thyroid cartilage, Thyrohyoid membrane

Longus capitis m.

Omohyoid m., sup. belly

Cricothyroid m., and lig.

Arch cricoid cartilage

Sternohyoid m.

Thyroid gland

Sternocleidomastoid m.

Scalenus medius m.

Scalenus post. m.

Omohyoid m., inf. belly

Clavicle

Deltoid m.

Cephalic v.

Pectoralis major m.

Scalenus ant. m.

Lesser supraclavicular fossa

Trachea, interclavicular lig.

Subclavius muscle, Costoclavicular lig.

Sternum

Serratus ant. m.

Ext. intercostal m.

Serratus ant. m.

Brachial plexus

Scalenus ant. m.

Scalenus medius m.

175

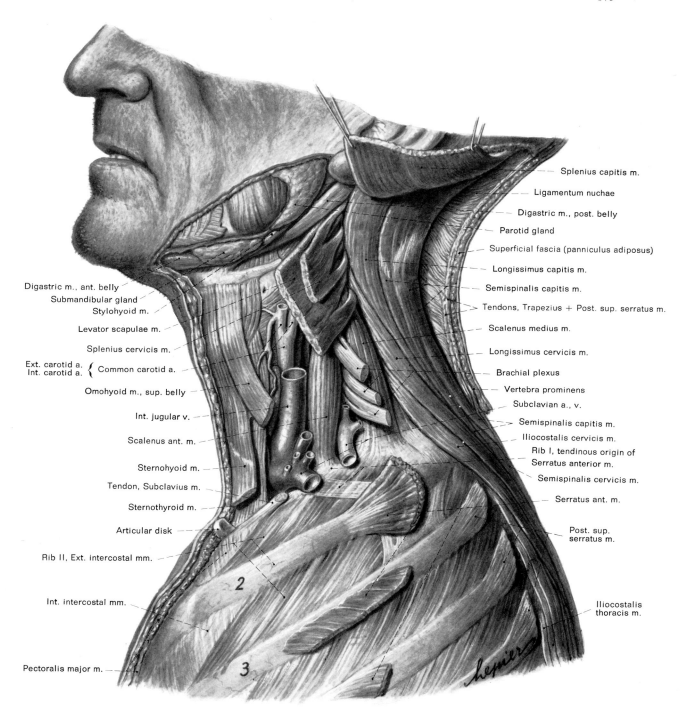

Digastric m., ant. belly
Submandibular gland
Stylohyoid m.
Levator scapulae m.
Splenius cervicis m.
Ext. carotid a.
Int. carotid a. { Common carotid a.
Omohyoid m., sup. belly
Int. jugular v.
Scalenus ant. m.
Sternohyoid m.
Tendon, Subclavius m.
Sternothyroid m.
Articular disk
Rib II, Ext. intercostal mm.
Int. intercostal mm.
Pectoralis major m.

Splenius capitis m.
Ligamentum nuchae
Digastric m., post. belly
Parotid gland
Superficial fascia (panniculus adiposus)
Longissimus capitis m.
Semispinalis capitis m.
Tendons, Trapezius + Post. sup. serratus m.
Scalenus medius m.
Longissimus cervicis m.
Brachial plexus
Vertebra prominens
Subclavian a., v.
Semispinalis capitis m.
Iliocostalis cervicis m.
Rib I, tendinous origin of Serratus anterior m.
Semispinalis cervicis m.
Serratus ant. m.
Post. sup. serratus m.
Iliocostalis thoracis m.

2

3

**Fig. 280.** Neck, upper thorax, deeper layers. Levator scapulae and Splenius cervicis muscles were cut in front. Observe the subclavian artery and brachial plexus in the scalene hiatus.

176

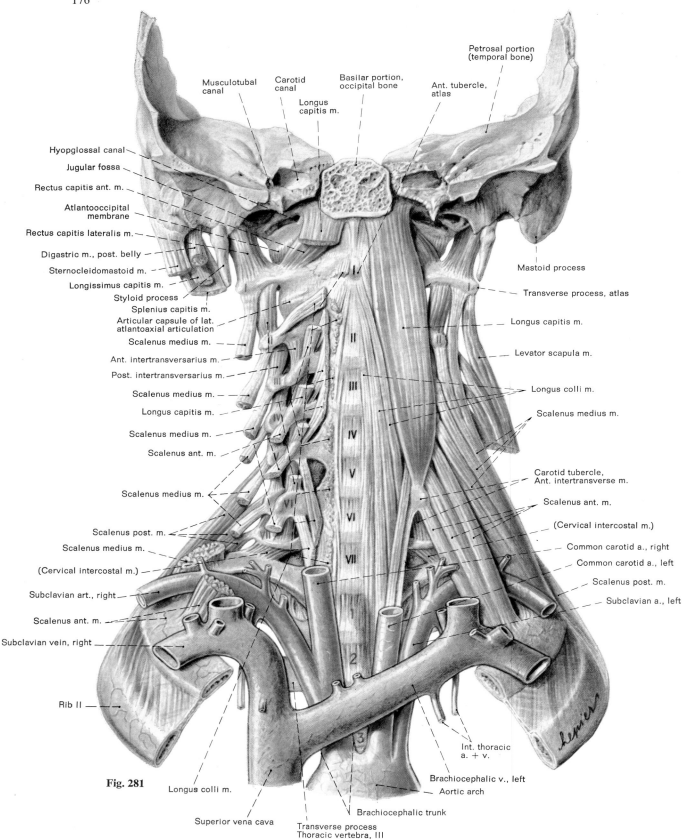

Hyopglossal canal

Jugular fossa

Rectus capitis ant. m.

Atlantooccipital membrane

Rectus capitis lateralis m.

Digastric m., post. belly

Sternocleidomastoid m.

Longissimus capitis m.

Styloid process

Splenius capitis m.

Articular capsule of lat. atlantoaxial articulation

Scalenus medius m.

Ant. intertransversarius m.

Post. intertransversarius m.

Scalenus medius m.

Longus capitis m.

Scalenus medius m.

Scalenus ant. m.

Scalenus medius m.

Scalenus post. m.

Scalenus medius m.

(Cervical intercostal m.)

Subclavian art., right

Scalenus ant. m.

Subclavian vein, right

Rib II

**Fig. 281**

Longus colli m.

Superior vena cava

Transverse process
Thoracic vertebra, III

Brachiocephalic trunk

Musculotubal canal

Carotid canal

Longus capitis m.

Basilar portion, occipital bone

Ant. tubercle, atlas

Petrosal portion (temporal bone)

Mastoid process

Transverse process, atlas

Longus capitis m.

Levator scapula m.

Longus colli m.

Scalenus medius m.

Carotid tubercle, Ant. intertransverse m.

Scalenus ant. m.

(Cervical intercostal m.)

Common carotid a., right

Common carotid a., left

Scalenus post. m.

Subclavian a., left

Int. thoracic a. + v.

Brachiocephalic v., left

Aortic arch

## Lateral Vertebral Group (Prevertebral) of Deep Cervical Muscles (Figs. 269, 281)

| Name | Origin | Insertion |
|---|---|---|
| 1. Scalenus anterior muscle | Anterior tubercles of transverse processes of 3rd to 6th cervical vertebrae | Scalene tubercle on 1st rib |
| 2. Scalenus medius muscle | Posterior tubercles of transverse processes of last six cervical vertebrae | Cranial surface of 1st rib, dorsal to subclavian groove |
| 3. Scalenus posterior muscle | Posterior tubercles of transverse processes of last three cervical vertebrae | Outer surface of 2nd rib |

*Nerve:* Cervical plexus (and brachial plexus)

*Action:* Scalene muscles, acting together, elevate 1st and 2nd ribs or flex the vertebral column (muscles of inspiration); acting one side at a time, they bend neck to side

## Anterior Vertebral Group (Prevertebral) of Deep Cervical Muscles (Fig. 281)

| Name | Origin | Insertion |
|---|---|---|
| **1. Longus colli muscle** | | |
| Vertical portion | Body of first 3 thoracic and last 3 cervical vertebrae | Bodies of cervical vertebrae $C_2$–$C_4$ |
| Superior oblique | Anterior tubercle of transverse process of cervical vertebrae $C_3$–$C_5$ | Tubercle on anterior arch of the atlas and body of next cervical vertebra |
| Inferior oblique | Anterior surface of bodies of first 2 or 3 thoracic vertebrae | Anterior tubercles of the transverse processes of 5th and 6th cervical vertebrae |
| **2. Longus capitis muscle** | Anterior tubercle of transverse processes of 3rd–6th cervical vertebrae | Inferior border of basilar part of occipital bone |
| **3. Rectus capitis anterior muscle** | Lateral mass of atlas and root of its transverse process | as above |

*Nerve:* Cervical plexus

*Action:* Bend the cervical vertebral column or the head forward, by unilateral innervation, incline and rotate the head toward the same side

**Fig. 281.** Deep cervical muscles after removal of the cervical viscera. Ventral view. Cervical vertebrae: I–VII; upper thoracic vertebrae: 1–3. The base of the skull cut off almost frontally near the level of the basilar portion. First and second ribs were cut near the bone-cartilage junction. The superior vena cava and arch of the aorta are shown with their large trunks: the brachiocephalic trunk, the common carotid artery, the left subclavian artery with its passage through the scalene hiatus.

178

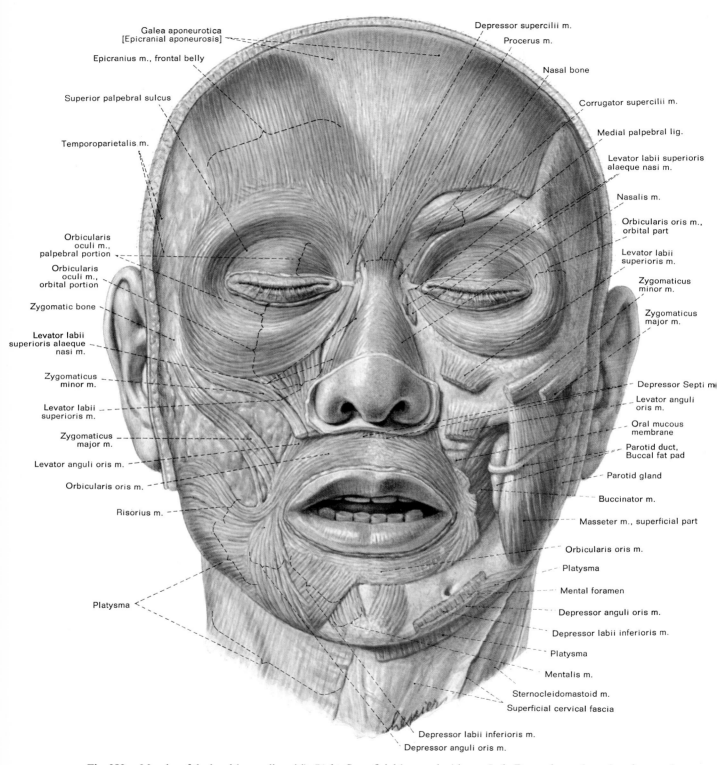

Galea aponeurotica [Epicranial aponeurosis]

Epicranius m., frontal belly

Superior palpebral sulcus

Temporoparietalis m.

Orbicularis oculi m., palpebral portion

Orbicularis oculi m., orbital portion

Zygomatic bone

Levator labii superioris alaeque nasi m.

Zygomaticus minor m.

Levator labii superioris m.

Zygomaticus major m.

Levator anguli oris m.

Orbicularis oris m.

Risorius m.

Platysma

Depressor supercilii m.

Procerus m.

Nasal bone

Corrugator supercilii m.

Medial palpebral lig.

Levator labii superioris alaeque nasi m.

Nasalis m.

Orbicularis oris m., orbital part

Levator labii superioris m.

Zygomaticus minor m.

Zygomaticus major m.

Depressor Septi m

Levator anguli oris m.

Oral mucous membrane

Parotid duct, Buccal fat pad

Parotid gland

Buccinator m.

Masseter m., superficial part

Orbicularis oris m.

Platysma

Mental foramen

Depressor anguli oris m.

Depressor labii inferioris m.

Platysma

Mentalis m.

Sternocleidomastoid m.

Superficial cervical fascia

Depressor labii inferioris m.

Depressor anguli oris m.

**Fig. 282.** Muscles of the head (musculi capiti). *Right:* Superficial (expression) layer. *Left:* Deeper layers (muscles of expression and chewing) of the facial muscles.

### Muscles of the Eyelids  (Fig. 282)

| Name | Origin | Insertion |
|---|---|---|
| **1. Orbicularis oculi muscle** | | |
| Orbital portion | Frontal process of maxilla; medial angle of eye; medial palpebral lig. | Surrounds orbital opening as a sphincter, some fibers go to eyebrow |
| Palpebral portion | Medial palpebral ligament | Lateral palpebral raphe |
| Lacrimal portion | Posterior lacrimal crest | Tarsus of each eyelid |
| **2. Depressor supercilii muscles** | Nasal process of frontal bone | Skin of eyebrow |

*Nerve:*   Facial nerve, temporal and zygomatic branches

*Action:*   Closes lids, compresses lacrimal sac, moves eyebrows

| | | |
|---|---|---|
| **3. Corrugator supercilii muscle** | Nasal process of frontal bone | Skin of eyebrow |
| **4. Procerus muscle** | Bridge of nose and lateral nasal cartilage | Skin of forehead between eyebrows |

*Nerve:*   Facial nerve, temporal branch

*Action:*   Acts upon skin of forehead (glabella) and eyebrows

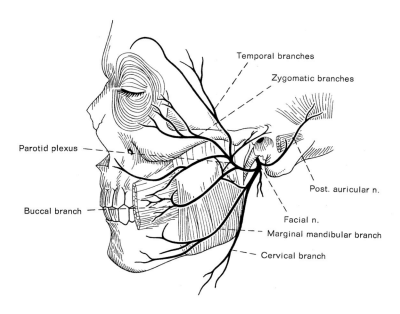

**Fig. 283.**   Nerve supply for the facial musculature (temporal, zygomatic, buccal, mandibular, and cervical branches). (Feneis, 1967).

## Epicranius Muscles  (Figs. 282, 284)

| Name | Origin | Insertion |
|------|--------|-----------|
| **Occipitofrontalis muscle, Frontal belly:** | Supraorbital margin, skin of forehead and eyebrows | Galea aponeurotica |
| **Occipitofrontalis muscle, Occipital belly:** | Supreme nuchal line | Galea aponeurotica |
| **Temporoparietalis muscle** | Superficial lamina, temporal fascia near ear | On skin and temporal fascia above and in front of ear |

*Nerve:*   Facial nerve

*Action:*   Moves scalp, wrinkles forehead

## Muscles of the Nose  (Figs. 282, 284)

**1. Nasalis muscle**

| | | |
|------|--------|-----------|
| **Transverse part:** | Area over canine teeth (the maxilla) | Aponeurosis over bridge of nose |
| **Alar part:** | Area over the lateral incisors (alar cartilage) | Skin at tip of nose |
| **2. Depressor septi muscle** | Incisive fossa of maxilla | Alar cartilage and septum of nose |

*Nerve:*   Facial nerve

*Action:*   Slightly moves nose, namely, ala of the nose (dilates and contracts nostrils)

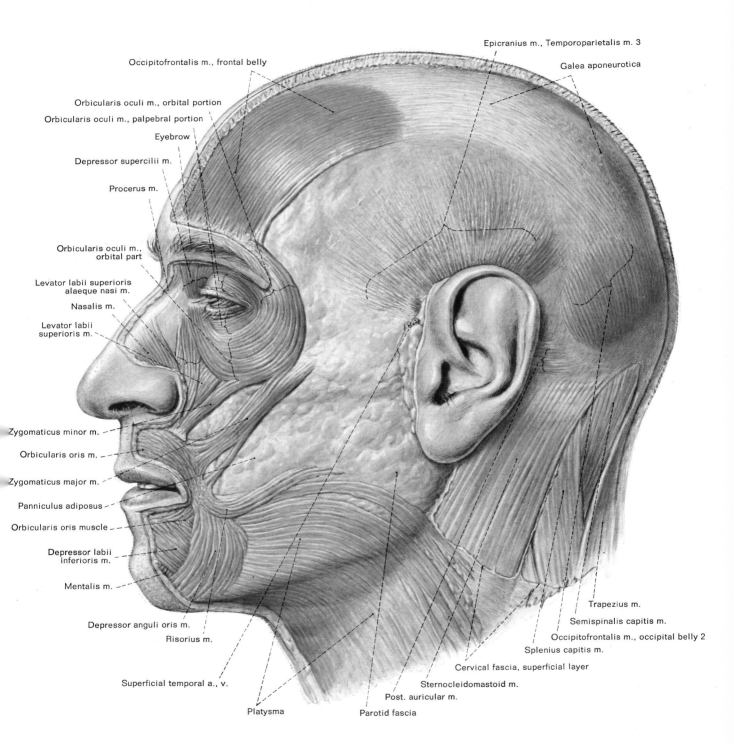

Epicranius m., Temporoparietalis m. 3

Galea aponeurotica

Occipitofrontalis m., frontal belly

Orbicularis oculi m., orbital portion

Orbicularis oculi m., palpebral portion

Eyebrow

Depressor supercilii m.

Procerus m.

Orbicularis oculi m., orbital part

Levator labii superioris alaeque nasi m.

Nasalis m.

Levator labii superioris m.

Zygomaticus minor m.

Orbicularis oris m.

Zygomaticus major m.

Panniculus adiposus

Orbicularis oris muscle

Depressor labii inferioris m.

Mentalis m.

Depressor anguli oris m.

Risorius m.

Superficial temporal a., v.

Platysma

Parotid fascia

Post. auricular m.

Sternocleidomastoid m.

Cervical fascia, superficial layer

Splenius capitis m.

Occipitofrontalis m., occipital belly 2

Semispinalis capitis m.

Trapezius m.

**Fig. 284.** Lateral aspect of the head with mimetic musculature and superficial layers of the cervical musculature. The three parts of the Epicranial muscles are designated 1, 2, 3.

182

## Muscles of the Oral Region (Figs. 282-286)

| Name | *Origin* | *Insertion* |
|---|---|---|
| **1. Levator labii superioris alaeque nasi muscle** | Frontal process of maxilla | Ala of nose and upper lip |
| **2. Levator labii superioris muscle** | Infraorbital margin | Ala of nose and upper lip |
| **3. Zygomaticus minor muscle** | Malar surface of zygomatic bone | Near angle of mouth |
| **4. Zygomaticus major muscle** | Lateral surface of zygomatic bone | Angle of mouth |
| **5. Risorius muscle** (a part of the Platysma) | Masseteric fascia | Angle of mouth |
| **6. Depressor anguli oris muscle** | Oblique line of mandible | Angle of mouth; lower lip |
| **7. Levator anguli oris muscle** | Canine fossa of maxilla | Musculature of upper lip; angle of mouth |
| **8. Depressor labii inferioris muscle** | Mandible between symphysis and mental foramen | Lower lip |
| **9. Orbicularis oris muscle** | The following specifications: Marginal part: fibers blended with adjacent muscles Labial part: fibers restricted to lips | Protrudes and shapes lips |
| **10. Buccinator muscle** | Outer surface of mandible; alveolar process of maxilla; pterygomandibular raphe | Angle of mouth and lips; its interlacing fibers contribute to Orbicularis oris m. |
| **11. Mentalis muscle** | Incisive fossa of mandible | Skin of chin |

*Nerve:* Facial nerve (Fig. 283)

*Action:* Moves lips, ala of nose, cheeks, skin of chin. Risorius: draws angle of mouth laterally (smiling)

183

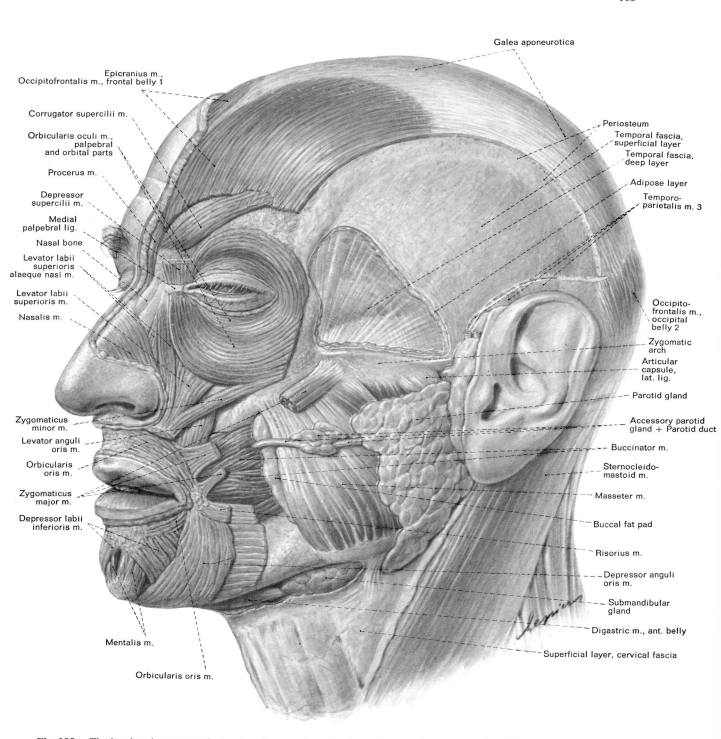

**Fig. 285.** The head and upper cervical region from the left side. Mimetic musculature, part of the Masseter muscles, salivary glands, the Sternocleidomastoid muscle and some of the upper cervical muscles. The three parts of the Epicranius muscle designated 1, 2, 3.

## Muscles of Mastication  (Figs. 286, 287, 289)

The muscles of mastication are invested by fasciae. They are the only cranial muscles resembling the true skeletal muscles with distinct separate muscles with well defined fascia. These 4 muscles (Masseter, Temporal and both Pterygoid muscles) move the mandible in the temporomandibular articulation.

| Name | Origin | Insertion |
|---|---|---|
| **1. Masseter muscle**<br>Superficial portion | Zygomatic process of maxilla; lower margin of zygomatic arch | Angle and ramus of mandible; base of coronoid process |
| Deep portion | From posterior part of lower margin and medial surface of zygomatic arch | |

*Nerve:*  Masseteric nerve from mandibular division of trigeminal nerve

*Action:*  Closes jaws, elevates mandible

| Name | Origin | Insertion |
|---|---|---|
| **2. Temporal muscle** | Temporal fossa and temporal fascia | Anterior border and medial surface of coronoid process of mandible |

*Nerve:*  Deep temporal nerves from mandibular division of trigeminal

*Action:*  Elevates mandible (closes jaws); posterior fibers retract mandible

| Name | Origin | Insertion |
|---|---|---|
| **3. Lateral pterygoid muscle** | *Main lower head:* Lateral surface of lateral pterygoid lamina<br>*Accessory upper head:* Infratemporal surface of great wing of sphenoid | Pterygoid fovea of condyloid process of mandible; articular disk of temporo-mandibular joint |
| **4. Medial pterygoid muscle** | Pterygoid fossa; pyramidal process of palatine bone; lateral lamina of pterygoid process | Medial surface and angle of mandible; opposite the masseter muscle (on pterygoid tuberosity) |

*Nerve:*  Lateral and medial pterygoid nerves, respectively, from mandibular division of trigeminal

*Action:*  Opens jaws, protrudes mandible, moves mandible from side to side, grinding motion (lateral); closes jaws (medial)

**Fig. 286.**  Lateral view of head and upper neck muscles with mimetic and masticator muscles. The external ear and part of the zygomatic arch were removed. A wide piece of the upper half of the Sternocleidomastoid was removed to display the large vessels. The Masseter muscle was partly removed to display its tendinous insertions between the muscle bundles. A few mimetic muscles were cut off near their origins.

185

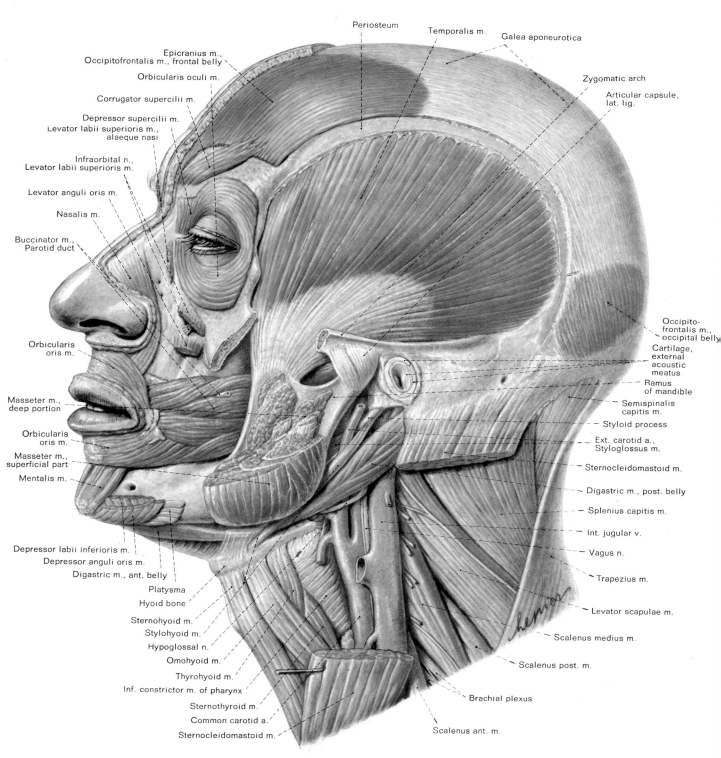

Periosteum

Temporalis m.

Galea aponeurotica

Epicranius m.,
Occipitofrontalis m., frontal belly

Orbicularis oculi m.

Corrugator supercilii m.

Zygomatic arch

Articular capsule,
lat. lig.

Depressor supercilii m.
Levator labii superioris m.,
alaeque nasi

Infraorbital n.,
Levator labii superioris m.

Levator anguli oris m.

Nasalis m.

Buccinator m.,
Parotid duct

Orbicularis
oris m.

Masseter m.,
deep portion

Orbicularis
oris m.

Masseter m.,
superficial part

Mentalis m.

Depressor labii inferioris m.

Depressor anguli oris m.

Digastric m., ant. belly

Platysma

Hyoid bone

Sternohyoid m.

Stylohyoid m.

Hypoglossal n.

Omohyoid m.

Thyrohyoid m.

Inf. constrictor m. of pharynx

Sternothyroid m.

Common carotid a.

Sternocleidomastoid m.

Occipito-
frontalis m.,
occipital belly

Cartilage,
external
acoustic
meatus

Ramus
of mandible

Semispinalis
capitis m.

Styloid process

Ext. carotid a.,
Styloglossus m.

Sternocleidomastoid m.

Digastric m., post. belly

Splenius capitis m.

Int. jugular v.

Vagus n.

Trapezius m.

Levator scapulae m.

Scalenus medius m.

Scalenus post. m.

Brachial plexus

Scalenus ant. m.

**Fig. 286**

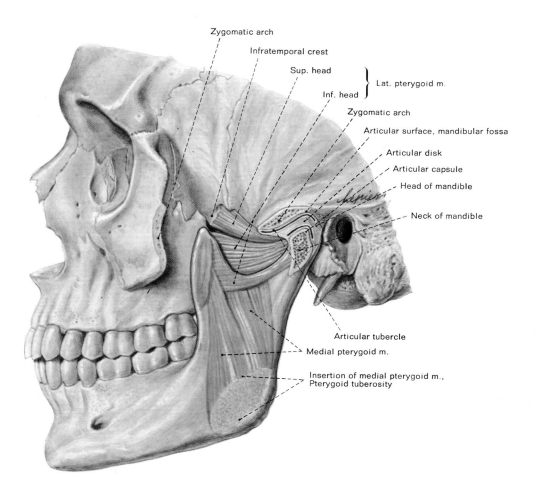

**Fig. 287.** Mandibular articulation. The temporomandibular joint was opened. The cut was made near the articular tubercle in a sagittal direction so that the neck of the mandible and the capsular ligament may be seen with the articular disk. The ramus of the mandible is displayed as being transparent in order to show the origin and course of the Lateral and Medial pterygoid muscles.

187

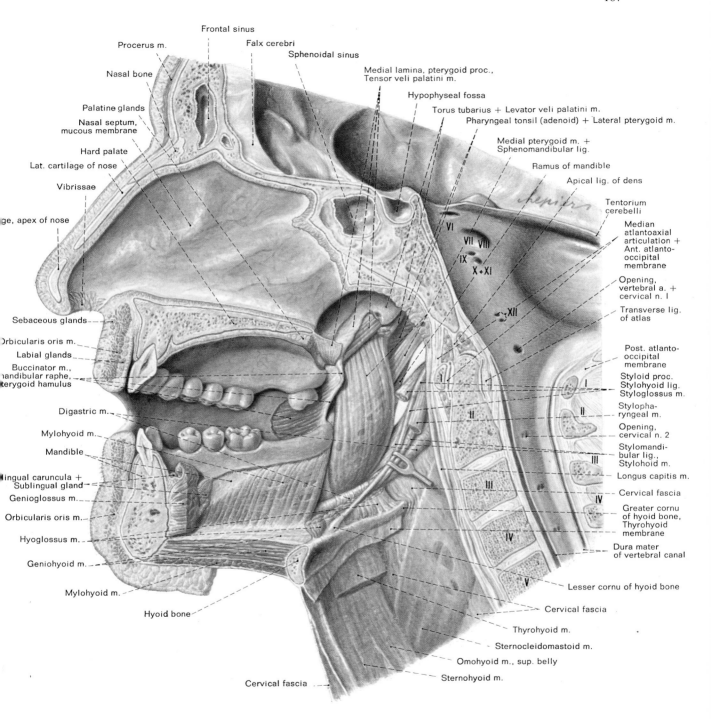

Frontal sinus

Procerus m.

Falx cerebri

Nasal bone

Sphenoidal sinus

Medial lamina, pterygoid proc.,
Tensor veli palatini m.

Hypophyseal fossa

Palatine glands

Torus tubarius + Levator veli palatini m.

Nasal septum,
mucous membrane

Pharyngeal tonsil (adenoid) + Lateral pterygoid m.

Medial pterygoid m. +
Sphenomandibular lig.

Hard palate

Ramus of mandible

Lat. cartilage of nose

Apical lig. of dens

Vibrissae

Tentorium
cerebelli

ge, apex of nose

Median
atlantoaxial
articulation +
Ant. atlanto-
occipital
membrane

VI

VII VIII

IX

X + XI

Opening,
vertebral a. +
cervical n. I

Sebaceous glands

XII

Transverse lig.
of atlas

Orbicularis oris m.

Post. atlanto-
occipital
membrane

Labial glands

Styloid proc.
Stylohyoid lig.
Styloglossus m.

Buccinator m.,
mandibular raphe,
pterygoid hamulus

I

Stylopha-
ryngeal m.

Digastric m.

II

II

Opening,
cervical n. 2

Mylohyoid m.

Stylomandi-
bular lig.,
Stylohoid m.

Mandible

III

Longus capitis m.

lingual caruncula +
Sublingual gland

III

Cervical fascia

Genioglossus m.

IV

Greater cornu
of hyoid bone,
Thyrohyoid
membrane

Orbicularis oris m.

Hyoglossus m.

IV

Dura mater
of vertebral canal

Geniohyoid m.

Mylohyoid m.

V

Lesser cornu of hyoid bone

Hyoid bone

Cervical fascia

Thyrohyoid m.

Sternocleidomastoid m.

Omohyoid m., sup. belly

Cervical fascia

Sternohyoid m.

**Fig. 288.** Paramedian sagittal section through the face and neck. The nasal and oral cavities, as well as some muscles of the floor of the mouth and upper cervical region are displayed. Cervical vertebrae, I-V. The points of exits of the cranial nerves through the dura mater, VI–XII.

188

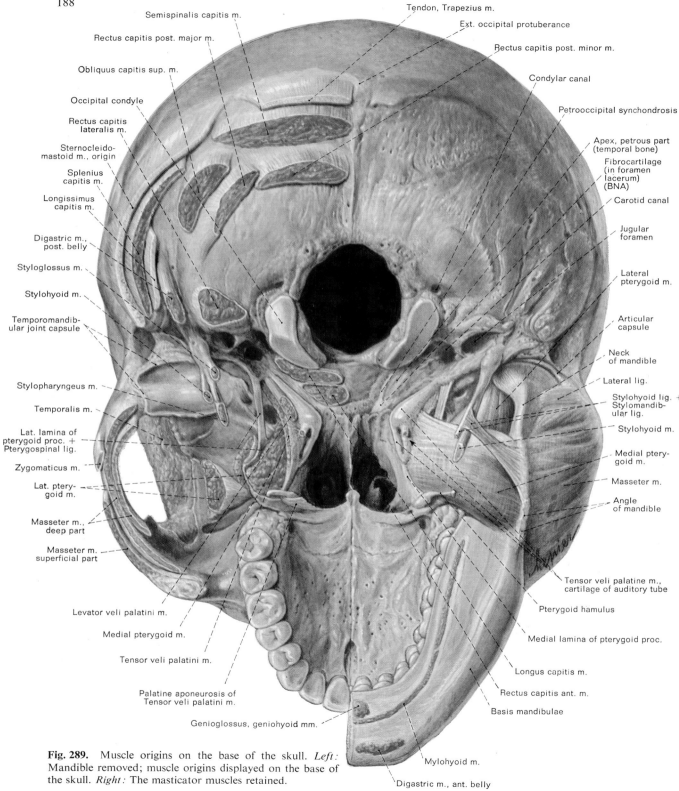

**Fig. 289.** Muscle origins on the base of the skull. *Left:* Mandible removed; muscle origins displayed on the base of the skull. *Right:* The masticator muscles retained.

# Myology

*Muscles of the Upper Limb*

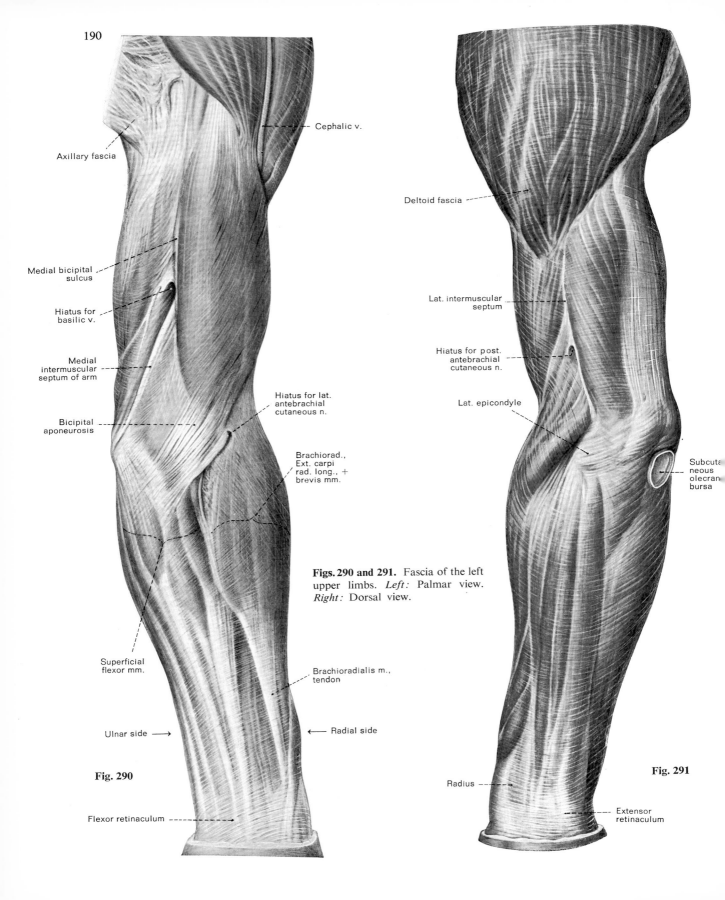

Axillary fascia

Cephalic v.

Medial bicipital sulcus

Hiatus for basilic v.

Medial intermuscular septum of arm

Bicipital aponeurosis

Hiatus for lat. antebrachial cutaneous n.

Brachiorad., Ext. carpi rad. long., + brevis mm.

Superficial flexor mm.

Brachioradialis m., tendon

Ulnar side →

← Radial side

Fig. 290

Flexor retinaculum

Deltoid fascia

Lat. intermuscular septum

Hiatus for post. antebrachial cutaneous n.

Lat. epicondyle

Subcutaneous olecranon bursa

**Figs. 290 and 291.** Fascia of the left upper limbs. *Left:* Palmar view. *Right:* Dorsal view.

Radius

Fig. 291

Extensor retinaculum

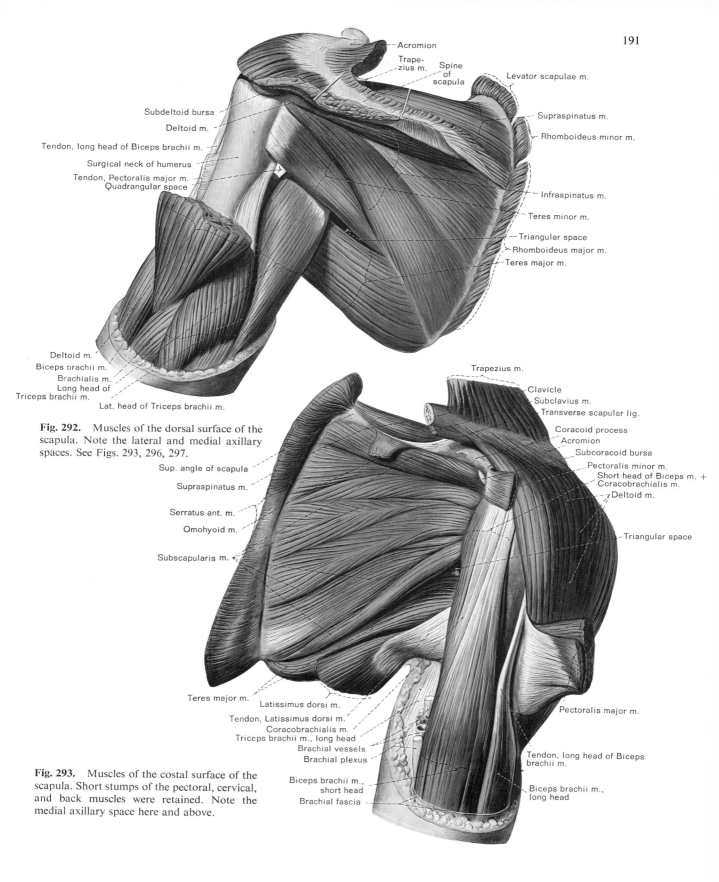

**Fig. 292.** Muscles of the dorsal surface of the scapula. Note the lateral and medial axillary spaces. See Figs. 293, 296, 297.

**Fig. 293.** Muscles of the costal surface of the scapula. Short stumps of the pectoral, cervical, and back muscles were retained. Note the medial axillary space here and above.

Acromion
Trape-zius m.
Spine of scapula
Levator scapulae m.
Supraspinatus m.
Rhomboideus minor m.
Subdeltoid bursa
Deltoid m.
Tendon, long head of Biceps brachii m.
Surgical neck of humerus
Tendon, Pectoralis major m.
Quadrangular space
Infraspinatus m.
Teres minor m.
Triangular space
Rhomboideus major m.
Teres major m.
Deltoid m.
Biceps brachii m.
Brachialis m.
Long head of Triceps brachii m.
Lat. head of Triceps brachii m.

Trapezius m.
Clavicle
Subclavius m.
Transverse scapular lig.
Coracoid process
Acromion
Subcoracoid bursa
Pectoralis minor m.
Short head of Biceps m. + Coracobrachialis m.
Deltoid m.
Triangular space
Sup. angle of scapula
Supraspinatus m.
Serratus ant. m.
Omohyoid m.
Subscapularis m.
Pectoralis major m.
Teres major m.
Latissimus dorsi m.
Tendon, Latissimus dorsi m.
Coracobrachialis m.
Triceps brachii m., long head
Brachial vessels
Brachial plexus
Biceps brachii m., short head
Brachial fascia
Tendon, long head of Biceps brachii m.
Biceps brachii m., long head

192

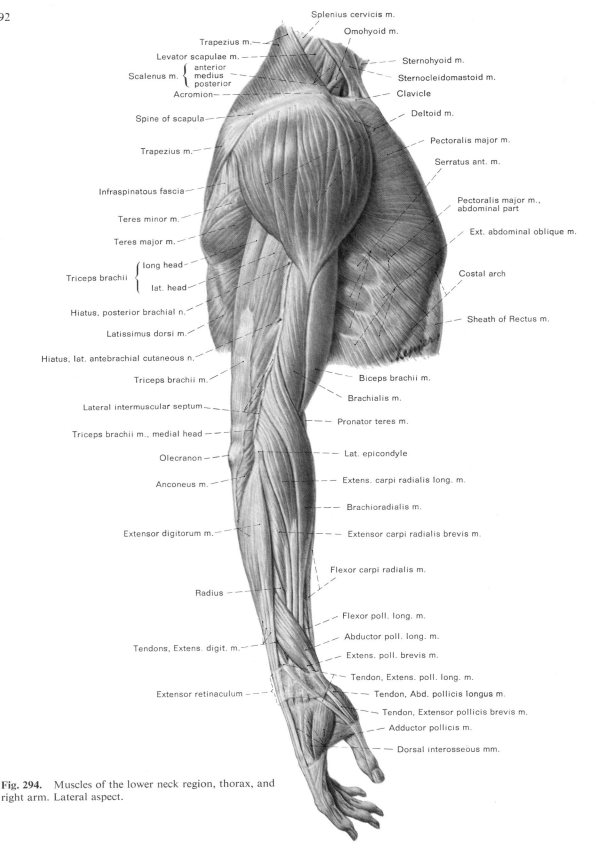

Splenius cervicis m.
Omohyoid m.
Trapezius m.
Levator scapulae m.
Scalenus m. { anterior medius posterior }
Sternohyoid m.
Sternocleidomastoid m.
Acromion
Clavicle
Spine of scapula
Deltoid m.
Trapezius m.
Pectoralis major m.
Serratus ant. m.
Infraspinatous fascia
Pectoralis major m., abdominal part
Teres minor m.
Ext. abdominal oblique m.
Teres major m.
Triceps brachii { long head lat. head }
Costal arch
Hiatus, posterior brachial n.
Sheath of Rectus m.
Latissimus dorsi m.
Hiatus, lat. antebrachial cutaneous n.
Triceps brachii m.
Biceps brachii m.
Brachialis m.
Lateral intermuscular septum
Pronator teres m.
Triceps brachii m., medial head
Olecranon
Lat. epicondyle
Anconeus m.
Extens. carpi radialis long. m.
Brachioradialis m.
Extensor digitorum m.
Extensor carpi radialis brevis m.
Flexor carpi radialis m.
Radius
Flexor poll. long. m.
Abductor poll. long. m.
Extens. poll. brevis m.
Tendon, Extens. poll. long. m.
Tendons, Extens. digit. m.
Tendon, Abd. pollicis longus m.
Tendon, Extensor pollicis brevis m.
Extensor retinaculum
Adductor pollicis m.
Dorsal interosseous mm.

**Fig. 294.** Muscles of the lower neck region, thorax, and right arm. Lateral aspect.

## Extensor Muscle of the Upper Arm (Figs. 294-296, 302, 308, 313)

| Name | Origin | Insertion |
|---|---|---|
| **Triceps brachii muscle**<br>*Long head:* (Operates 2 joints) | Infraglendoidal tubercle of scapula | Verticle muscle fibers running distalward to the olecranon |
| *Lateral head:* (Operates 1 joint) | Lateral and dorsal side of humerus, lateral 2/3 of lateral intermuscular septum | Joins the common tendon of insertion to the olecranon |
| *Medial head:* (Operates 1 joint) | Dorsal side of humerus, lateral and distal to radial groove; medial and lateral intermuscular septa | Posterior aspect of olecranon and into deep fascia on both sides of the forearm |
| **Anconeus muscle**<br>(Situated in the forearm) | Lateral epicondyle of humerus. Developmentally, it appears to be a part of the Triceps brachii m. | Posterior surface of ulna, slightly distal to olecranon |

*Nerve:*   Radial nerve (C 7, 8)

*Action:*   Extends forearm; adducts and extends arm, braces extended elbow joint (when pushing an object)

**Quadrangular and triangular spaces:**
1. *Quadrangular Space:* Bounded by tendon of long head of Triceps brachii, medially; Teres major, inferiorly; the humerus, laterally; Teres minor and capsule of shoulder joint, superiorly (Fig. 292).
   Transmits: Axillary nerve, posterior humeral circumflex vessels.
2. *Triangular space:* Bounded by Teres minor, superiorly; Teres major, inferiorly; long head of the Triceps, laterally (Fig. 292).
   Transmits: Circumflex scapular artery.

**Fig. 295.**   The Deltoid muscle and muscles of the left upper arm. Dorsalateral view.

**Fig. 296.**   Muscles of the left upper arm, deeper layer. Dorsolateral view. The Deltoid muscle has been removed except for attachments. The antebrachial fascia was removed where it covered the Anconeus muscle; the Teres minor and lateral head of the Triceps brachii were cut and reflected.
+ the lateral axillary space, quadrangular; beneath is the medial axillary space, triangular.

196

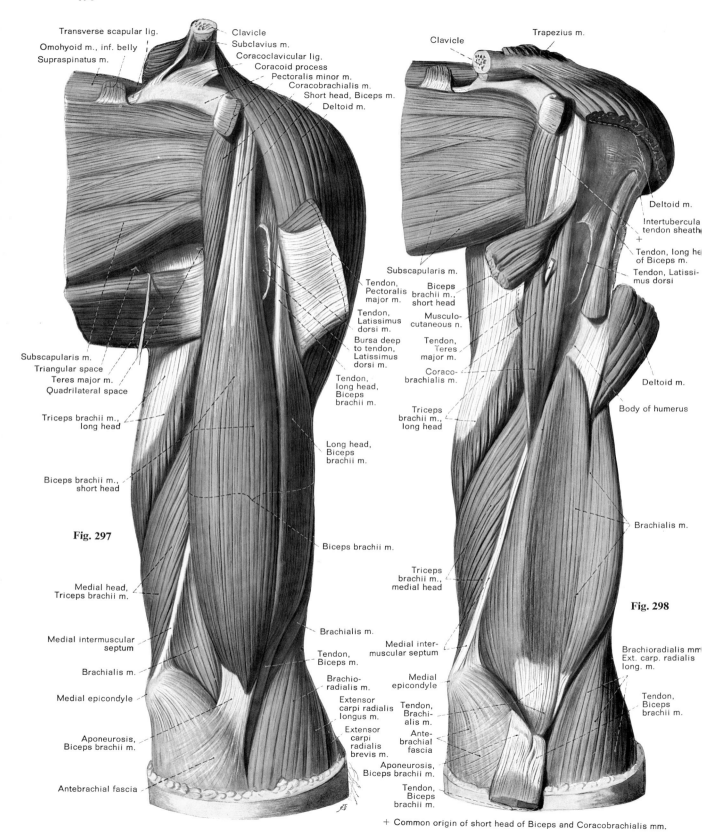

Transverse scapular lig.
Omohyoid m., inf. belly
Supraspinatus m.

Clavicle
Subclavius m.
Coracoclavicular lig.
Coracoid process
Pectoralis minor m.
Coracobrachialis m.
Short head, Biceps m.
Deltoid m.

Clavicle

Trapezius m.

Deltoid m.
Intertubercular
tendon sheath
+
Tendon, long head
of Biceps m.
Tendon, Latissi-
mus dorsi

Subscapularis m.

Tendon,
Pectoralis
major m.

Tendon,
Latissimus
dorsi m.

Bursa deep
to tendon,
Latissimus
dorsi m.

Tendon,
long head,
Biceps
brachii m.

Biceps
brachii m.,
short head

Musculo-
cutaneous n.

Tendon,
Teres
major m.

Coraco-
brachialis m.

Triceps
brachii m.,
long head

Deltoid m.

Body of humerus

Subscapularis m.
Triangular space
Teres major m.
Quadrilateral space

Triceps brachii m.,
long head

Biceps brachii m.,
short head

**Fig. 297**

Long head,
Biceps
brachii m.

Brachialis m.

Medial head,
Triceps brachii m.

Triceps
brachii m.,
medial head

**Fig. 298**

Medial intermuscular
septum

Biceps brachii m.

Brachialis m.

Medial epicondyle

Brachialis m.
Tendon,
Biceps m.
Brachio-
radialis m.
Extensor
carpi radialis
longus m.
Extensor
carpi
radialis
brevis m.

Medial inter-
muscular septum

Medial
epicondyle

Tendon,
Brachi-
alis m.

Ante-
brachial
fascia

Brachioradialis mm
Ext. carp. radialis
long. m.

Tendon,
Biceps
brachii m.

Aponeurosis,
Biceps brachii m.

Antebrachial fascia

Aponeurosis,
Biceps brachii m.

Tendon,
Biceps
brachii m.

+ Common origin of short head of Biceps and Coracobrachialis mm.

## Flexor Surface of the Muscles of the Arm (Figs. 294, 297, 298, 300, 303, 312)

| Name | | Origin | Insertion |
|---|---|---|---|
| **1. Biceps brachii muscle** (Operates 2 joints) | *Long head:* | Tendon through shoulder joint to supraglenoid tubercle of scapula (long tendon) | Posterior half of radial tuberosity. Bicipital aponeurosis to antebrachial fascia |
| | *Short head:* | Short tendon from tip of coracoid process of scapula | |

*Action:*  Flexes and supinates the forearm. Tenses antebrachial fascia. Long head aids in flexion of the shoulder joint and holds head of humerus in place

| | | | |
|---|---|---|---|
| **2. Coracobrachialis muscle** (sometimes pierced by musculo-cutaneous nerve) | | Tip of the coracoid process (fused with short head of biceps) | Ventral and medial side of humerus near middle of shaft |

*Action:*  Flexes and adducts the arm

| | | | |
|---|---|---|---|
| **3. Brachialis muscle** (Operates 1 joint) | | Distal half of anterior aspect of humerus and the medial and lateral intermuscular septa | Tuberosity of ulna (short tendon) and rough impression on anterior surface of coronoid process |

*Action:*  Primary flexor of forearm

*Nerve:*  Musculocutaneous nerve for all three muscles

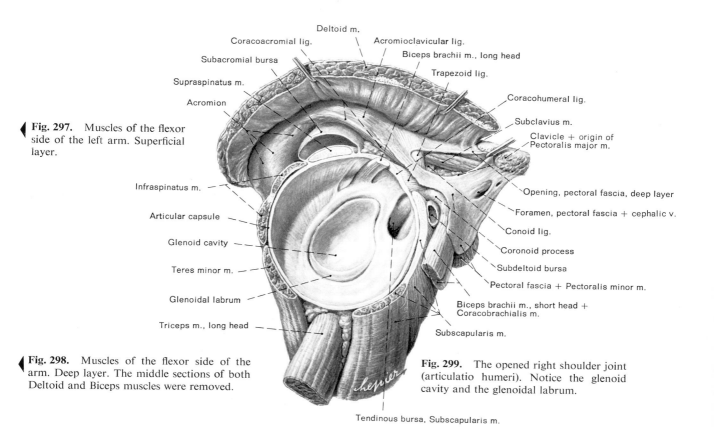

**Fig. 297.** Muscles of the flexor side of the left arm. Superficial layer.

**Fig. 298.** Muscles of the flexor side of the arm. Deep layer. The middle sections of both Deltoid and Biceps muscles were removed.

**Fig. 299.** The opened right shoulder joint (articulatio humeri). Notice the glenoid cavity and the glenoidal labrum.

Deltoid m.
Coracoacromial lig.
Acromioclavicular lig.
Biceps brachii m., long head
Subacromial bursa
Trapezoid lig.
Supraspinatus m.
Coracohumeral lig.
Acromion
Subclavius m.
Clavicle + origin of Pectoralis major m.
Infraspinatus m.
Opening, pectoral fascia, deep layer
Articular capsule
Foramen, pectoral fascia + cephalic v.
Glenoid cavity
Conoid lig.
Coronoid process
Teres minor m.
Subdeltoid bursa
Glenoidal labrum
Pectoral fascia + Pectoralis minor m.
Biceps brachii m., short head + Coracobrachialis m.
Triceps m., long head
Subscapularis m.
Tendinous bursa, Subscapularis m.

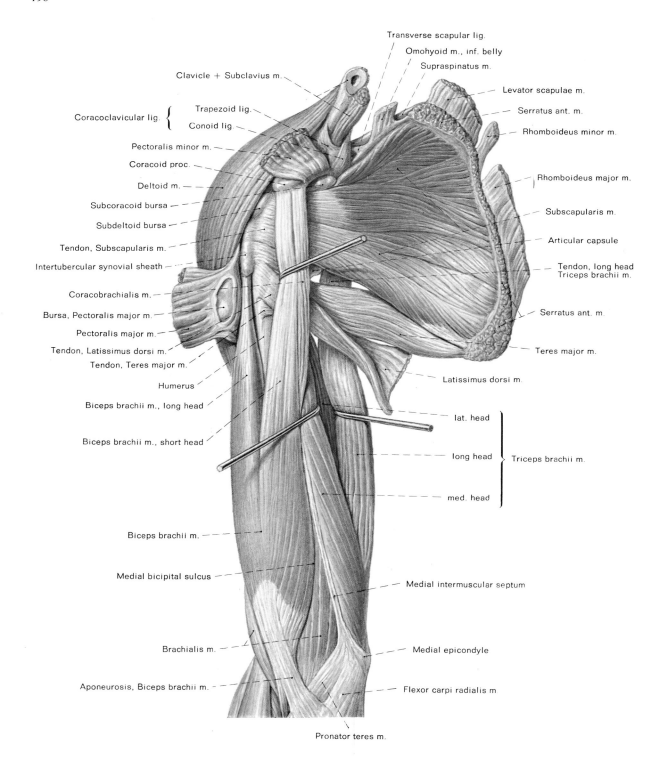

Transverse scapular lig.

Omohyoid m., inf. belly

Supraspinatus m.

Clavicle + Subclavius m.

Levator scapulae m.

Serratus ant. m.

Coracoclavicular lig. {

Trapezoid lig.

Conoid lig.

Rhomboideus minor m.

Pectoralis minor m.

Coracoid proc.

Deltoid m.

Rhomboideus major m.

Subcoracoid bursa

Subscapularis m.

Subdeltoid bursa

Articular capsule

Tendon, Subscapularis m.

Tendon, long head
Triceps brachii m.

Intertubercular synovial sheath

Coracobrachialis m.

Serratus ant. m.

Bursa, Pectoralis major m.

Pectoralis major m.

Teres major m.

Tendon, Latissimus dorsi m.

Tendon, Teres major m.

Latissimus dorsi m.

Humerus

Biceps brachii m., long head

lat. head

Biceps brachii m., short head

long head    Triceps brachii m.

med. head

Biceps brachii m.

Medial bicipital sulcus

Medial intermuscular septum

Brachialis m.

Medial epicondyle

Aponeurosis, Biceps brachii m.

Flexor carpi radialis m

Pronator teres m.

**Fig. 300.** The muscles of the costal surface of the scapula and muscles of the flexor side of the upper arm. Superficial layer.

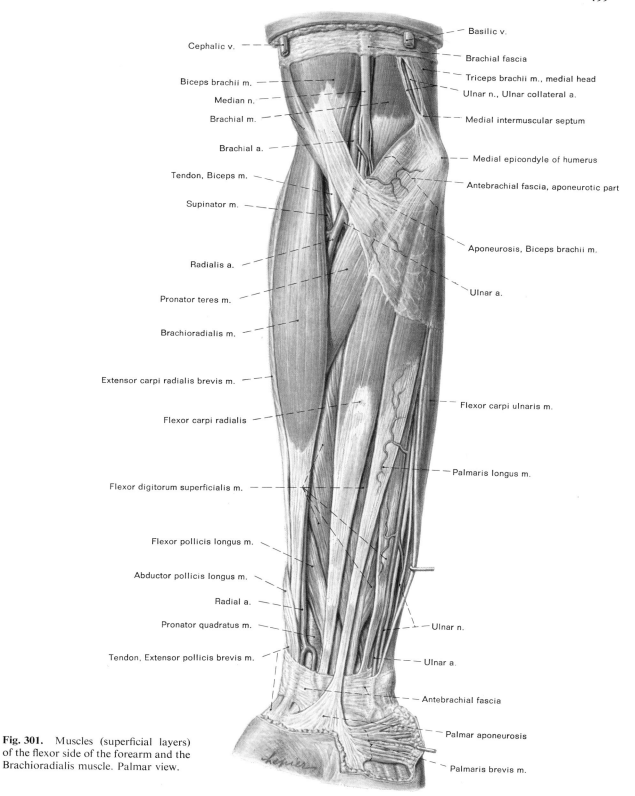

Cephalic v.

Biceps brachii m.

Median n.

Brachial m.

Brachial a.

Tendon, Biceps m.

Supinator m.

Radialis a.

Pronator teres m.

Brachioradialis m.

Extensor carpi radialis brevis m.

Flexor carpi radialis

Flexor digitorum superficialis m.

Flexor pollicis longus m.

Abductor pollicis longus m.

Radial a.

Pronator quadratus m.

Tendon, Extensor pollicis brevis m.

Basilic v.

Brachial fascia

Triceps brachii m., medial head

Ulnar n., Ulnar collateral a.

Medial intermuscular septum

Medial epicondyle of humerus

Antebrachial fascia, aponeurotic part

Aponeurosis, Biceps brachii m.

Ulnar a.

Flexor carpi ulnaris m.

Palmaris longus m.

Ulnar n.

Ulnar a.

Antebrachial fascia

Palmar aponeurosis

Palmaris brevis m.

**Fig. 301.** Muscles (superficial layers) of the flexor side of the forearm and the Brachioradialis muscle. Palmar view.

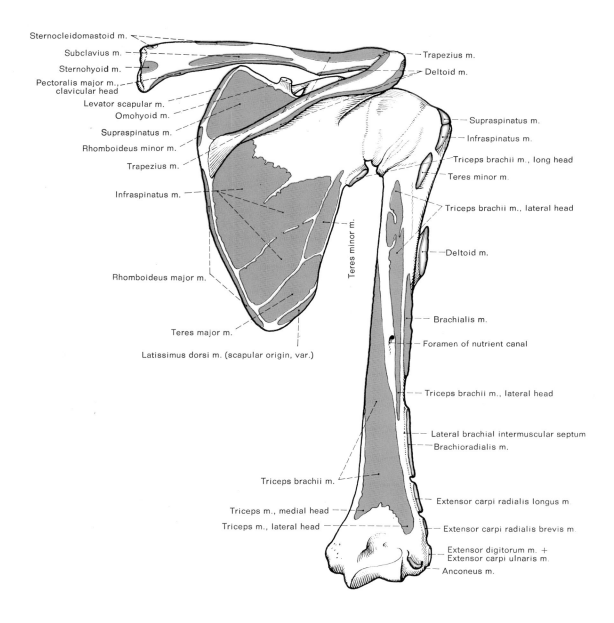

Sternocleidomastoid m.

Subclavius m.

Sternohyoid m.

Pectoralis major m., clavicular head

Levator scapular m.

Omohyoid m.

Supraspinatus m.

Rhomboideus minor m.

Trapezius m.

Infraspinatus m.

Rhomboideus major m.

Teres major m.

Latissimus dorsi m. (scapular origin, var.)

Triceps brachii m.

Triceps m., medial head

Triceps m., lateral head

Trapezius m.

Deltoid m.

Supraspinatus m.

Infraspinatus m.

Triceps brachii m., long head

Teres minor m.

Triceps brachii m., lateral head

Deltoid m.

Brachialis m.

Foramen of nutrient canal

Triceps brachii m., lateral head

Lateral brachial intermuscular septum

Brachioradialis m.

Extensor carpi radialis longus m.

Extensor carpi radialis brevis m.

Extensor digitorum m. + Extensor carpi ulnaris m.

Anconeus m.

Teres minor m.

**Fig. 302.** Diagram of muscle origins and insertions of clavicle, scapula, and humerus. Dorsal view of right upper limb.

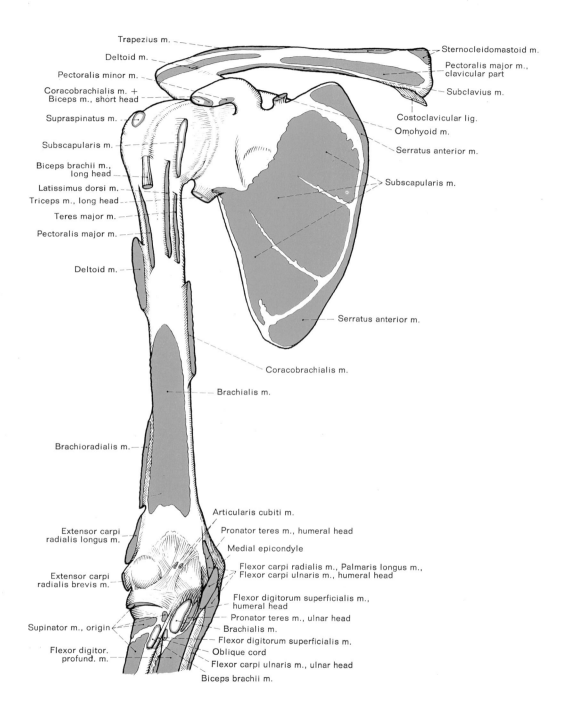

**Fig. 303.** Diagram of muscle origins and insertions on the clavicle, scapula, humerus, and cranial end of the ulna and radius. Ventral view of the right upper limb.

202

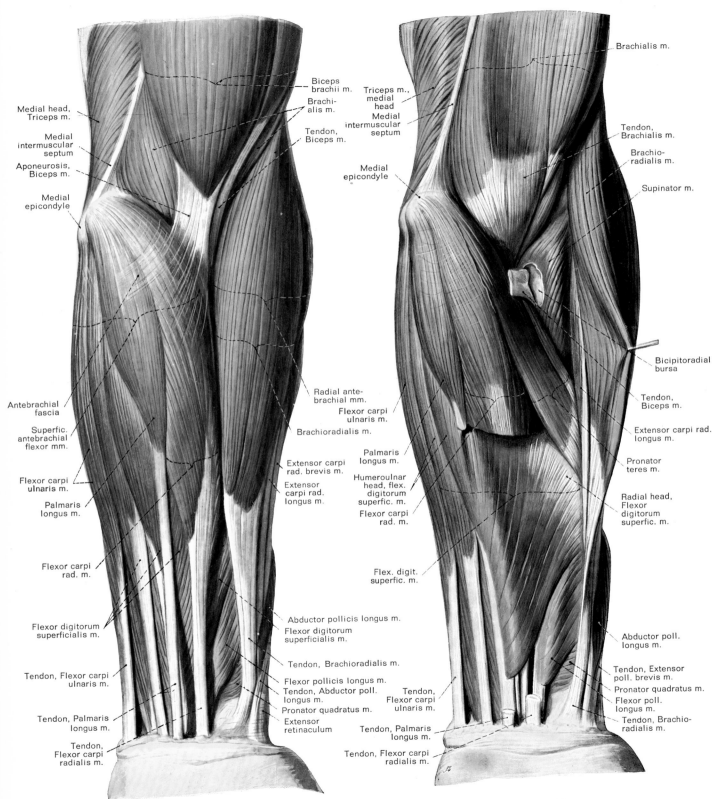

Medial head,
Triceps m.

Medial
intermuscular
septum

Aponeurosis,
Biceps m.

Medial
epicondyle

Antebrachial
fascia

Superfic.
antebrachial
flexor mm.

Flexor carpi
ulnaris m.

Palmaris
longus m.

Flexor carpi
rad. m.

Flexor digitorum
superficialis m.

Tendon, Flexor carpi
ulnaris m.

Tendon, Palmaris
longus m.

Tendon,
Flexor carpi
radialis m.

Biceps
brachii m.
Brachi-
alis m.

Tendon,
Biceps m.

Radial ante-
brachial mm.
Flexor carpi
ulnaris m.
Brachioradialis m.

Extensor carpi
rad. brevis m.
Extensor
carpi rad.
longus m.

Abductor pollicis longus m.
Flexor digitorum
superficialis m.
Tendon, Brachioradialis m.
Flexor pollicis longus m.
Tendon, Abductor poll.
longus m.
Pronator quadratus m.
Extensor
retinaculum

**Fig. 304**

Brachialis m.

Triceps m.,
medial
head
Medial
intermuscular
septum

Medial
epicondyle

Tendon,
Brachialis m.
Brachio-
radialis m.

Supinator m.

Bicipitoradial
bursa

Tendon,
Biceps m.

Extensor carpi rad.
longus m.

Pronator
teres m.

Radial head,
Flexor
digitorum
superfic. m.

Palmaris
longus m.
Humeroulnar
head, flex.
digitorum
superfic. m.
Flexor carpi
rad. m.

Flex. digit.
superfic. m.

Abductor poll.
longus m.

Tendon, Extensor
poll. brevis m.
Pronator quadratus m.
Flexor poll.
longus m.
Tendon, Brachio-
radialis m.

Tendon,
Flexor carpi
ulnaris m.
Tendon, Palmaris
longus m.
Tendon, Flexor carpi
radialis m.

**Fig. 305**

## Flexor Muscles of Forearm, Superficial Group (Figs. 301, 304, 305, 312, 315, 318)

| Name | Origin | Insertion |
| --- | --- | --- |
| **1. Pronator teres muscle** | | |
| *Humeral head* (strong) | Medial epicondyle of the humerus, antebrachial fascia | On the lateral and dorsal surface of radius (middle $1/3$) |
| *Ulnar head* (weak) | Coronoid process of ulna | |
| *Nerve:* Median nerve (passes through between the two heads) | | |
| *Action:* Pronates and flexes the forearm | | |
| **2. Flexor carpi radialis muscle** | Medial epicondyle of humerus and antebrachial fascia | Base of 2nd metacarpal bone, palmar surface |
| *Nerve:* Median nerve | | |
| *Action:* Flexes wrist and elbow; abducts wrist, pronates forearm | | |
| **3. Palmaris longus muscle** (inconstant) | Medial epicondyle of humerus; antebrachial fascia | Palmar aponeurosis |
| *Nerve:* Median nerve | | |
| *Action:* Tenses palmar aponeurosis; weak flexor of elbow and wrist | | |
| **4. Flexor digitorum superficialis muscle** | | |
| *Humeroulnar head:* | Medial epicondyle of humerus and coronoid process of ulna | 4 long tendons to the middle phalanges of fingers 2 to 5 |
| *Radial head:* | Upper half, anterior border of radius | |
| *Nerve:* Median nerve C 7, 8; T 1 | | |
| *Action:* Flexes middle phalanges of 4 medial fingers; assists in flexion of forearm; medial abduction of hand | | |
| **5. Flexor carpi ulnaris muscle** | | |
| *Humeral head:* | Medial epicondyle of the humerus | Pisiform bone and, by ligaments, to 5th metacarpal and hamate bones |
| *Ulnar head:* | Olecranon and, via the antebrachial fascia, posterior border of ulna | |
| *Nerve:* Ulnar nerve (C 7, 8; T 1) | | |
| *Action:* Flexes and adducts wrist joint; flexor of elbow | | |

**Fig. 304.** Flexor muscles of the left forearm, superficial layer. Palmar view.

**Fig. 305.** The same, after severing the Palmaris longus and Flexor carpi radialis muscles.

204

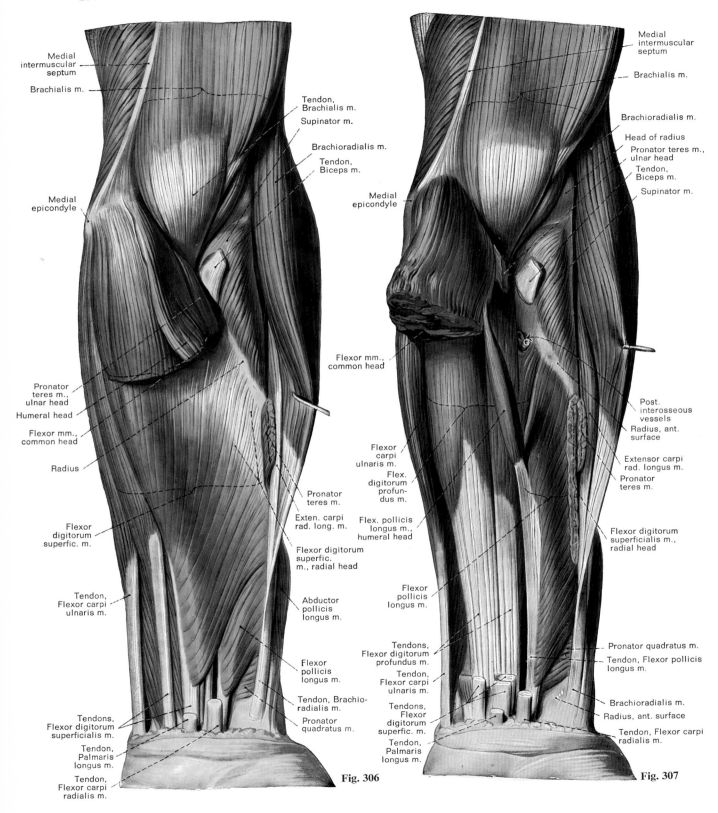

Medial intermuscular septum

Brachialis m.

Medial epicondyle

Pronator teres m., ulnar head

Humeral head

Flexor mm., common head

Radius

Flexor digitorum superfic. m.

Tendon, Flexor carpi ulnaris m.

Tendons, Flexor digitorum superficialis m.

Tendon, Palmaris longus m.

Tendon, Flexor carpi radialis m.

Tendon, Brachialis m.

Supinator m.

Brachioradialis m.

Tendon, Biceps m.

Pronator teres m.

Exten. carpi rad. long. m.

Flexor digitorum superfic. m., radial head

Abductor pollicis longus m.

Flexor pollicis longus m.

Tendon, Brachioradialis m.

Pronator quadratus m.

**Fig. 306**

Medial intermuscular septum

Brachialis m.

Brachioradialis m.

Head of radius

Pronator teres m., ulnar head

Tendon, Biceps m.

Supinator m.

Medial epicondyle

Flexor mm., common head

Flexor carpi ulnaris m.

Flex. digitorum profundus m.

Flex. pollicis longus m., humeral head

Flexor pollicis longus m.

Tendons, Flexor digitorum profundus m.

Tendon, Flexor carpi ulnaris m.

Tendons, Flexor digitorum superfic. m.

Tendon, Palmaris longus m.

Post. interosseous vessels

Radius, ant. surface

Extensor carpi rad. longus m.

Pronator teres m.

Flexor digitorum superficialis m., radial head

Pronator quadratus m.

Tendon, Flexor pollicis longus m.

Brachioradialis m.

Radius, ant. surface

Tendon, Flexor carpi radialis m.

**Fig. 307**

## Flexor Muscles of the Forearm, Deep Group (Figs. 306, 307, 312)

| Name | Origin | Insertion |
| --- | --- | --- |
| **1. Flexor digitorum profundus muscle** | Anterior and medial surfaces of ulna; interosseous membrane | Distal phalanges of fingers 2 to 5 |

*Nerve:* Ulnar nerve for ulnar side, median nerve for radial side (C 7, 8; T 1)

*Action:* Flexes joints of fingers 2 to 5 (especially the terminal phalanges but also the other phalanges) and wrist joint

| Name | Origin | Insertion |
| --- | --- | --- |
| **2. Flexor pollicis longus muscle** *Radial head* (the main part) | Anterior surface of radius; adjacent part of interosseous membrane | Terminal phalanx of thumb |
| *Humeral head* | Coronoid process of ulna or medial epicondyle of humerus | |

*Nerve:* Anterior interosseous branch of median nerve (C 8; T 1)

*Action:* Flexes terminal phalanx of thumb; aids in flexion of proximal phalanx and adduction of metacarpal

| Name | Origin | Insertion |
| --- | --- | --- |
| **3. Pronator quadratus muscle** | Anterior surface of ulna, distal ¼ | Anterior surface of distal fourth of radius |

*Nerve:* Anterior interosseous branch of median nerve (C 8; T 1)

*Action:* Pronates the hand

**Fig. 306.** Flexor muscles of the left forearm, middle layer. Pronator teres, Flexor carpi radialis, and the Palmaris longus muscles were divided to display the Flexor digitorum superficialis muscle; the Brachioradialis muscle was pulled back laterally.

**Fig. 307.** Deep layers of the flexor muscles of the left forearm. All superficial flexor muscles were cut and partially resected with the exception of the Flexor carpi ulnaris muscle.

206

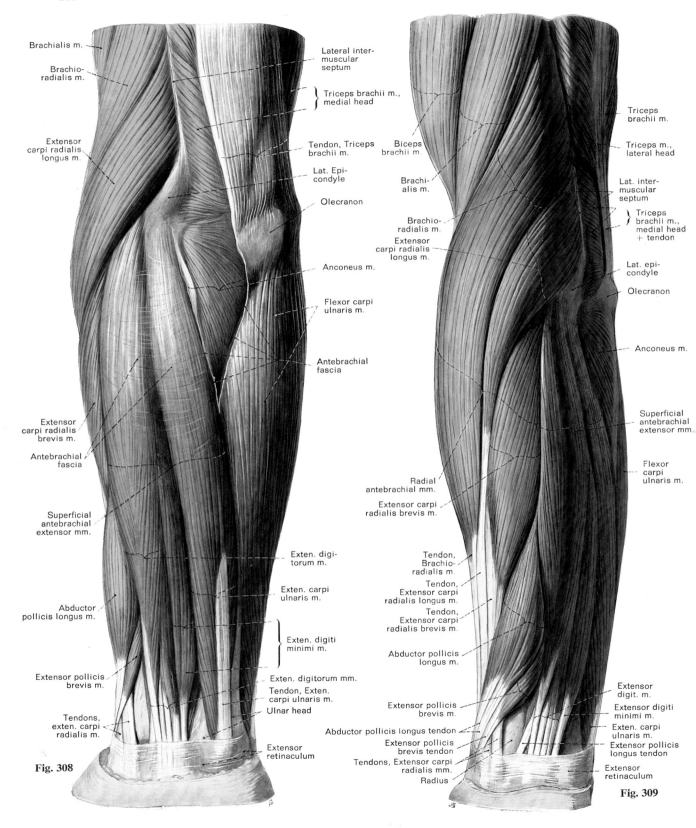

Brachialis m.

Brachio-
radialis m.

Extensor
carpi radialis
longus m.

Extensor
carpi radialis
brevis m.

Antebrachial
fascia

Superficial
antebrachial
extensor mm.

Abductor
pollicis longus m.

Extensor pollicis
brevis m.

Tendons,
exten. carpi
radialis m.

Fig. 308

Lateral inter-
muscular
septum

Triceps brachii m.,
medial head

Tendon, Triceps
brachii m.

Lat. Epi-
condyle

Olecranon

Anconeus m.

Flexor carpi
ulnaris m.

Antebrachial
fascia

Exten. digi-
torum m.

Exten. carpi
ulnaris m.

Exten. digiti
minimi m.

Exten. digitorum mm.

Tendon, Exten.
carpi ulnaris m.

Ulnar head

Extensor
retinaculum

Triceps
brachii m.

Triceps m.,
lateral head

Biceps
brachii m.

Brachi-
alis m.

Lat. inter-
muscular
septum

Brachio-
radialis m.

Triceps
brachii m.,
medial head
+ tendon

Extensor
carpi radialis
longus m.

Lat. epi-
condyle

Olecranon

Anconeus m.

Superficial
antebrachial
extensor mm.

Flexor
carpi
ulnaris m.

Radial
antebrachial mm.

Extensor carpi
radialis brevis m.

Tendon,
Brachio-
radialis m.

Tendon,
Extensor carpi
radialis longus m.

Tendon,
Extensor carpi
radialis brevis m.

Abductor pollicis
longus m.

Extensor pollicis
brevis m.

Abductor pollicis longus tendon

Extensor pollicis
brevis tendon

Tendons, Extensor carpi
radialis mm.

Radius

Extensor
digit. m.

Extensor digiti
minimi m.

Exten. carpi
ulnaris m.

Extensor pollicis
longus tendon

Extensor
retinaculum

Fig. 309

## Extensor Muscles of the Forearm  (Figs. 302-304, 308, 309, 312, 313)

| Name | Origin | Insertion |
|---|---|---|
| **1. Brachioradialis muscle** | Lateral supracondylar ridge of humerus; lateral intermuscular septum | Proximal end of styloid process of radius |

*Nerve:*  Radial nerve (C 5, 6)

*Action:*  Flexes forearm; pronates forearm if supinated; supinates, if forearm is pronated

| Name | Origin | Insertion |
|---|---|---|
| **2. Extensor carpi radialis longus m.** | Distal $\frac{1}{3}$ of lateral supracondylar ridge of humerus and lateral intermuscular septum | Base of 2nd metacarpal bone |
| **3. Extensor carpi radialis brevis m.** | Lateral epicondyle of humerus | Base of 3rd metacarpal bone |

*Nerve:*  Radial nerve (C 6, 7)

*Action:*  Extends and abducts the hand

## Superficial Layers of Extensor Muscles  (Figs. 308, 309, 316)

| Name | Origin | Insertion |
|---|---|---|
| **1. Extensor digitorum muscle** | Lateral epicondyle of humerus; antebrachial fascia | By 4 tendons to middle and distal phalanges of the fingers |
| **2. Extensor digiti minimi muscle** | | Joins extensor tendon to little finger |

*Nerve:*  Deep radial nerve (C 6, 7, 8)

*Action:*  Extends the little finger (proximal phalanges, in particular); indirectly the entire hand, also medial abduction

| Name | Origin | Insertion |
|---|---|---|
| **3. Extensor carpi ulnaris muscle** Separated from above by an intermuscular septum | Lateral epicondyle of humerus; antebrachial fascia | Base of 5th metacarpal, dorsal surface |

*Nerve:*  Deep radial nerve (C 6, 7, 8)

*Action:*  Extends (slightly) and adducts hand

**Fig. 308.**  Superficial group of extensor muscles of the left forearm and the distal part of the arm. Dorsal view.

**Fig. 309.**  Superficial muscles of the left forearm and the distal part of the arm. As seen from the lateral (radial) side.

208

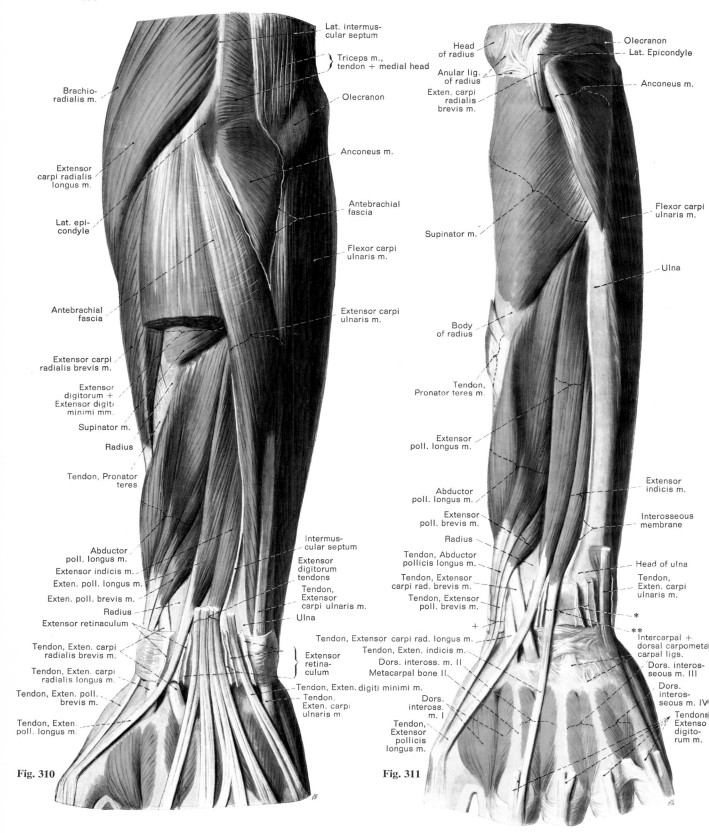

Fig. 310

Fig. 311

**Extensor Muscles of the Forearm** (continued) **and Supinator Muscle (Figs. 310, 311, 313, 316)**

| Name | Origin | Insertion |
|---|---|---|
| **1. Abductor pollicis longus muscle** | Posterior surface of ulna and radius; interosseous membrane | Base of 1st metacarpal of thumb, radial side |
| **2. Extensor pollicis brevis muscle** | Posterior surface of radius; interosseous membrane | Base of proximal phalanx of thumb |

*Nerve:* Deep radial nerve

*Action:* Abducts thumb; extends 1st phalanx of thumb, and abducts hand

| Name | Origin | Insertion |
|---|---|---|
| **1. Extensor pollicis longus muscle** | Posterior surface of ulna; interosseous membrane | Distal phalanx of thumb |
| **2. Extensor indicis muscle** | | Dorsal extensor expansion to 1st phalanx of index finger |

*Nerve:* Deep radial nerve (C 6, 7, 8)

*Action:* Extends thumb and index finger, somewhat adducts index finger

| Name | Origin | Insertion |
|---|---|---|
| **Supinator muscle** (Figs. 306, 311–313) Two layers (superficial and deep) between which the deep branch of radial nerve lies | Lateral epicondyle of humerus; radial collateral ligament; anular ligament of radius; supinator crest of ulna | Lateral surface and posterior border of radius, proximal and distal to tuberosity of radius |

*Nerve:* Deep radial nerve (C 6)

*Action:* Supinates hand and forearm

**Fig. 310.** Extensor muscles of the left forearm. Dorsal view. The Extensor digitorum and Digiti minimi were severed; the tendon compartments of the Extensor retinaculum were partly opened: 1. the Extensor digiti minimi; 2. Extensor digitorum and Extensor indicis; 3. the Extensor pollicis longus.

**Fig. 311.** Deep layer of extensor muscles of the left forearm. Dorsolateral view. The superficial layer of the extensors and the muscles of the radial group were removed with the exception of the tendon stumps. The tendon compartments of the Extensor retinaculum were completely opened: * the Extensor digiti minimi; ** Extensor digitorum and Extensor indicis muscles; + Abductor pollicis longus and Extensor pollicis brevis muscles.

210

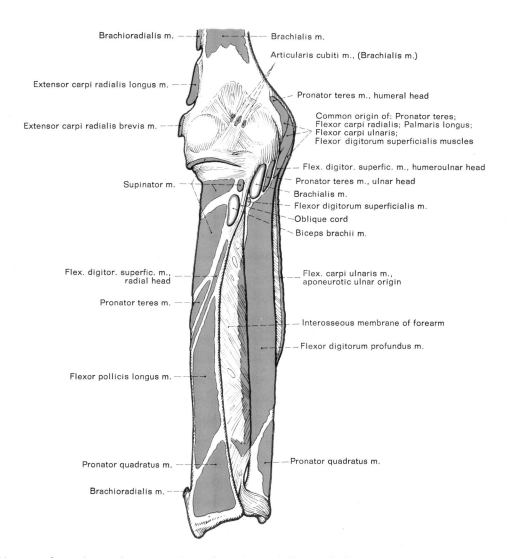

Brachioradialis m.

Brachialis m.

Articularis cubiti m., (Brachialis m.)

Extensor carpi radialis longus m.

Pronator teres m., humeral head

Common origin of: Pronator teres;
Flexor carpi radialis; Palmaris longus;
Flexor carpi ulnaris;
Flexor digitorum superficialis muscles

Extensor carpi radialis brevis m.

Flex. digitor. superfic. m., humeroulnar head

Pronator teres m., ulnar head

Brachialis m.

Supinator m.

Flexor digitorum superficialis m.

Oblique cord

Biceps brachii m.

Flex. digitor. superfic. m.,
radial head

Flex. carpi ulnaris m.,
aponeurotic ulnar origin

Pronator teres m.

Interosseous membrane of forearm

Flexor digitorum profundus m.

Flexor pollicis longus m.

Pronator quadratus m.

Pronator quadratus m.

Brachioradialis m.

**Fig. 312.** Diagram of muscle attachments to the radius, ulna, and distal end of the humerus. Anterior or palmar view of right arm (2/3).

211

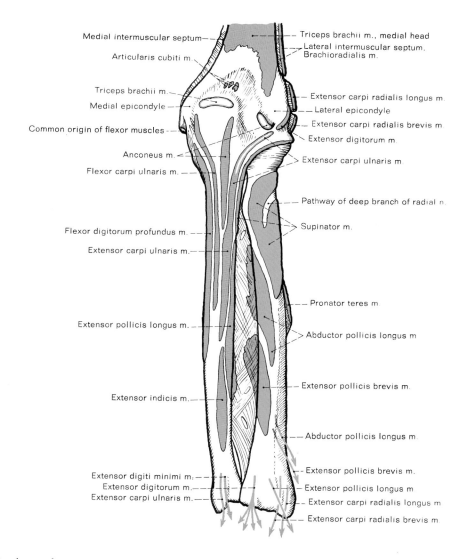

Medial intermuscular septum

Articularis cubiti m.

Triceps brachii m.

Medial epicondyle

Common origin of flexor muscles

Anconeus m.

Flexor carpi ulnaris m.

Flexor digitorum profundus m.

Extensor carpi ulnaris m.

Extensor pollicis longus m.

Extensor indicis m.

Extensor digiti minimi m.
Extensor digitorum m.
Extensor carpi ulnaris m.

Triceps brachii m., medial head

Lateral intermuscular septum.
Brachioradialis m.

Extensor carpi radialis longus m.
Lateral epicondyle
Extensor carpi radialis brevis m.
Extensor digitorum m.
Extensor carpi ulnaris m.

Pathway of deep branch of radial n.

Supinator m.

Pronator teres m.

Abductor pollicis longus m.

Extensor pollicis brevis m.

Abductor pollicis longus m.

Extensor pollicis brevis m.
Extensor pollicis longus m.
Extensor carpi radialis longus m.
Extensor carpi radialis brevis m.

**Fig. 313.** Muscle attachments mapped out on the radius, ulna, and distal end of the humerus. Posterior or dorsal view of the right arm. Arrows at distal end of the ulna and radius indicate the tendon compartments.

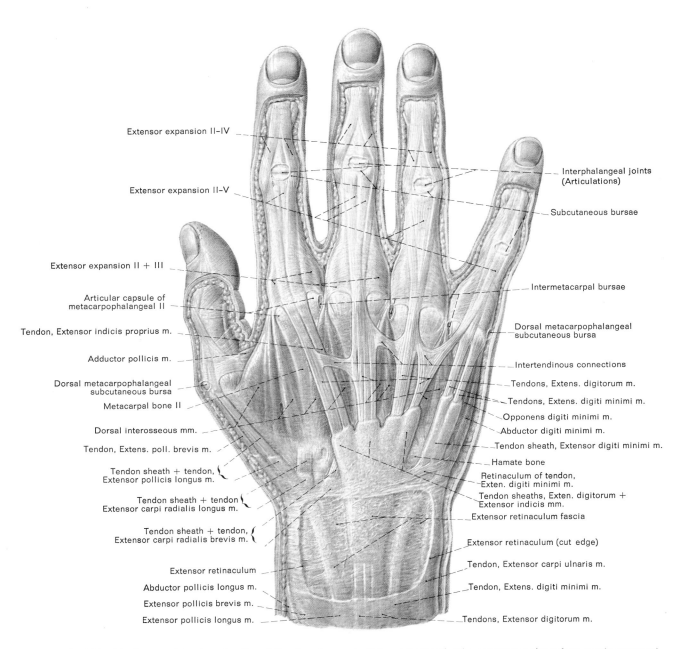

Extensor expansion II–IV

Extensor expansion II–V

Extensor expansion II + III

Articular capsule of
metacarpophalangeal II

Tendon, Extensor indicis proprius m.

Adductor pollicis m.

Dorsal metacarpophalangeal
subcutaneous bursa

Metacarpal bone II

Dorsal interosseous mm.

Tendon, Extens. poll. brevis m.

Tendon sheath + tendon,
Extensor pollicis longus m.

Tendon sheath + tendon
Extensor carpi radialis longus m.

Tendon sheath + tendon,
Extensor carpi radialis brevis m.

Extensor retinaculum

Abductor pollicis longus m.

Extensor pollicis brevis m.

Extensor pollicis longus m.

Interphalangeal joints
(Articulations)

Subcutaneous bursae

Intermetacarpal bursae

Dorsal metacarpophalangeal
subcutaneous bursa

Intertendinous connections

Tendons, Extens. digitorum m.

Tendons, Extens. digiti minimi m.

Opponens digiti minimi m.

Abductor digiti minimi m.

Tendon sheath, Extensor digiti minimi m.

Hamate bone

Retinaculum of tendon,
Exten. digiti minimi m.

Tendon sheaths, Exten. digitorum +
Extensor indicis mm.

Extensor retinaculum fascia

Extensor retinaculum (cut edge)

Tendon, Extensor carpi ulnaris m.

Tendon, Extens. digiti minimi m.

Tendons, Extensor digitorum m.

**Fig. 314.** Tendons and tendon sheaths of the dorsal aspect of the right hand. The extensor retinaculum partly removed.

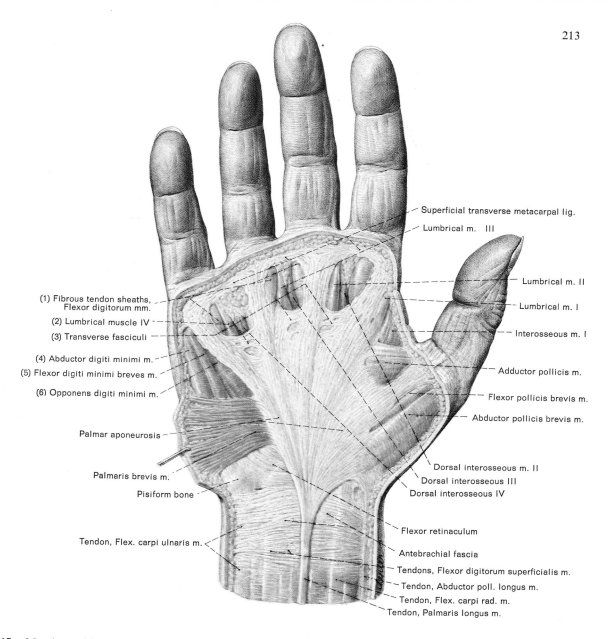

Superficial transverse metacarpal lig.

Lumbrical m. III

Lumbrical m. II

Lumbrical m. I

Interosseous m. I

Adductor pollicis m.

Flexor pollicis brevis m.

Abductor pollicis brevis m.

Dorsal interosseous m. II

Dorsal interosseous III

Dorsal interosseous IV

Flexor retinaculum

Antebrachial fascia

Tendons, Flexor digitorum superficialis m.

Tendon, Abductor poll. longus m.

Tendon, Flex. carpi rad. m.

Tendon, Palmaris longus m.

(1) Fibrous tendon sheaths, Flexor digitorum mm.

(2) Lumbrical muscle IV

(3) Transverse fasciculi

(4) Abductor digiti minimi m.

(5) Flexor digiti minimi breves m.

(6) Opponens digiti minimi m.

Palmar aponeurosis

Palmaris brevis m.

Pisiform bone

Tendon, Flex. carpi ulnaris m.

**Fig. 315.** Muscles and fascia of the right palm. The interossei muscles, the palmar aponeurosis and Palmaris brevis muscle after removal of the skin and subcutaneous fatty tissues of the palm of the hand.

| Name | Origin | Insertion |
|---|---|---|
| **Palmaris brevis muscle**<br>Cutaneous muscle, numerous separated fasciculi | Palmar aponeurosis, medial margin | Skin over medial border of palm |

*Nerve:* Ulnar nerve, superficial branch (C 8)

*Action:* Tenses skin of medial side of palm

214

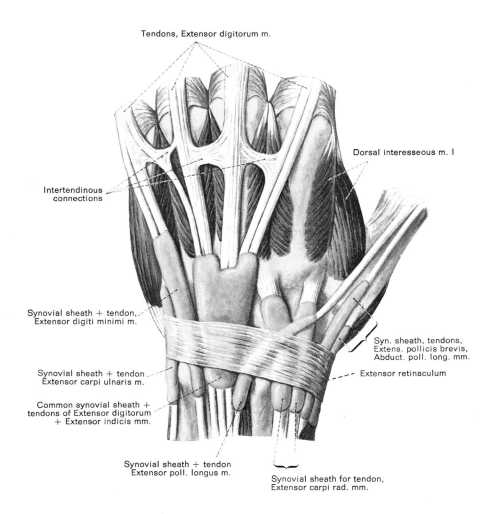

Tendons, Extensor digitorum m.

Dorsal interesseous m. I

Intertendinous connections

Synovial sheath + tendon, Extensor digiti minimi m.

Syn. sheath, tendons, Extens. pollicis brevis, Abduct. poll. long. mm.

Synovial sheath + tendon Extensor carpi ulnaris m.

Extensor retinaculum

Common synovial sheath + tendons of Extensor digitorum + Extensor indicis mm.

Synovial sheath + tendon Extensor poll. longus m.

Synovial sheath for tendon, Extensor carpi rad. mm.

**Fig. 316.** Semidiagram of the tendons and tendon sheaths of the extensor tendons of the dorsal aspect of the hand and wrist. The tendon sheaths (vaginae synoviales) for the tendons of the Extensor pollicis brevis and Abductor pollicis longus muscles as well as those of the Extensor carpi longus and brevis muscles are mostly or partly held in common. Six tendon compartments hold tendons in position on the dorsum of the hand: (1) the most lateral or radial, the tendons of the Abductor pollicis longus and the Extensor pollicis brevis muscles; (2) the tendons of the Extensor carpi radialis longus and brevis muscles; (3) the tendon of the Extensor pollicis longus; (4) the tendons of the Extensor digitorum and Extensor indicis muscles; (5) the tendon of the Extensor digiti minimi; and (6) the most medial or ulnar, the tendon of the Extensor carpi ulnaris muscle.

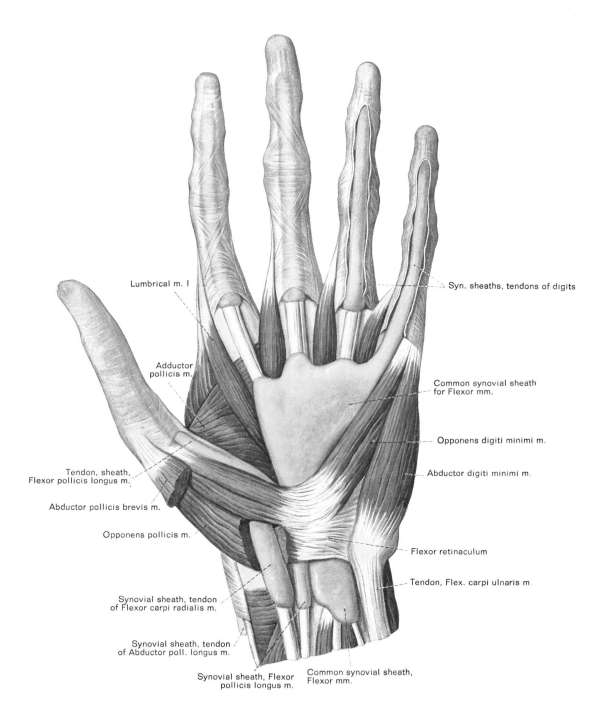

Lumbrical m. I

Adductor
pollicis m.

Tendon, sheath,
Flexor pollicis longus m.

Abductor pollicis brevis m.

Opponens pollicis m.

Synovial sheath, tendon
of Flexor carpi radialis m.

Synovial sheath, tendon
of Abductor poll. longus m.

Synovial sheath, Flexor
pollicis longus m.

Syn. sheaths, tendons of digits

Common synovial sheath
for Flexor mm.

Opponens digiti minimi m.

Abductor digiti minimi m.

Flexor retinaculum

Tendon, Flex. carpi ulnaris m.

Common synovial sheath,
Flexor mm.

**Fig. 317.** Semidiagram of the synovial sheaths of the tendons of the palmar aspect of the left hand and wrist. The synovial tendon sheath of the Flexor carpi radialis muscle has been exposed by removing a short segment of the muscles of the thenar eminence. The ligamentous fibrous sheath of the 4th and 5th fingers were split. The tendon sheaths were displayed by injecting them with a blue latex. In the living, they are filled with a clear, colorless fluid.

216

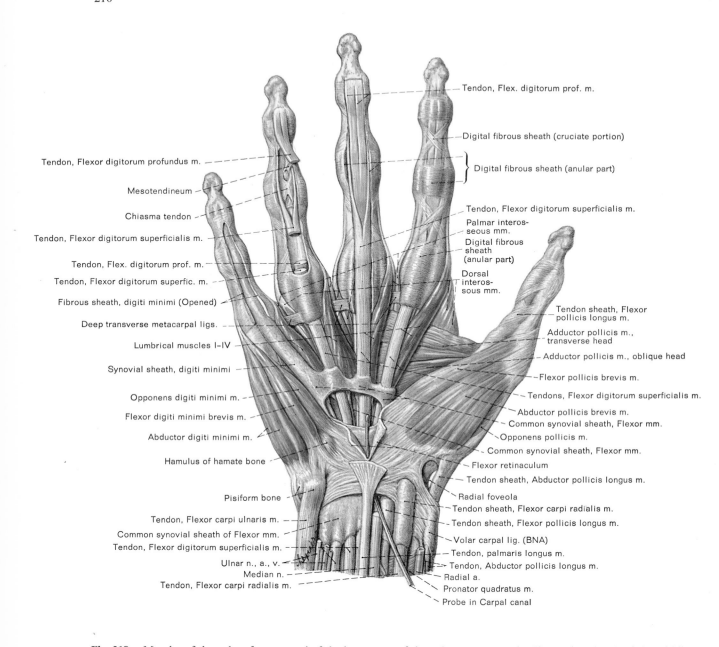

Tendon, Flex. digitorum prof. m.

Digital fibrous sheath (cruciate portion)

Digital fibrous sheath (anular part)

Tendon, Flexor digitorum profundus m.

Mesotendineum

Chiasma tendon

Tendon, Flexor digitorum superficialis m.

Tendon, Flex. digitorum prof. m.

Tendon, Flexor digitorum superfic. m.

Fibrous sheath, digiti minimi (Opened)

Deep transverse metacarpal ligs.

Lumbrical muscles I–IV

Synovial sheath, digiti minimi

Opponens digiti minimi m.

Flexor digiti minimi brevis m.

Abductor digiti minimi m.

Hamulus of hamate bone

Pisiform bone

Tendon, Flexor carpi ulnaris m.

Common synovial sheath of Flexor mm.

Tendon, Flexor digitorum superficialis m.

Ulnar n., a., v.

Median n.

Tendon, Flexor carpi radialis m.

Tendon, Flexor digitorum superficialis m.

Palmar interos-
seous mm.

Digital fibrous
sheath
(anular part)

Dorsal
interos-
sous mm.

Tendon sheath, Flexor
pollicis longus m.

Adductor pollicis m.,
transverse head

Adductor pollicis m., oblique head

Flexor pollicis brevis m.

Tendons, Flexor digitorum superficialis m.

Abductor pollicis brevis m.

Common synovial sheath, Flexor mm.

Opponens pollicis m.

Common synovial sheath, Flexor mm.

Flexor retinaculum

Tendon sheath, Abductor pollicis longus m.

Radial foveola

Tendon sheath, Flexor carpi radialis m.

Tendon sheath, Flexor pollicis longus m.

Volar carpal lig. (BNA)

Tendon, palmaris longus m.

Tendon, Abductor pollicis longus m.

Radial a.

Pronator quadratus m.

Probe in Carpal canal

**Fig. 318.** Muscles of the palm after removal of the larger part of the palmar aponeurosis. The tendon sheath of the middle finger was split along its entire length. The flexor retinaculum was partially opened.

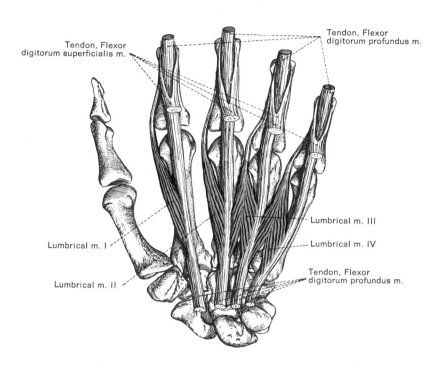

**Fig. 319.** Diagram of the lumbrical muscles. Palmar view of the left hand.

## Lumbrical Muscles of the Hand (Figs. 319, 320)

| | |
|---|---|
| *Origin:* | Tendons of Flexor digitorum profundus muscle |
| *Insertion:* | Dorsal aponeurosis of the proximal phalanx of fingers II to V |
| *Nerve:* | Two lateral lumbricals: Median nerve<br>Two medial lumbricals: Ulnar nerve |
| *Action:* | Flexes the metacarpophalangeal joints; extends the two distal phalanges |

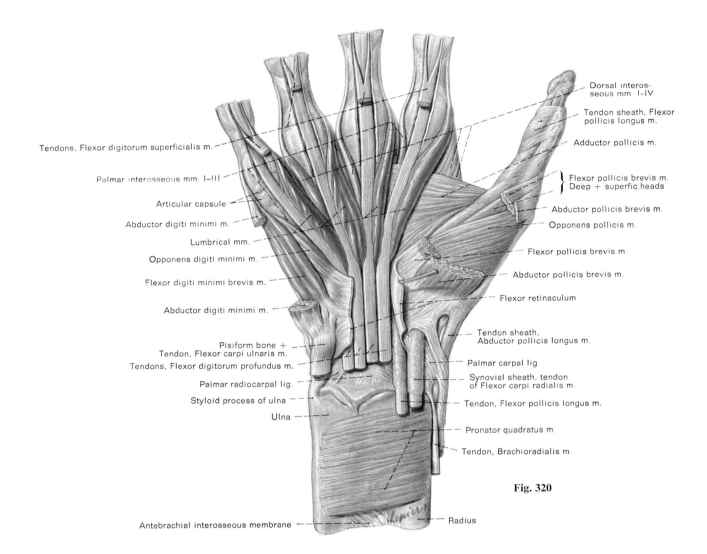

Dorsal interos-
seous mm I–IV

Tendon sheath, Flexor
pollicis longus m.

Adductor pollicis m.

Flexor pollicis brevis m.
Deep + superfic.heads

Abductor pollicis brevis m.

Opponens pollicis m.

Flexor pollicis brevis m.

Abductor pollicis brevis m.

Flexor retinaculum

Tendon sheath,
Abductor pollicis longus m.

Palmar carpal lig

Synovial sheath, tendon
of Flexor carpi radialis m.

Tendon, Flexor pollicis longus m.

Pronator quadratus m.

Tendon, Brachioradialis m.

Fig. 320

Radius

Tendons, Flexor digitorum superficialis m.

Palmar interosseous mm. I–III

Articular capsule

Abductor digiti minimi m.

Lumbrical mm.

Opponens digiti minimi m.

Flexor digiti minimi brevis m.

Abductor digiti minimi m.

Pisiform bone +
Tendon, Flexor carpi ulnaris m.

Tendons, Flexor digitorum profundus m.

Palmar radiocarpal lig.

Styloid process of ulna

Ulna

Antebrachial interosseous membrane

### Muscles of the Hypothenar Eminence (Figs. 318, 320, 321, 325, 326)

| Name | Origin | Insertion |
| --- | --- | --- |
| **1. Abductor digiti minimi muscle** | Pisiform bone and tendon of Flexor carpi ulnaris | Proximal phalanx of little finger, ulnar side |
| **2. Flexor digiti minimi brevis m.** (variable) | Flexor retinaculum, hamulus of hamate bone | Ulnar side of proximal phalanx of little finger |
| **3. Opponens digiti minimi muscle** | Flexor retinaculum; hook of hamate bone | Ulnar margin of 5th metacarpal |

*Nerve:*    Ulnar nerve, deep branch (C 8; T 1)

*Action:*    As their names indicate: Abducts and reflexes little finger; Opponens digiti minimi muscle also rotates 5th metacarpal and brings it out of plane of palm to meet the thumb and cup the hand

**Fig. 320.**    Deeper layers of the musculature of the palm and the Pronator quadratus muscle. The Flexor retinaculum was severed. The flexor tendons of fingers 2–5 were severed to display the Lumbrical muscles. The muscles of the thenar and hypothenar eminences were partly removed.

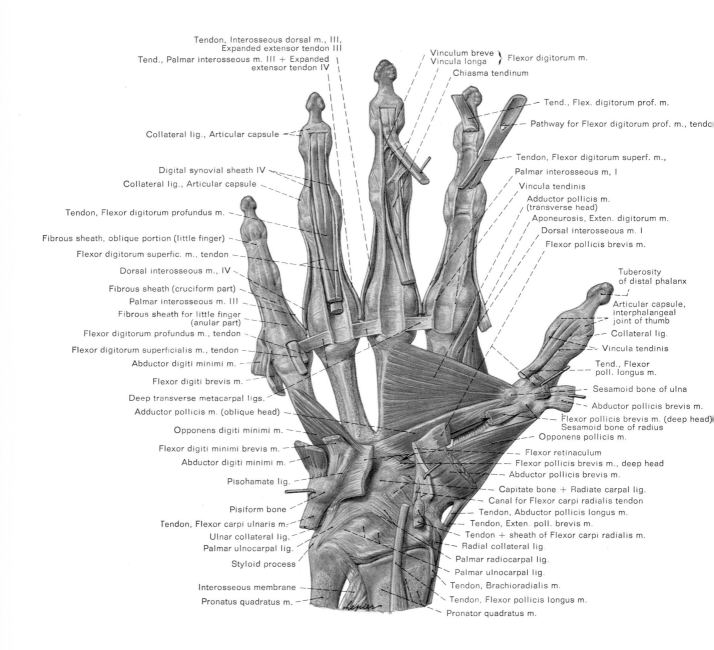

Tendon, Interosseous dorsal m., III,
Expanded extensor tendon III

Tend., Palmar interosseous m. III + Expanded
extensor tendon IV

Vinculum breve ⎱
Vincula longa ⎰ Flexor digitorum m.

Chiasma tendinum

Tend., Flex. digitorum prof. m.

Pathway for Flexor digitorum prof. m., tendo

Collateral lig., Articular capsule

Tendon, Flexor digitorum superf. m.,

Palmar interosseous m, I

Digital synovial sheath IV

Vincula tendinis

Collateral lig., Articular capsule

Adductor pollicis m.
(transverse head)

Aponeurosis, Exten. digitorum m.

Tendon, Flexor digitorum profundus m.

Dorsal interosseous m. I

Flexor pollicis brevis m.

Fibrous sheath, oblique portion (little finger)

Flexor digitorum superfic. m., tendon

Tuberosity
of distal phalanx

Dorsal interosseous m., IV

Articular capsule,
interphalangeal
joint of thumb

Fibrous sheath (cruciform part)

Palmar interosseous m. III

Collateral lig.

Fibrous sheath for little finger
(anular part)

Vincula tendinis

Flexor digitorum profundus m., tendon

Tend., Flexor
poll. longus m.

Flexor digitorum superficialis m., tendon

Abductor digiti minimi m.

Sesamoid bone of ulna

Flexor digiti brevis m.

Abductor pollicis brevis m.

Deep transverse metacarpal ligs.

Flexor pollicis brevis m. (deep head)

Adductor pollicis m. (oblique head)

Sesamoid bone of radius

Opponens pollicis m.

Opponens digiti minimi m.

Flexor digiti minimi brevis m.

Flexor retinaculum

Abductor digiti minimi m.

Flexor pollicis brevis m., deep head

Abductor pollicis brevis m.

Pisohamate lig.

Capitate bone + Radiate carpal lig.

Canal for Flexor carpi radialis tendon

Pisiform bone

Tendon, Abductor pollicis longus m.

Tendon, Exten. poll. brevis m.

Tendon, Flexor carpi ulnaris m.

Tendon + sheath of Flexor carpi radialis m.

Ulnar collateral lig.

Radial collateral lig.

Palmar ulnocarpal lig.

Palmar radiocarpal lig.

Palmar ulnocarpal lig.

Styloid process

Tendon, Brachioradialis m.

Interosseous membrane

Tendon, Flexor pollicis longus m.

Pronatus quadratus m.

Pronator quadratus m.

**Fig. 321.** Deepest layer of the musculature of the palm. The carpal canal was opened by cutting the flexor retinaculum. The origin and insertion of the Pronator quadratus muscle was severed at the distal end of the radius and ulna. The tendon of the Flexor pollicis longus was kept in place. The flexor tendons of the fingers (after opening the tendon sheaths) were dissected to their insertion.

## Muscles of the Thenar Eminence (Figs. 318, 320, 321, 325, 326)

The superficial layer of the thenar eminence is formed by the Abductor pollicis brevis, Opponens pollicis muscles, and the superficial or lateral portion of the Flexor pollicis brevis muscle. The deep layers of the thenar eminence muscles are composed of the deep or medial portion of the Flexor pollicis brevis and the Adductor pollicis muscles.

| Name | Origin | Insertion |
|---|---|---|
| **1. Abductor pollicis brevis muscle** | Flexor retinaculum; tuberosity of scaphoid; ridge of trapezium | Radial side, proximal phalanx of thumb |
| *Nerve:* Median nerve | | |
| *Action:* Abducts thumb | | |
| **2. Opponens pollicis muscle** | Flexor retinaculum; ridge of trapezium | Entire length of radial border of 1st metacarpal of thumb |
| *Nerve:* Medial nerve (C 6, 7, [8, T 1]) | | |
| *Action:* Opposes thumb to other fingers, abducts, flexes, rotates first metacarpal | | |
| **3. Flexor pollicis brevis muscle** | | |
|     *Superficial portion* | Flexor retinaculum | Radial side of proximal phalanx of thumb; lateral sesamoid bone |
|     *Deeper portion* | Ridge of trapezium | |
| *Nerve:* Lateral portion: Median nerve (C 6, 7). Deep or medial portion: Ulnar nerve, deep branch (C 8, T 1) | | |
| *Action:* Flexes proximal phalanx of thumb | | |
| **4. Adductor pollicis muscle** | | |
|     a) *Oblique head* | a) Capitate bone; bases of 2nd and 3rd metacarpals | Medial (ulnar) side of proximal phalanx of thumb, sesamoid bone |
|     b) *Transverse head* | b) Anterior surface of 3rd metacarpal | |
| *Nerve:* Ulnar nerve, deep palmar branch (C 8; T 1) | | |
| *Action:* Adducts the thumb; aids in opposition | | |

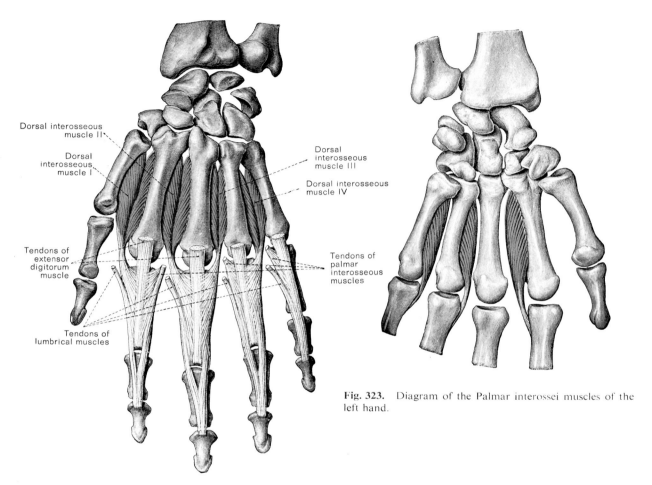

Dorsal interosseous
muscle II

Dorsal
interosseous
muscle I

Dorsal
interosseous
muscle III

Dorsal interosseous
muscle IV

Tendons of
extensor
digitorum
muscle

Tendons of
palmar
interosseous
muscles

Tendons of
lumbrical muscles

**Fig. 322.** Diagram of the Dorsal interossei muscles and expanded extensor tendons of the fingers of the left hand.

**Fig. 323.** Diagram of the Palmar interossei muscles of the left hand.

**Dorsal and Palmar Interossei Muscles (Figs. 316, 322-326)**

| | |
|---|---|
| *Nerve:* | Ulnar nerve |
| *Action:* | Dorsal interossei muscles abduct; the Palmar interoseii adduct the fingers |

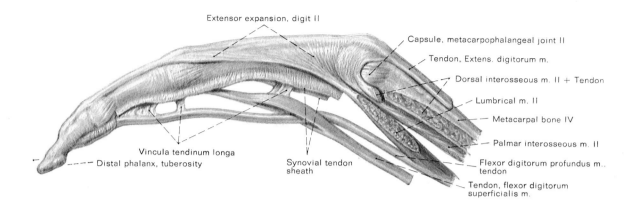

**Fig. 324.** Index finger of the right hand with the dorsal aponeurosis as well as the tendons of its flexor and extensor muscles.

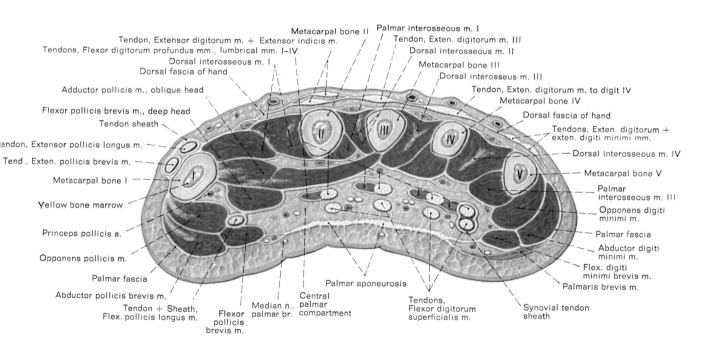

**Fig. 325.** Cross section of the right hand in the region of the metacarpal bones (I–V).

224

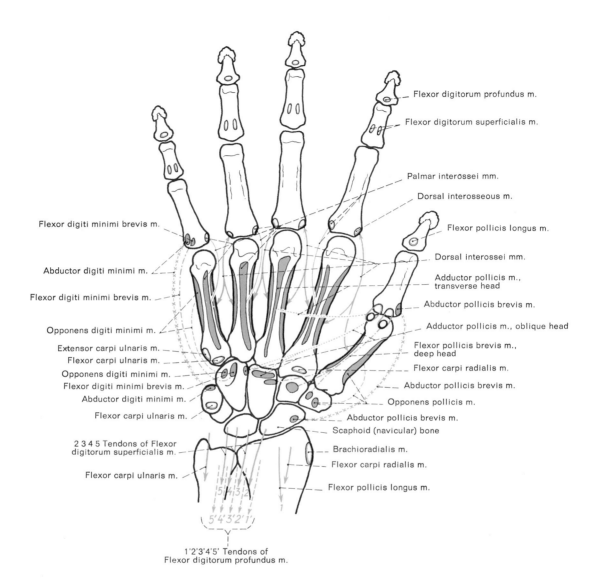

Flexor digitorum profundus m.

Flexor digitorum superficialis m.

Palmar interossei mm.

Dorsal interosseous m.

Flexor pollicis longus m.

Dorsal interossei mm.

Adductor pollicis m., transverse head

Abductor pollicis brevis m.

Adductor pollicis m., oblique head

Flexor pollicis brevis m., deep head

Flexor carpi radialis m.

Abductor pollicis brevis m.

Opponens pollicis m.

Abductor pollicis brevis m.

Scaphoid (navicular) bone

Brachioradialis m.

Flexor carpi radialis m.

Flexor pollicis longus m.

Flexor digiti minimi brevis m.

Abductor digiti minimi m.

Flexor digiti minimi brevis m.

Opponens digiti minimi m.

Extensor carpi ulnaris m.

Flexor carpi ulnaris m.

Opponens digiti minimi m.

Flexor digiti minimi brevis m.

Abductor digiti minimi m.

Flexor carpi ulnaris m.

2 3 4 5 Tendons of Flexor digitorum superficialis m.

Flexor carpi ulnaris m.

5 4 3 2

5' 4' 3' 2' 1'

1'2'3'4'5' Tendons of Flexor digitorum profundus m.

**Fig. 326.** Muscle origins and insertions mapped out on the palmar aspect of the right hand and wrist. The tendon sheath of the radiocarpal articulation (1–7, two are not numbered) shown by the proximal placed arrows.

The tendons of the Flexor digitorum superficialis m. (2–5): solid red arrows. The tendons of the Flexor digitorum profundus m. (1'–5'): broken red arrows.

# Myology

---

*Muscles of the Lower Limb*

226

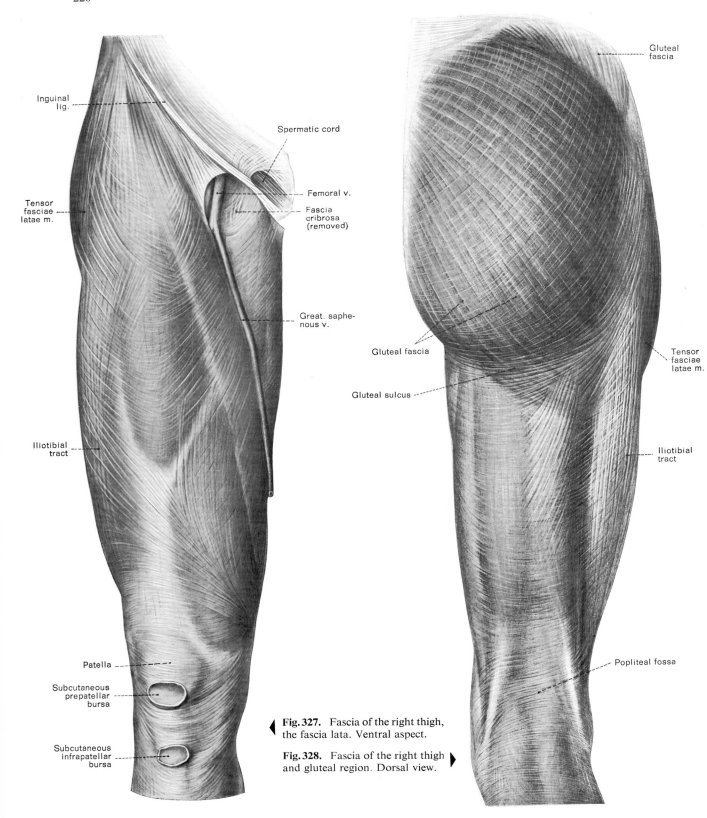

Inguinal lig.

Tensor fasciae latae m.

Iliotibial tract

Patella

Subcutaneous prepatellar bursa

Subcutaneous infrapatellar bursa

Spermatic cord

Femoral v.

Fascia cribrosa (removed)

Great. saphenous v.

Gluteal fascia

Gluteal fascia

Gluteal sulcus

Tensor fasciae latae m.

Iliotibial tract

Popliteal fossa

◄ **Fig. 327.** Fascia of the right thigh, the fascia lata. Ventral aspect.

**Fig. 328.** Fascia of the right thigh and gluteal region. Dorsal view. ►

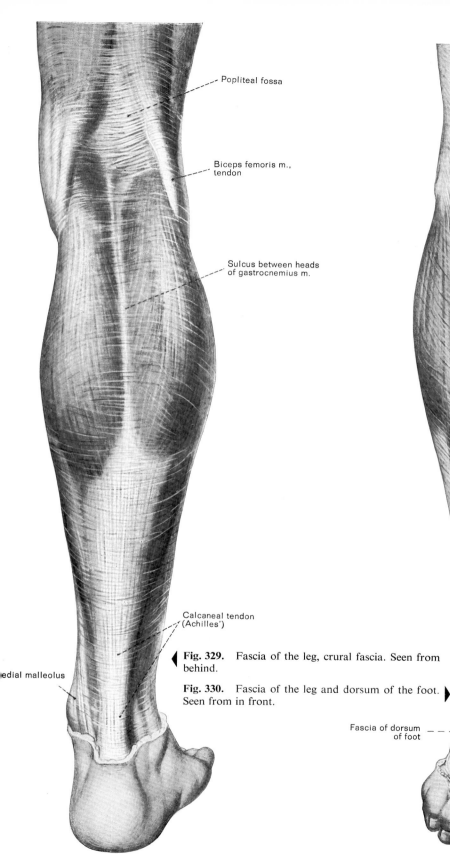

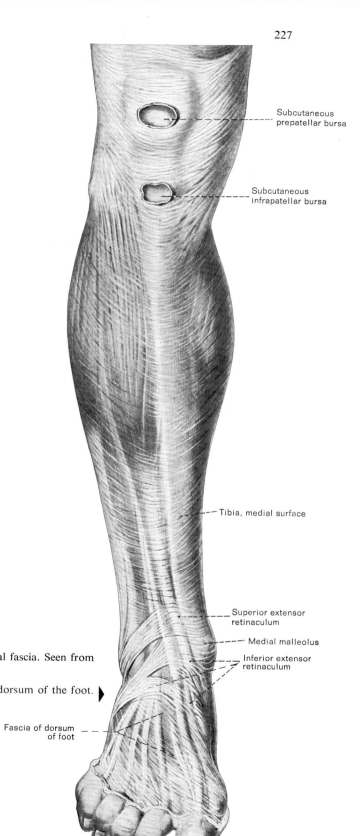

227

Popliteal fossa

Biceps femoris m.,
tendon

Sulcus between heads
of gastrocnemius m.

Subcutaneous
prepatellar bursa

Subcutaneous
infrapatellar bursa

Tibia, medial surface

Superior extensor
retinaculum

Medial malleolus

Inferior extensor
retinaculum

Calcaneal tendon
(Achilles')

Fascia of dorsum
of foot

Medial malleolus

**Fig. 329.** Fascia of the leg, crural fascia. Seen from behind.

**Fig. 330.** Fascia of the leg and dorsum of the foot. Seen from in front.

228

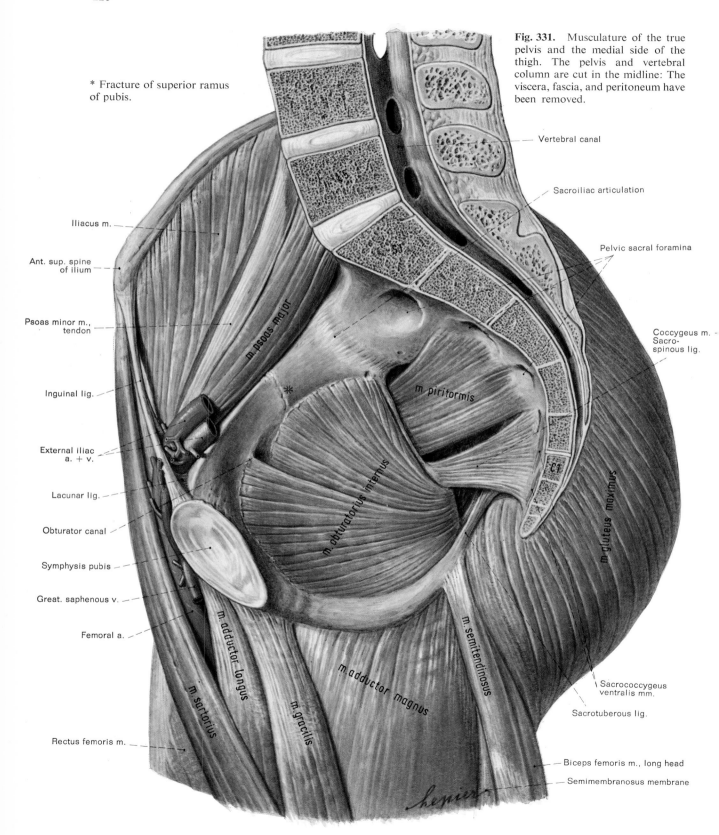

* Fracture of superior ramus of pubis.

**Fig. 331.** Musculature of the true pelvis and the medial side of the thigh. The pelvis and vertebral column are cut in the midline: The viscera, fascia, and peritoneum have been removed.

Vertebral canal

Sacroiliac articulation

Pelvic sacral foramina

Iliacus m.

Ant. sup. spine of ilium

Psoas minor m., tendon

Inguinal lig.

External iliac a. + v.

Lacunar lig.

Obturator canal

Symphysis pubis

Great. saphenous v.

Femoral a.

Rectus femoris m.

Coccygeus m.
Sacro-spinous lig.

m. psoas major

m. piriformis

m. obturatorius internus

m. gluteus maximus

C1

m. adductor longus

m. sartorius

m. gracilis

m. adductor magnus

m. semitendinosus

Sacrococcygeus ventralis mm.

Sacrotuberous lig.

Biceps femoris m., long head

Semimembranosus membrane

L5

S1

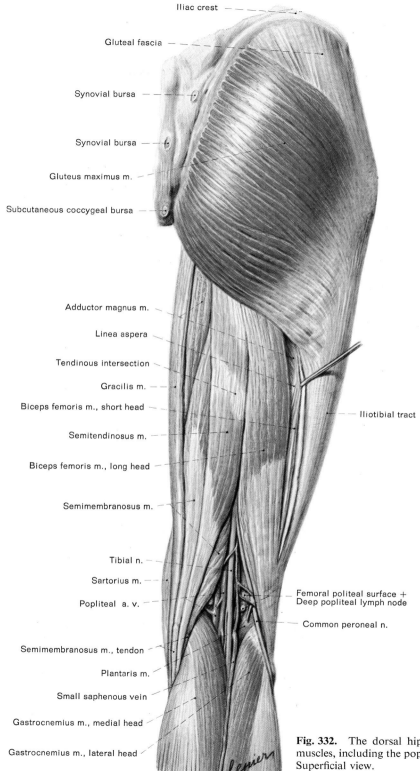

Iliac crest

Gluteal fascia

Synovial bursa

Synovial bursa

Gluteus maximus m.

Subcutaneous coccygeal bursa

Adductor magnus m.

Linea aspera

Tendinous intersection

Gracilis m.

Biceps femoris m., short head

Semitendinosus m.

Biceps femoris m., long head

Semimembranosus m.

Tibial n.

Sartorius m.

Popliteal a. v.

Semimembranosus m., tendon

Plantaris m.

Small saphenous vein

Gastrocnemius m., medial head

Gastrocnemius m., lateral head

Iliotibial tract

Femoral popliteal surface +
Deep popliteal lymph node

Common peroneal n.

**Fig. 332.** The dorsal hip and thigh muscles, including the popliteal fossa. Superficial view.

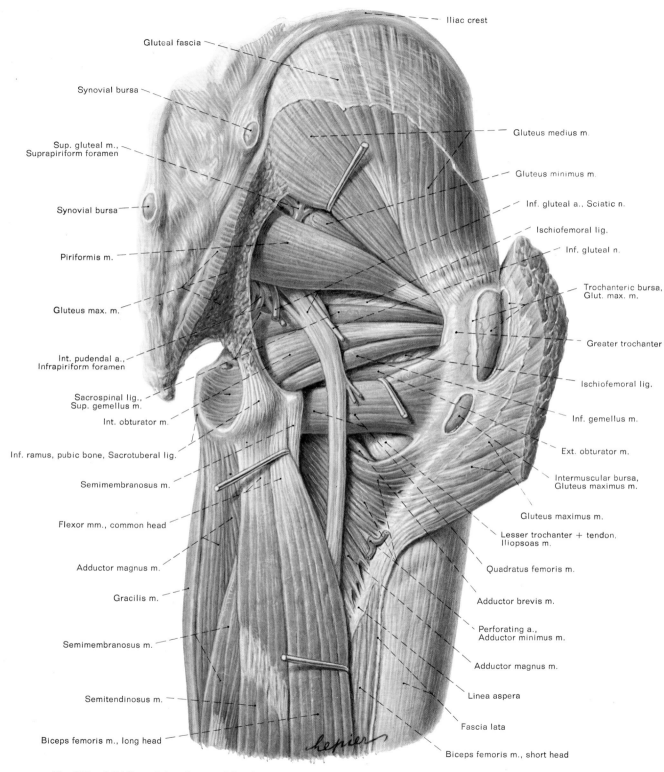

Iliac crest

Gluteal fascia

Synovial bursa

Gluteus medius m.

Sup. gluteal m.,
Suprapiriform foramen

Gluteus minimus m.

Synovial bursa

Inf. gluteal a., Sciatic n.

Ischiofemoral lig.

Piriformis m.

Inf. gluteal n.

Trochanteric bursa,
Glut. max. m.

Gluteus max. m.

Greater trochanter

Int. pudendal a.,
Infrapiriform foramen

Ischiofemoral lig.

Sacrospinal lig.,
Sup. gemellus m.

Inf. gemellus m.

Int. obturator m.

Ext. obturator m.

Inf. ramus, pubic bone, Sacrotuberal lig.

Intermuscular bursa,
Gluteus maximus m.

Semimembranosus m.

Gluteus maximus m.

Flexor mm., common head

Lesser trochanter + tendon,
Iliopsoas m.

Adductor magnus m.

Quadratus femoris m.

Gracilis m.

Adductor brevis m.

Semimembranosus m.

Perforating a.,
Adductor minimus m.

Adductor magnus m.

Semitendinosus m.

Linea aspera

Fascia lata

Biceps femoris m., long head

Biceps femoris m., short head

**Fig. 333.** Middle and deep layers of the gluteal region and a superficial layer of the flexors on the thigh. The Gluteus maximus muscle is severed and reflected.

## Dorsal Hip Muscles of Gluteal Region (Figs. 331, 338-340)

| Name | Origin | Insertion |
|---|---|---|
| **1. Gluteus maximus muscle** (powerful, with coarse fasciculi) | Posterior gluteal line of the ilium; posterior aspect of sacrum, side of coccyx, sacrotuberous ligament | Gluteal tuberosity of femur and iliotibial tract of fascia lata |

*Nerve:* Inferior gluteal nerve (L 5; S 1, 2)

*Action:* Extensor and powerful lateral rotator of thigh; inferior fibers assist in adduction of thigh; balances trunk on femur; fibers to iliotibial tract braces knee joint

| | | |
|---|---|---|
| **2. Gluteus medius muscle** | External aspect of ilium; between anterior and posterior gluteal lines; gluteal aponeurosis | Oblique ridge on lateral surface of greater trochanter of femur |

*Nerve:* Superior gluteal nerve (L 4, 5; S 1)

*Action:* Abducts femur, posterior fibers extend and rotate laterally, anterior fibers flex and rotate medially

| | | |
|---|---|---|
| **3. Gluteus minimus muscle** | Outer aspect of ilium between anterior and inferior gluteal lines | Tip (tendinous) of greater trochanter of femur and capsule of hip joint |

*Nerve:* Superior gluteal nerve (L 4, 5; S 1)

*Action:* Rotates thigh medially, abducts femur and, to some extent, flexes it

| | | |
|---|---|---|
| **4. Piriformis muscle** | Pelvic surface of sacrum, lateral to sacral foramina 2, 3, and 4 | A long tendon to upper border of greater trochanter of the femur |

*Nerve:* Sciatic nerve or direct branches from the sacral plexus (S 1, 2)

*Action:* Rotates femur laterally; assists in abduction

| | | |
|---|---|---|
| **5. Internal obturator muscle** | Margin of obturator foramen; obturator membrane | Medial surface of greater trochanter of femur, proximal to trochanteric fossa |
| **6. Superior gemellus muscle** | Ischial spine | With tendon of Internal obturator muscle to greater trochanter |
| **7. Inferior gemellus muscle** | Ischial tuberosity | |

*Nerve:* Direct branches from the sacral plexus

*Action:* Rotates femur laterally, Internal obturator m. extends and abducts when femur is flexed

| | | |
|---|---|---|
| **8. Quadratus femoris muscle** | Lateral border of ischial tuberosity | Quadrate line of femur extending down to intertrochanteric crest |

*Nerve:* Sciatic nerve, branch from sacral plexus (L 4, 5; S 1)

*Action:* Rotates femur laterally and helps in adduction

| | | |
|---|---|---|
| **9. Tensor fasciae latae muscle** | Iliac crest; anterior superior iliac spine | Iliotibial tract of fascia lata |

*Nerve:* Superior gluteal nerve (L 4, 5; S 1)

*Action:* Tenses fascia lata; assists in flexion, abduction, and medial rotation of femur

232

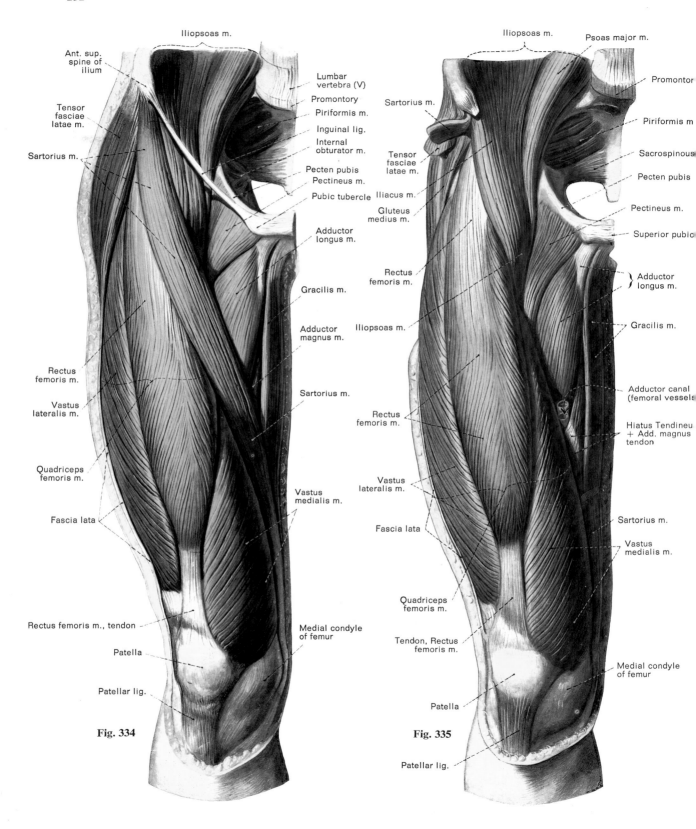

Iliopsoas m.

Ant. sup. spine of ilium

Tensor fasciae latae m.

Sartorius m.

Lumbar vertebra (V)

Promontory

Piriformis m.

Inguinal lig.

Internal obturator m.

Pecten pubis

Pectineus m.

Pubic tubercle

Adductor longus m.

Gracilis m.

Adductor magnus m.

Rectus femoris m.

Vastus lateralis m.

Sartorius m.

Quadriceps femoris m.

Fascia lata

Vastus medialis m.

Rectus femoris m., tendon

Medial condyle of femur

Patella

Patellar lig.

Fig. 334

Iliopsoas m.

Psoas major m.

Promontor

Sartorius m.

Piriformis m.

Sacrospinous

Tensor fasciae latae m.

Pecten pubis

Iliacus m.

Pectineus m.

Gluteus medius m.

Superior pubic

Rectus femoris m.

Adductor longus m.

Iliopsoas m.

Gracilis m.

Rectus femoris m.

Adductor canal (femoral vessels

Hiatus Tendineu + Add. magnus tendon

Vastus lateralis m.

Fascia lata

Sartorius m.

Vastus medialis m.

Quadriceps femoris m.

Tendon, Rectus femoris m.

Medial condyle of femur

Patella

Patellar lig.

Fig. 335

33

## Anterior Femoral Muscles (Figs. 334-336)

| Name | Origin | Insertion |
|---|---|---|
| **Sartorius muscle** | Anterior superior iliac spine | Medial margin of tibial tuberosity |

*Nerve:*　Femoral nerve (L 2, 3)

*Action:*　Flexes, laterally rotates, abducts thigh; flexes leg; rotates leg medially in knee joint when leg is flexed

**Quadriceps femoris muscle (Extensor muscles)**

| Name | Origin | Insertion |
|---|---|---|
| **Rectus femoris muscle**<br>(operates 2 joints)<br>Straight (anterior) head | Tendon from anterior inferior spine of ilium | The common tendon of the Quadriceps femoris muscle (which is the most powerful muscle in the entire human body) attaches to the cranial, medial, and lateral margins of the patella and, through intermediation of the patellar ligament, is inserted on the tibial tuberosity |
| Reflected (posterior) head | Cranial margin of acetabulum | |
| **Vastas medialis muscle** | Medial lip of linea aspera; intertrochanteric line (distal end thicker than proximal) | |
| **Vastas lateralis muscle** | Lateral lip of linea aspera as far proximally as greater trochanter | |
| **Vastas intermedius muscle** | Anterior and lateral surfaces of the shaft of the femur; lateral intermuscular septum | |
| **Articularis genus muscle** | From anterior surface of femur | Synovial membrane of knee joint |

*Nerve:*　Femoral nerve (L 2, 3, 4)

*Action:*　Extends leg. Rectus femoris aids in flexion of hip joint; Articularis genus muscle draws articular capsule proximally

### The Lacuna of the Inguinal Region:

The inguinal ligament stretches from the anterior superior spine of the ilium to the symphysis pubis. The two lacuna are between the inguinal ligament and the pelvic bones and are separated by the iliopectineal arch as follows:
1. *Lacuna of muscles:* lateral for the passage of the Iliopsoas muscle and femoral nerve.
2. *Lacuna of vessels:* medial, for the passage of the femoral vessels and lymph vessels of the femoral triangle.
Boundaries: Ventrally, inguinal ligament; dorsally, periosteum of the bone; medially, the lacunar ligament.
Topographical arrangement: Lymph vessels are entirely medial; then the femoral vein and, laterally, the femoral artery.

**Femoral hernia:** The inner aperture, through which a hernia passes, is a weak space between the femoral vein and the lacunar ligament. It is filled with lymph vessels and connective tissue. The outer aperture through which a hernia passes is the hiatus saphenous (fossa ovalis) of the fascia lata for the entrance of the great saphenous vein and the superficial lymph vessels.

**Fig. 334.**　The muscles of the ventral side of the right thigh. Superficial layer. The inguinal ligament is retained to show its attachments.

**Fig. 335.**　Muscles of the ventral side of the right thigh. The Sartorius muscle and the inguinal ligament have been removed.

234

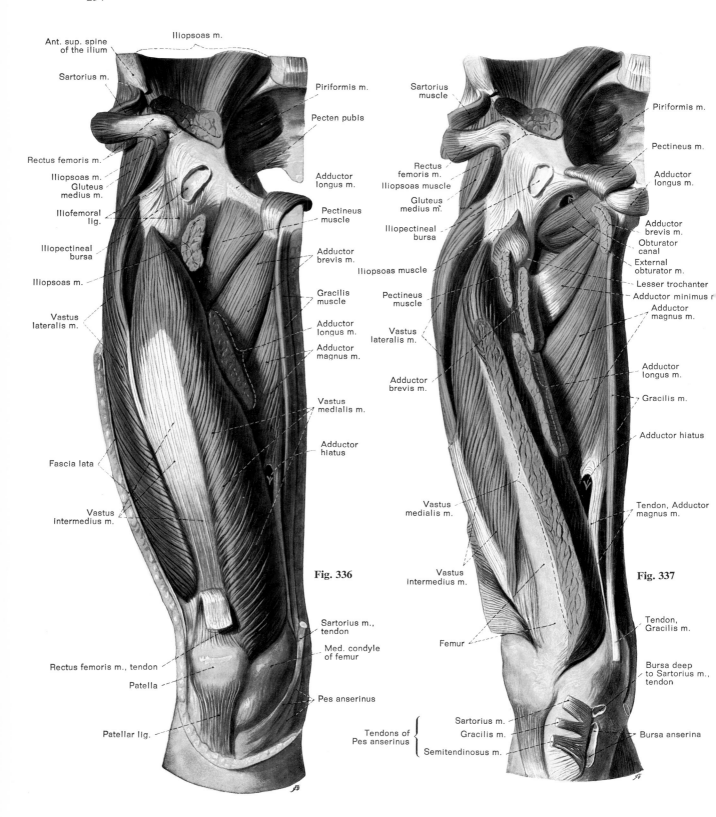

Ant. sup. spine of the ilium

Iliopsoas m.

Sartorius m.

Piriformis m.

Pecten pubis

Rectus femoris m.

Iliopsoas m.
Gluteus medius m.

Iliofemoral lig.

Iliopectineal bursa

Adductor longus m.

Pectineus muscle

Iliopsoas m.

Adductor brevis m.

Vastus lateralis m.

Gracilis muscle

Adductor longus m.

Adductor magnus m.

Fascia lata

Vastus intermedius m.

Vastus medialis m.

Adductor hiatus

**Fig. 336**

Sartorius m., tendon

Med. condyle of femur

Rectus femoris m., tendon

Patella

Pes anserinus

Patellar lig.

Sartorius muscle

Piriformis m.

Pectineus m.

Rectus femoris m.

Iliopsoas muscle

Gluteus medius m.

Iliopectineal bursa

Adductor longus m.

Adductor brevis m.

Obturator canal

External obturator m.

Lesser trochanter

Adductor minimus r

Pectineus muscle

Iliopsoas muscle

Vastus lateralis m.

Adductor brevis m.

Adductor magnus m.

Adductor longus m.

Gracilis m.

Adductor hiatus

Vastus medialis m.

Tendon, Adductor magnus m.

Vastus intermedius m.

**Fig. 337**

Femur

Tendon, Gracilis m.

Bursa deep to Sartorius m., tendon

Tendons of Pes anserinus

Sartorius m.

Gracilis m.

Semitendinosus m.

Bursa anserina

## Medial Femoral Muscles (Adductor) (Figs. 338, 339, 344, 345, 352)

| Name | Origin | Insertion |
|---|---|---|
| **1. Pectineus muscle** | Pecten of pubis | Pectineal line of femur |
| *Nerve:* Femoral nerve (L 2, 3) and the accessory obturator nerve | | |
| *Action:* Adducts the thigh; also aids in flexion and lateral rotation in the hip joint | | |
| **2. Adductor longus muscle** | Tendon from the border of superior and inferior pubic rami near symphysis | Middle third of medial lip of linea aspera |
| *Nerve:* Obturator nerve | | |
| *Action:* Adducts, aids flexion, and rotates thigh laterally | | |
| **3. Gracilis muscle** (forms middle tendon of pes anserinus) | Flat tendon from inferior ramus of pubis near symphysis | Long tendon on medial borders of the shaft of the tibia near the tibial tuberosity (pes anserinus) |
| *Nerve:* Obturator nerve (L 3, 4) | | |
| *Action:* Adducts thigh, aids in flexion of the knee; rotates the leg medially | | |
| **4. Adductor brevis muscle** | Inferior pubic ramus | Proximal third of medial lip of linea aspera; and pectineal line |
| *Nerve:* Obturator nerve (L 3, 4) | | |
| *Action:* Adducts thigh, aids in flexion and in lateral rotation of the thigh | | |
| **5. Adductor magnus muscle*** (This and also the Adductor brevis m., lie in deeper layers than 1 to 3 above) | Lower part of inferior pubic ramus; ramus of ischium; ischial tuberosity | Fleshy: proximal 2/3 of linea aspera, medial lip, gluteal tuberosity Tendinous: Medial epicondyle of femur (*hiatus tendineus*) |
| *Nerve:* Obturator (L 3, 4) nerve and sciatic (L 4, 5; S 1) nerve | | |
| *Action:* Powerful adductor of thigh; aids in flexion and assists in lateral rotation in hip joint. Lower portion of muscle extends the thigh and rotates it medially | | |
| **6. Obturator externus muscle** | Medial margin of obturator foramen; outer surface of obturator membrane | Trochanteric fossa of femur |
| *Nerve:* Obturator nerve (L 3, 4) | | |
| *Action:* Rotates femur laterally; also aids in flexing the hip joint | | |

* The proximal, almost transverse part of the Adductor magnus muscle was formerly called (BNA) the Adductor minimus muscle. It works somewhat irregularly from the main muscle and aids in the lateral rotation of the hip joint.

**Fig. 336.** Middle layer of muscles of the ventral surface of the thigh. The Sartorius, Iliopsoas, Rectus femoris, and Adductor longus muscles were partially resected.

**Fig. 337.** Deep layers of muscles of the ventral surface of the thigh. Preparation same as in 336, in addition, the Pectineus, Adductor brevis, Vastas medialis, and Gracilis muscles were cut.

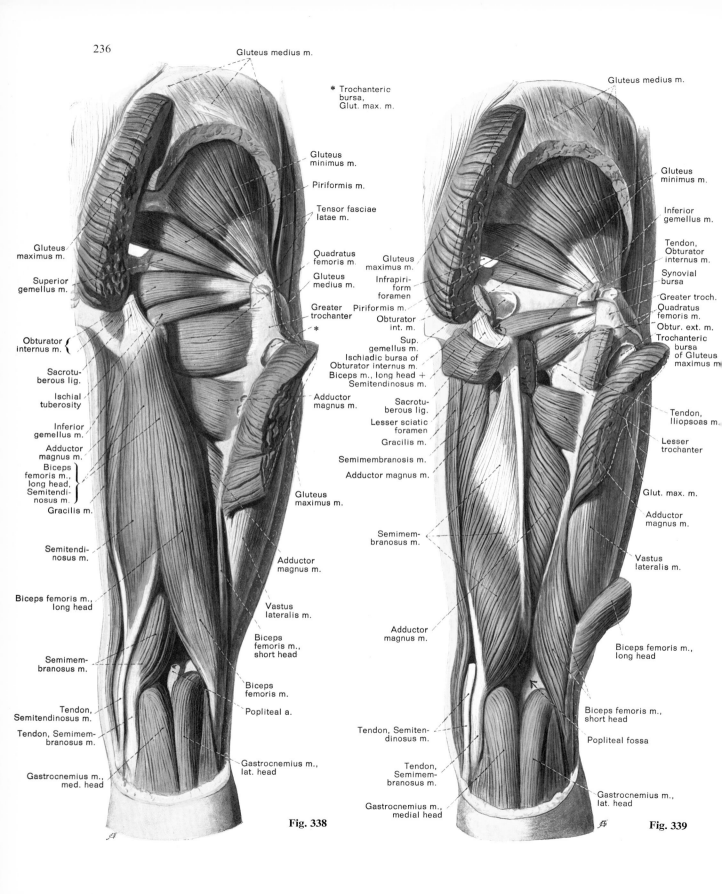

Gluteus medius m.

* Trochanteric
bursa,
Glut. max. m.

Gluteus
minimus m.

Piriformis m.

Tensor fasciae
latae m.

Quadratus
femoris m.

Gluteus
maximus m.

Infrapiri-
form
foramen

Greater
trochanter

Obturator
int. m.

*

Sup.
gemellus m.

Ischiadic bursa of
Obturator internus m.

Biceps m., long head +
Semitendinosus m.

Sacrotu-
berous lig.

Lesser sciatic
foramen

Gracilis m.

Semimembranosis m.

Adductor magnus m.

Semimem-
branosus m.

Adductor
magnus m.

Tendon, Semiten-
dinosus m.

Tendon,
Semimem-
branosus m.

Gastrocnemius m.,
medial head

Gluteus
maximus m.

Superior
gemellus m.

Obturator
internus m.

Sacrotu-
berous lig.

Ischial
tuberosity

Inferior
gemellus m.

Adductor
magnus m.

Biceps
femoris m.,
long head,
Semitendi-
nosus m.

Gracilis m.

Semitendi-
nosus m.

Biceps femoris m.,
long head

Semimem-
branosus m.

Tendon,
Semitendinosus m.

Tendon, Semimem-
branosus m.

Gastrocnemius m.,
med. head

Gluteus
medius m.

Piriformis m.

Greater
trochanter

Adductor
magnus m.

Gluteus
maximus m.

Adductor
magnus m.

Vastus
lateralis m.

Biceps femoris m.,
short head

Biceps
femoris m.

Popliteal a.

Gastrocnemius m.,
lat. head

Gluteus medius m.

Gluteus
minimus m.

Inferior
gemellus m.

Tendon,
Obturator
internus m.

Synovial
bursa

Greater troch.

Quadratus
femoris m.

Obtur. ext. m.

Trochanteric
bursa
of Gluteus
maximus m

Tendon,
Iliopsoas m.

Lesser
trochanter

Glut. max. m.

Adductor
magnus m.

Vastus
lateralis m.

Biceps femoris m.,
long head

Biceps femoris m.,
short head

Popliteal fossa

Gastrocnemius m.,
lat. head

**Fig. 338**

**Fig. 339**

# The Posterior Femoral Muscles (Hamstring Muscles) (Flexors) (Figs. 338-345)

| Name | Origin | Insertion |
|---|---|---|
| **1. Biceps femoris muscle**<br>*Long head* – operates 2 joints | Ischial tuberosity (short tendon fuses with Semitendinosus muscle) | Head of fibula by strong tendon, lateral condyle of tibia (small slip) |
| *Short head* – operates 1 joint | Distal half of lateral lip of linea aspera | |

*Nerve:*  *Long head:* Tibial nerve (S 1–3)  *Short head:* Common peroneal nerve (L 5; S 1, 2)

*Action:*  Both heads flex the leg, then rotate it laterally; long head also extends the thigh

| | | |
|---|---|---|
| **2. Semitendinosus muscle**<br>(forms the 3rd tendon of the pes anserinus) (operates 2 joints) | Short tendon from ischial tuberosity, fused with the long head of the biceps muscle | Long tendon: the terminal ramification (pes anserinus) of the tendon takes place on medial margin of the tuberosity of the tibia |

*Nerve:*  Tibial nerve (L 4, 5; S 1, 2)

*Action:*  Extends thigh; flexes the leg (medial rotation)

| | | |
|---|---|---|
| **3. Semimembranosus muscle**<br>(operates 2 joints) | Ischial tuberosity (by broad tendon; in the inner space with No.1 and No.2 above and the Adductor magnus muscle) | Thick, short tendon on medial condyle of the tibia (via oblique popliteal ligament, to lateral condyle of the femur) |

*Nerve:*  Tibial nerve (L 5; S 1, 2)

*Action:*  Flexes the leg, medial rotation of the flexed leg; extends the thigh

**I. Greater sciatic foramen** (foramen ischiadicum majus). Boundaries: Greater sciatic notch (incisura ischiadica major), sacrospinal and sacrotuberous ligaments. The Piriformis muscle passes through this foramen.
1. Caudal to the Piriformis muscle (the infrapiriform foramen) is the passage for the sciatic nerve (n. ischiadicus), inferior gluteal vessels, the posterior femoral cutaneous nerve, the internal pudendal vessels, the pudendal nerve.
2. Cranial to the Piriformis muscle (suprapiriform foramen) is the passage of superior gluteal vessels and superior gluteal nerve.

**II. Lesser sciatic foramen** (foramen ischiadicum minus). Boundaries: Lesser sciatic notch (incisura ischiadica minor) sacrospinal and sacrotuberous ligaments transmit the internal pudendal vessels and nerve and the tendon of the Obturator internus and its nerve in the pudendal canal. The pudendal canal lies in the deep ischiorectal fossa and is formed from the fascia of the Obturator internus muscle (Fig. 272).

**Fig. 338.**  Deep layer of the dorsal muscles of the hip and superficial layers of the flexors on the thigh, the muscles of the popliteal fossa. The Gluteus maximus and medius muscles were transected and reflected.

**Fig. 339.**  Deep layer of posterior hip muscles and flexors of the thigh. Besides the Gluteus maximus and medius, the Quadratus femoris, Internal obturator, Biceps femoris (long head), and the Semitendinosus muscles were cut. (The latter was cleaned away so that only the terminal tendons remain.)

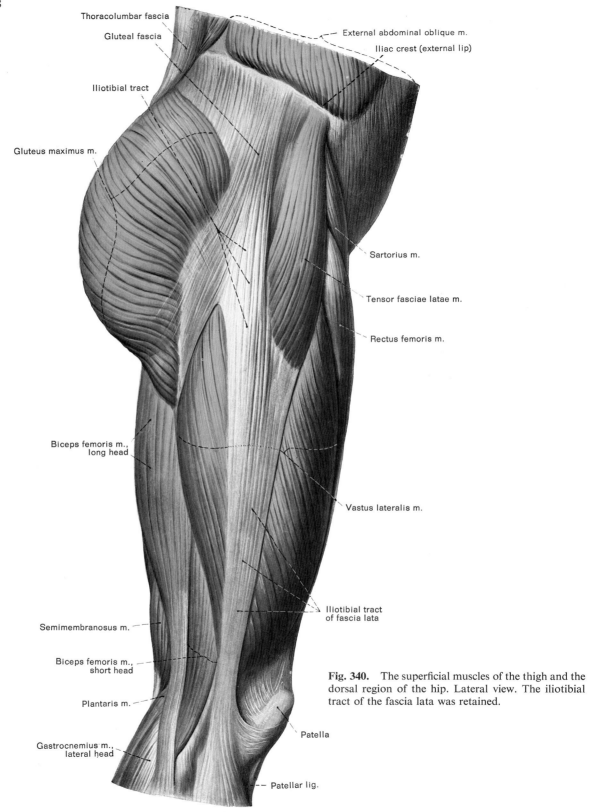

Thoracolumbar fascia

Gluteal fascia

Iliotibial tract

Gluteus maximus m.

External abdominal oblique m.

Iliac crest (external lip)

Sartorius m.

Tensor fasciae latae m.

Rectus femoris m.

Biceps femoris m.,
long head

Vastus lateralis m.

Iliotibial tract
of fascia lata

Semimembranosus m.

Biceps femoris m.,
short head

Plantaris m.

Gastrocnemius m.,
lateral head

Patella

Patellar lig.

**Fig. 340.** The superficial muscles of the thigh and the dorsal region of the hip. Lateral view. The iliotibial tract of the fascia lata was retained.

239

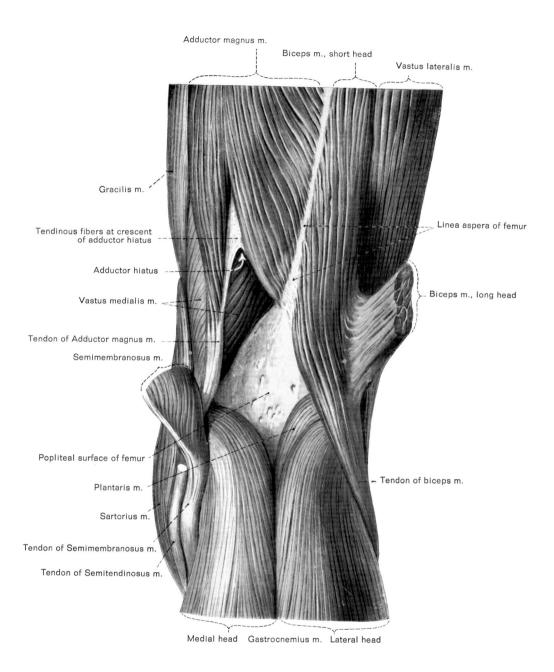

Adductor magnus m.

Biceps m., short head

Vastus lateralis m.

Gracilis m.

Tendinous fibers at crescent
of adductor hiatus

Adductor hiatus

Vastus medialis m.

Tendon of Adductor magnus m.

Semimembranosus m.

Popliteal surface of femur

Plantaris m.

Sartorius m.

Tendon of Semimembranosus m.

Tendon of Semitendinosus m.

Linea aspera of femur

Biceps m., long head

Tendon of biceps m.

Medial head    Gastrocnemius m.    Lateral head

**Fig. 341.**   The deep muscles of the popliteal fossa. Dorsal view. The Adductor magnus and the hiatus tendineus [adductorius] have been exposed by cutting the Semimembranosus, Semitendinosus, and the long head of the Biceps muscles.

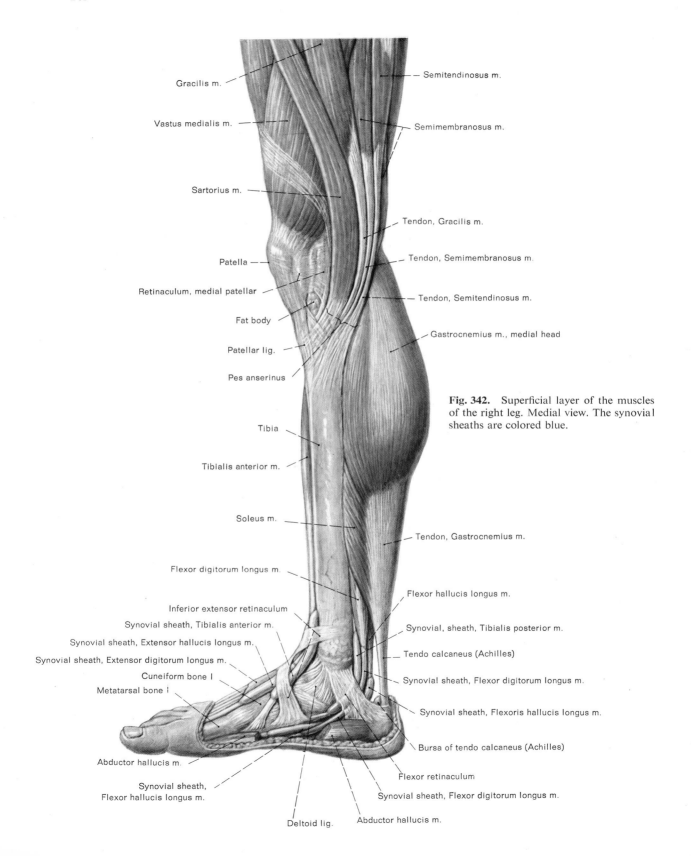

Gracilis m.

Semitendinosus m.

Vastus medialis m.

Semimembranosus m.

Sartorius m.

Tendon, Gracilis m.

Tendon, Semimembranosus m.

Patella

Tendon, Semitendinosus m.

Retinaculum, medial patellar

Fat body

Gastrocnemius m., medial head

Patellar lig.

Pes anserinus

**Fig. 342.** Superficial layer of the muscles of the right leg. Medial view. The synovial sheaths are colored blue.

Tibia

Tibialis anterior m.

Soleus m.

Tendon, Gastrocnemius m.

Flexor digitorum longus m.

Flexor hallucis longus m.

Inferior extensor retinaculum

Synovial sheath, Tibialis anterior m.

Synovial, sheath, Tibialis posterior m.

Synovial sheath, Extensor hallucis longus m.

Tendo calcaneus (Achilles)

Synovial sheath, Extensor digitorum longus m.

Synovial sheath, Flexor digitorum longus m.

Cuneiform bone I

Metatarsal bone I

Synovial sheath, Flexoris hallucis longus m.

Bursa of tendo calcaneus (Achilles)

Abductor hallucis m.

Flexor retinaculum

Synovial sheath, Flexor hallucis longus m.

Synovial sheath, Flexor digitorum longus m.

Deltoid lig.

Abductor hallucis m.

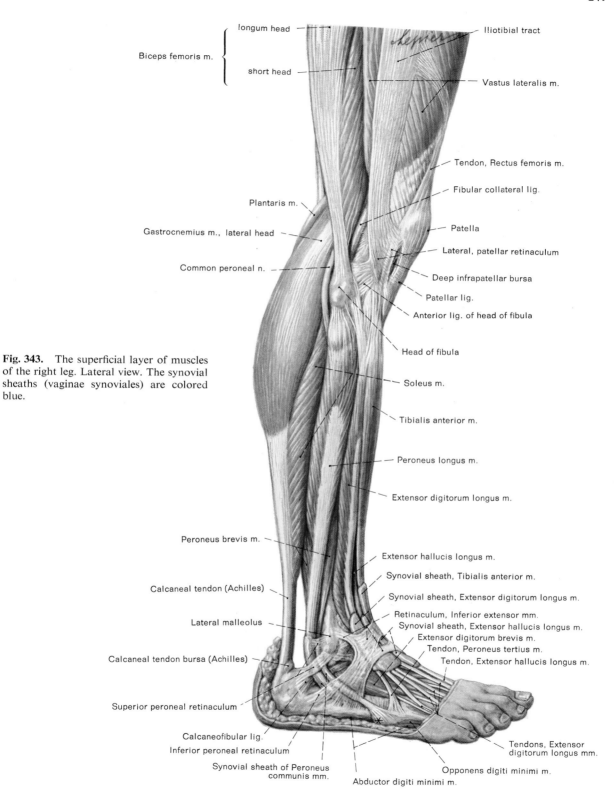

Biceps femoris m.
longum head
short head

Iliotibial tract

Vastus lateralis m.

Tendon, Rectus femoris m.

Fibular collateral lig.

Plantaris m.

Gastrocnemius m., lateral head

Common peroneal n.

Patella

Lateral, patellar retinaculum

Deep infrapatellar bursa

Patellar lig.

Anterior lig. of head of fibula

Head of fibula

**Fig. 343.** The superficial layer of muscles of the right leg. Lateral view. The synovial sheaths (vaginae synoviales) are colored blue.

Soleus m.

Tibialis anterior m.

Peroneus longus m.

Extensor digitorum longus m.

Peroneus brevis m.

Extensor hallucis longus m.

Synovial sheath, Tibialis anterior m.

Synovial sheath, Extensor digitorum longus m.

Calcaneal tendon (Achilles)

Retinaculum, Inferior extensor mm.

Synovial sheath, Extensor hallucis longus m.

Lateral malleolus

Extensor digitorum brevis m.

Tendon, Peroneus tertius m.

Tendon, Extensor hallucis longus m.

Calcaneal tendon bursa (Achilles)

Superior peroneal retinaculum

Calcaneofibular lig.

Inferior peroneal retinaculum

Synovial sheath of Peroneus communis mm.

Tendons, Extensor digitorum longus mm.

Opponens digiti minimi m.

Abductor digiti minimi m.

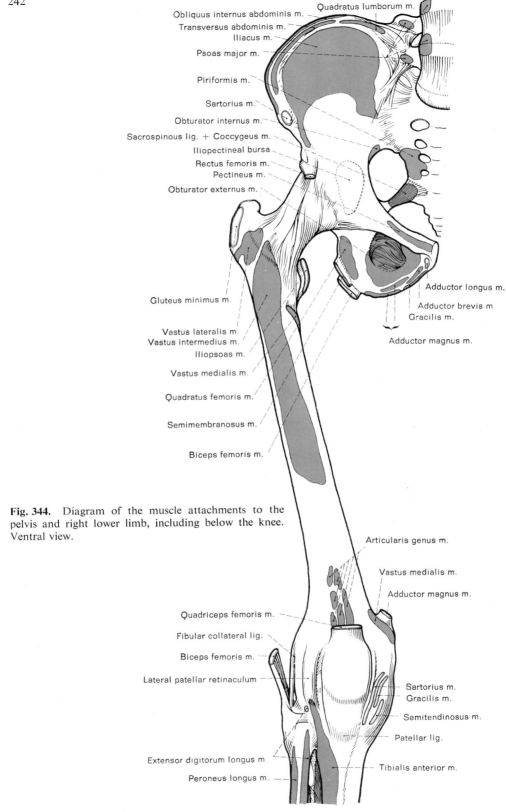

Quadratus lumborum m.
Obliquus internus abdominis m.
Transversus abdominis m.
Iliacus m.
Psoas major m.
Piriformis m.
Sartorius m.
Obturator internus m.
Sacrospinous lig. + Coccygeus m.
Iliopectineal bursa
Rectus femoris m.
Pectineus m.
Obturator externus m.
Adductor longus m.
Adductor brevis m
Gracilis m.
Gluteus minimus m.
Adductor magnus m.
Vastus lateralis m.
Vastus intermedius m.
Iliopsoas m.
Vastus medialis m.
Quadratus femoris m.
Semimembranosus m.
Biceps femoris m.

**Fig. 344.** Diagram of the muscle attachments to the pelvis and right lower limb, including below the knee. Ventral view.

Articularis genus m.
Vastus medialis m.
Adductor magnus m.
Quadriceps femoris m.
Fibular collateral lig.
Biceps femoris m.
Lateral patellar retinaculum
Sartorius m.
Gracilis m.
Semitendinosus m.
Patellar lig.
Extensor digitorum longus m.
Peroneus longus m.
Tibialis anterior m.

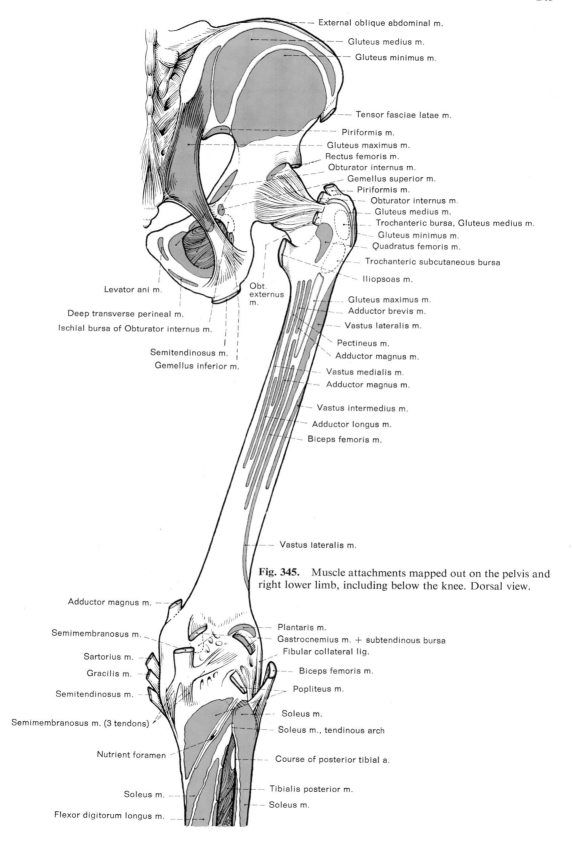

External oblique abdominal m.
Gluteus medius m.
Gluteus minimus m.

Tensor fasciae latae m.
Piriformis m.
Gluteus maximus m.
Rectus femoris m.
Obturator internus m.
Gemellus superior m.
Piriformis m.
Obturator internus m.
Gluteus medius m.
Trochanteric bursa, Gluteus medius m.
Gluteus minimus m.
Quadratus femoris m.
Trochanteric subcutaneous bursa
Iliopsoas m.
Gluteus maximus m.
Adductor brevis m.
Vastus lateralis m.
Pectineus m.
Adductor magnus m.
Vastus medialis m.
Adductor magnus m.
Vastus intermedius m.
Adductor longus m.
Biceps femoris m.

Levator ani m.
Obt. externus m.
Deep transverse perineal m.
Ischial bursa of Obturator internus m.
Semitendinosus m.
Gemellus inferior m.

Vastus lateralis m.

**Fig. 345.** Muscle attachments mapped out on the pelvis and right lower limb, including below the knee. Dorsal view.

Adductor magnus m.
Semimembranosus m.
Sartorius m.
Gracilis m.
Semitendinosus m.
Semimembranosus m. (3 tendons)
Nutrient foramen
Soleus m.
Flexor digitorum longus m.

Plantaris m.
Gastrocnemius m. + subtendinous bursa
Fibular collateral lig.
Biceps femoris m.
Popliteus m.
Soleus m.
Soleus m., tendinous arch
Course of posterior tibial a.
Tibialis posterior m.
Soleus m.

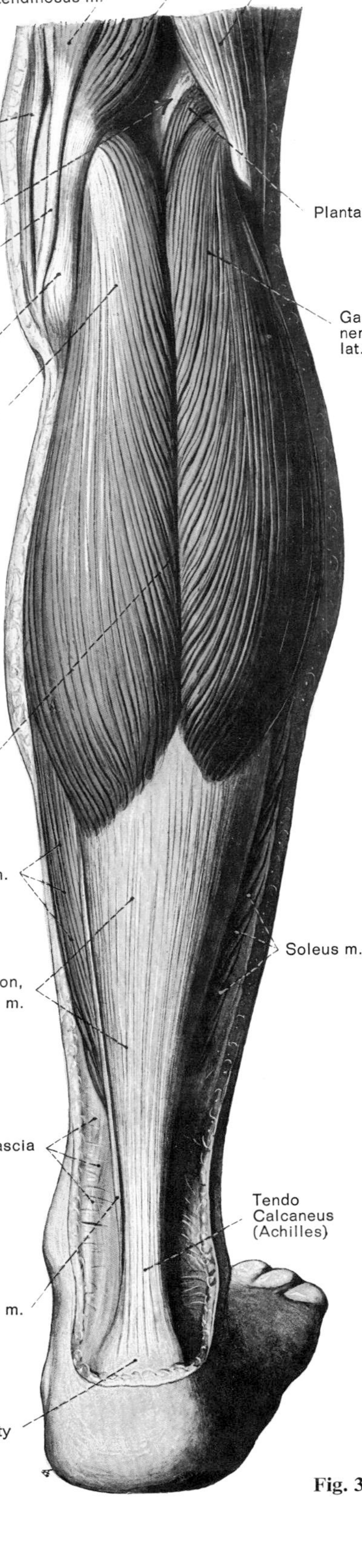

Semitendinosus m.

Semimem-
branosus m.

Biceps
femoris m.

Gracilis m.

Popliteal fossa

Tendon,
Semitendinosus m.

Tendon,
Semimembranosus m.

Gastrocnemius m.,
medial head

Plantaris m.

Gastroc-
nemius m.,
lat. head

Sulcus between heads
of Gastrocnemius m.

Soleus m.

Tendon,
Gastrocnemius m.

Soleus m.

Crural fascia

Tendo
Calcaneus
(Achilles)

Tendon, Plantaris m.

Calcaneal tuberosity

**Fig. 346**

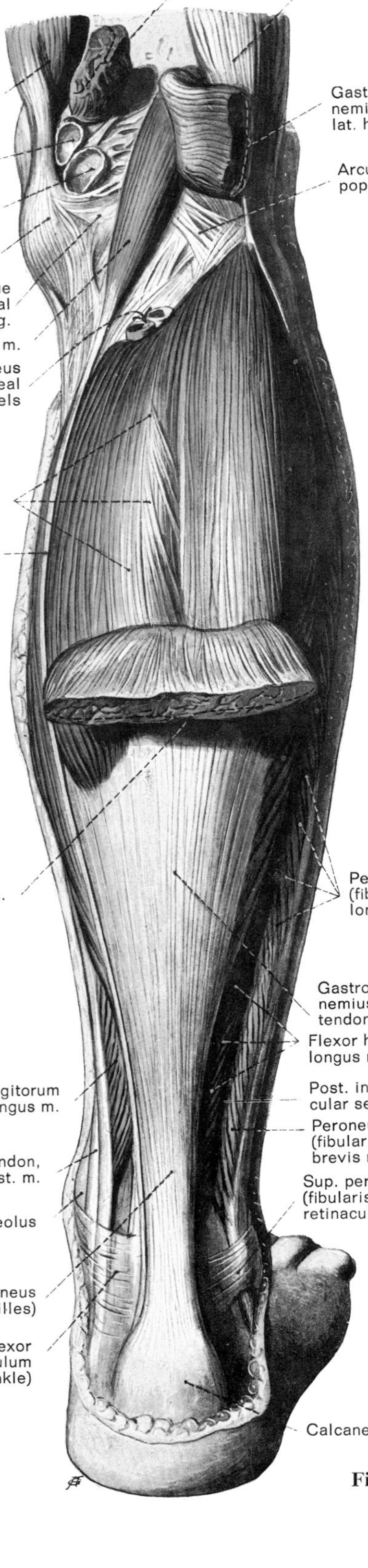

Gastrocnemius m., medial head

Biceps femoris m.

Semimembranosus m.

Gastroc-
nemius m.,
lat. head

Subtendinous bursa
of medial head of
Gastrocnemius m.

Arcuate
popliteal lig.

Bursa,
Semimem-
branosus m.

Medial condyle
of tibia

Oblique
popliteal
lig.

Plantaris m.

Arcus tendineus
+ Popliteal
vessels

Soleus m.

Plantaris m.,
tendon

Peroneus
(fibularis)
longus m.

Gastrocnemius m.

Gastroc-
nemius m.,
tendon

Flexor hallucis
longus m.

Post. intermus-
cular septa

Flexor digitorum
longus m.

Peroneus
(fibularis)
brevis m.

Tendon,
Tibialis post. m.

Sup. peroneal
(fibularis)
retinaculum

Medial malleolus

Tendo calcaneus
(Achilles)

Flexor
retinaculum
(ankle)

Calcaneal tuberosity

**Fig. 347**

## Muscles of the Posterior Compartment of the Leg (Figs. 341-343, 345-347)

| Name | Origin | Insertion |
|---|---|---|
| **1. Gastrocnemius muscle** | | |
| *Medial head* (Fig. 345) | Medial condyle of femur; capsule of knee | |
| *Lateral head* | Lateral condyle of femur; capsule of knee | Aponeurosis unites with the tendon of the Soleus muscle to form the tendo calcaneus |
| **2. Soleus muscle** (with Gastrocnemius, occasionally described as Triceps surae muscle) | Posterior surface of head and upper third of fibula; soleal line and middle third of medial border of tibia; tendinous arch (transverse intermuscular septum) between the tibia and fibula | |
| **3. Plantaris muscle** | Lateral condyle of femur | Posterior part of calcaneus in front or side of the calcaneal tendon (with long thin tendon) |

*Nerve:* Tibial nerve

*Action:* Plantar flexion of foot and tends to supinate it; Gastrocnemius muscle points the toe (with Plantaris); flexes knee; braces knee and ankle joints when standing

| Name | Origin | Insertion |
|---|---|---|
| **4. Popliteus muscle** | Tendon from lateral condyle of femur; somewhat from the oblique popliteal ligament | Posterior surface of tibia, proximal to soleal line (Fig. 353) |

*Nerve:* Tibial nerve

*Action:* Flexes leg; rotates femur medially to help unlock dead center

Note: The oblique origin of the Soleus muscle arises through a tendinous arch of the Soleus muscle fissure, through this the popliteal vessels and tibial nerve leave the popliteal space distally and arrive in the deep region of the calf.

**Fig. 346.** Superficial view of the muscular components of the calf.

**Fig. 347.** Second layer of the calf muscles. The Gastrocnemius is cut and reflected; the deeper layer of crural fascia was removed up to the retinacula.

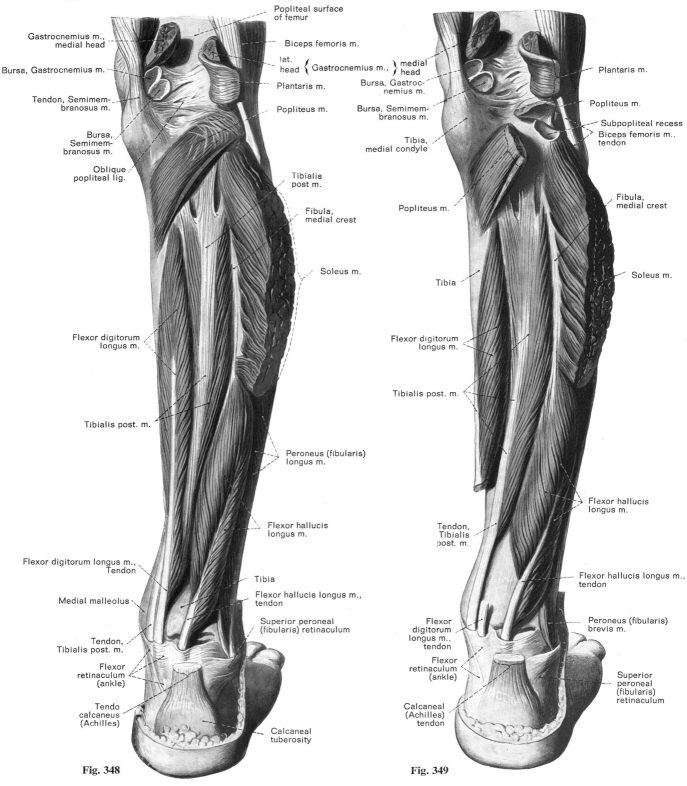

Popliteal surface
of femur

Gastrocnemius m.,
medial head

Bursa, Gastrocnemius m.

Tendon, Semimem-
branosus m.

Bursa,
Semimem-
branosus m.

Oblique
popliteal lig.

Biceps femoris m.

lat.
head { Gastrocnemius m., } medial
head

Plantaris m.

Popliteus m.

Tibialis
post m.

Fibula,
medial crest

Soleus m.

Flexor digitorum
longus m.

Tibialis post. m.

Peroneus (fibularis)
longus m.

Flexor hallucis
longus m.

Flexor digitorum longus m.,
Tendon

Medial malleolus

Tibia

Flexor hallucis longus m.,
tendon

Superior peroneal
(fibularis) retinaculum

Tendon,
Tibialis post. m.

Flexor
retinaculum
(ankle)

Tendo
calcaneus
(Achilles)

Calcaneal
tuberosity

**Fig. 348**

Plantaris m.

Bursa, Gastroc-
nemius m.

Bursa, Semimem-
branosus m.

Tibia,
medial condyle

Popliteus m.

Popliteus m.

Subpopliteal recess

Biceps femoris m.,
tendon

Fibula,
medial crest

Soleus m.

Tibia

Flexor digitorum
longus m.

Tibialis post. m.

Flexor hallucis
longus m.

Tendon,
Tibialis
post. m.

Flexor hallucis longus m.,
tendon

Flexor
digitorum
longus m.,
tendon

Peroneus (fibularis)
brevis m.

Flexor
retinaculum
(ankle)

Calcaneal
(Achilles)
tendon

Superior
peroneal
(fibularis)
retinaculum

**Fig. 349**

## Muscles of the Posterior Compartment of the Leg (Deep Layers) (Figs. 348, 349, 353)

| Name | *Origin* | *Insertion* |
|------|----------|-------------|
| **1. Tibialis posterior muscle** | Posterior surface of the tibia (proximal part), interosseous membrane of the leg, medial surface of the fibula | Tuberosity of navicular bone; plantar surface of the 3 cuneiforms, sustentaculum tali of the calcaneus, bases of metatarsals 2 to 4. (Fig. 354) |

*Action:*   Plantar flexes the foot, supinates (adducts and inverts)

| Name | *Origin* | *Insertion* |
|------|----------|-------------|
| **2. Flexor digitorum longus muscle** | Posterior surface and interosseus margin of the tibia, distal to soleal line with a tendinous arch from distal third of the fibula | By 4 tendons into bases of distal phalanges of toes 2 to 5 |

*Action:*   Flexes terminal phalanges of toes 2–5, assists in plantar flexion, supination and adduction of the foot

| Name | *Origin* | *Insertion* |
|------|----------|-------------|
| **3. Flexor hallucis longus muscle** | Distal $2/3$ of posterior surface and margin of fibula, interosseus membrane of the leg, posterior intermuscular septum | Base of terminal phalanx of big toe |

*Nerve:*   Tibial nerve for all three muscles

*Action:*   Flexes big toe, plantar flexion, supination, and adduction of foot

---

Note: The medial malleolar region contains from front to back: The tendons for the Tibialis posterior and Flexor digitorum longus muscles; the posterior tibial vessels, the tibial nerve and, deep dorsally, the tendon of the Flexor hallucis longus. A short tunnel is fashioned through the retinaculum, through which the structure of the deep calf region goes to the sole of the foot (Fig. 365).

The lateral malleolar region contains the tendons of the Peroneus longus and Peroneus brevis muscles, which are fixed by a superior and inferior retinaculum.

---

**Fig. 348.**   Deeper muscles of the posterior compartment of the leg. The Gastrocnemius, the Soleus, and the Plantaris muscles were removed or reflected.

**Fig. 349.**   Deepest layer of the muscular compartment of the calf. The Popliteus and Flexor digitorum longus muscles were transected.

248

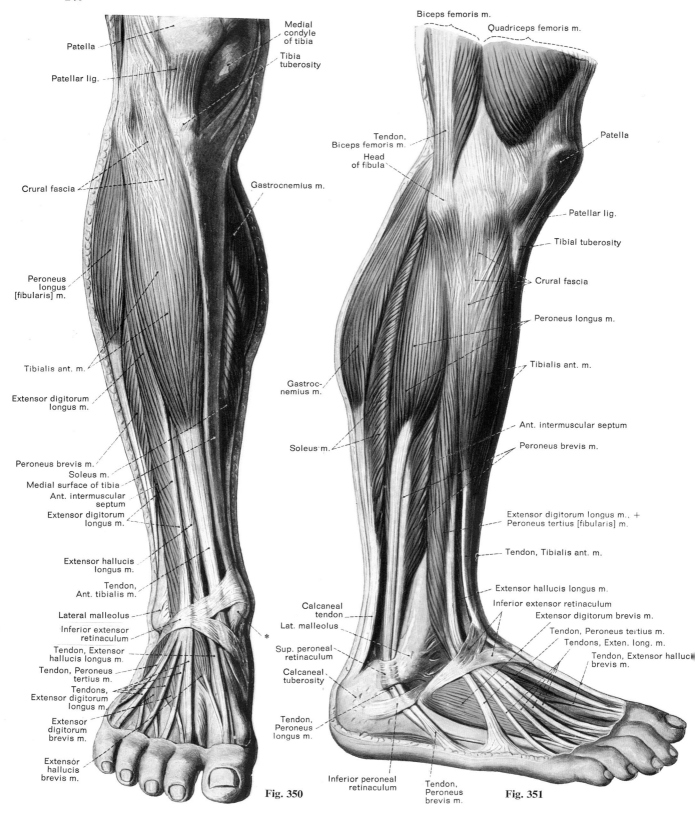

Patella

Patellar lig.

Crural fascia

Peroneus longus [fibularis] m.

Tibialis ant. m.

Extensor digitorum longus m.

Peroneus brevis m.

Soleus m.

Medial surface of tibia

Ant. intermuscular septum

Extensor digitorum longus m.

Extensor hallucis longus m.

Tendon, Ant. tibialis m.

Lateral malleolus

Inferior extensor retinaculum

Tendon, Extensor hallucis longus m.

Tendon, Peroneus tertius m.

Tendons, Extensor digitorum longus m.

Extensor digitorum brevis m.

Extensor hallucis brevis m.

Medial condyle of tibia

Tibia tuberosity

Gastrocnemius m.

Fig. 350

Biceps femoris m.

Quadriceps femoris m.

Tendon, Biceps femoris m.

Head of fibula

Gastrocnemius m.

Soleus m.

Calcaneal tendon

Lat. malleolus

Sup. peroneal retinaculum

Calcaneal tuberosity

Tendon, Peroneus longus m.

Inferior peroneal retinaculum

Tendon, Peroneus brevis m.

Patella

Patellar lig.

Tibial tuberosity

Crural fascia

Peroneus longus m.

Tibialis ant. m.

Ant. intermuscular septum

Peroneus brevis m.

Extensor digitorum longus m., + Peroneus tertius [fibularis] m.

Tendon, Tibialis ant. m.

Extensor hallucis longus m.

Inferior extensor retinaculum

Extensor digitorum brevis m.

Tendon, Peroneus tertius m.

Tendons, Exten. long. m.

Tendon, Extensor halluc. brevis m.

Fig. 351

## Muscles of the Anterior Compartment of the Leg (Figs. 350-352, 364)

| Name | Origin | Insertion |
|---|---|---|
| **1. Tibialis anterior muscle**<br>With long tendon running under the retinaculum of the superior and inferior extensor muscles | Lateral condyle; upper half of lateral surface of tibia; interosseous membrane; crural fascia | Base of 1st metatarsal (medial edge); medial cuneiform (I) (plantar surface) |

*Nerve:* Branch of deep peroneal (fibularis) nerve (L 4, 5; S 1)

*Action:* Dorsally flexes and supinates (adducts and inverts) the foot

| Name | Origin | Insertion |
|---|---|---|
| **2. Extensor hallucis longus muscle** | Middle half of fibular and interosseous membrane; crural fascia | Base of distal phalanx of great toe |
| **3. Extensor digitorum longus muscle**<br>Tendon fixed by the retinacula of the superior and inferior | Lateral condyle of tibia; proximal ¾ of fibula; interosseous membrane; crural fascia, anterior intermuscular septum of leg | Tendons to 2nd and terminal phalanges of 4 lateral toes |
| **4. Peroneus (fibularis) tertius muscle** | Distal third of shaft of fibula; interosseous membrane | Dorsal surface, fifth metatarsal bone (flat tendon) |

*Nerve:* Deep peroneal (fibular) nerve (L 4, 5; S 1)

*Action:* Extends toes; dorsiflexes ankle joint at the same time the Extensor digitorum longus muscle pronates and abducts the foot; also the Extensor hallucis longus muscle supinates the foot

## Muscles of the Lateral Compartment of the Leg (Figs. 350, 351, 353, 365)

| Name | Origin | Insertion |
|---|---|---|
| **1. Peroneus (fibularis) longus muscle**<br>The tendon is a cartilaginous thickening at the tuberosity of the cuboid bone | Head and upper ²/₃ of lateral surface and posterior margin of fibula; intermuscular septa | Long tendon ends on lateral side of the base of the 1st metatarsal bone and the lateral side of the medial cuneiform (Fig. 354) |
| **2. Peroneus brevis muscle** | Distal ²/₃ of the lateral surface and anterior margin of the fibula, intermuscular septa | Tuberosity at the base of the 5th metatarsal, tendon strip to little toe (Fig. 357) |

*Nerve:* Superficial peroneal (fibularis) nerve

*Action:* Pronates (everts and abducts) and plantar flexes the foot

**Fig. 350.** Muscles of the anterior compartments of the leg and the dorsum of the foot. The superior extensor retinaculum was removed; the inferior extensor retinaculum was retained. *Med. malleolus

**Fig. 351.** Muscles of the lower leg and dorsum of the foot, seen from the lateral side. The fascia was removed as far as the retinacula.

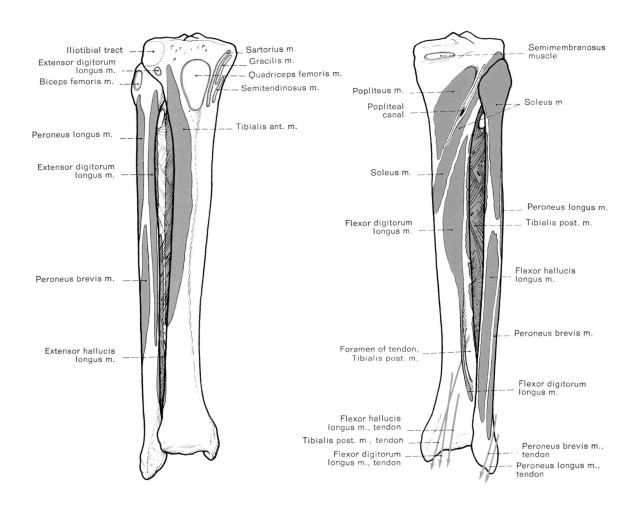

Iliotibial tract

Extensor digitorum longus m.

Biceps femoris m.

Peroneus longus m.

Extensor digitorum longus m.

Peroneus brevis m.

Extensor hallucis longus m.

Sartorius m.

Gracilis m.

Quadriceps femoris m.

Semitendinosus m.

Tibialis ant. m.

Semimembranosus muscle

Popliteus m.

Popliteal canal

Soleus m.

Flexor digitorum longus m.

Foramen of tendon, Tibialis post. m.

Flexor hallucis longus m., tendon

Tibialis post. m., tendon

Flexor digitorum longus m., tendon

Soleus m.

Peroneus longus m.

Tibialis post. m.

Flexor hallucis longus m.

Peroneus brevis m.

Flexor digitorum longus m.

Peroneus brevis m., tendon

Peroneus longus m., tendon

**Figs. 352 and 353.** Diagram of the muscle origins and insertions on the right tibia and fibula. Fig. 352. Ventral aspect. Fig. 353. Dorsal aspect.

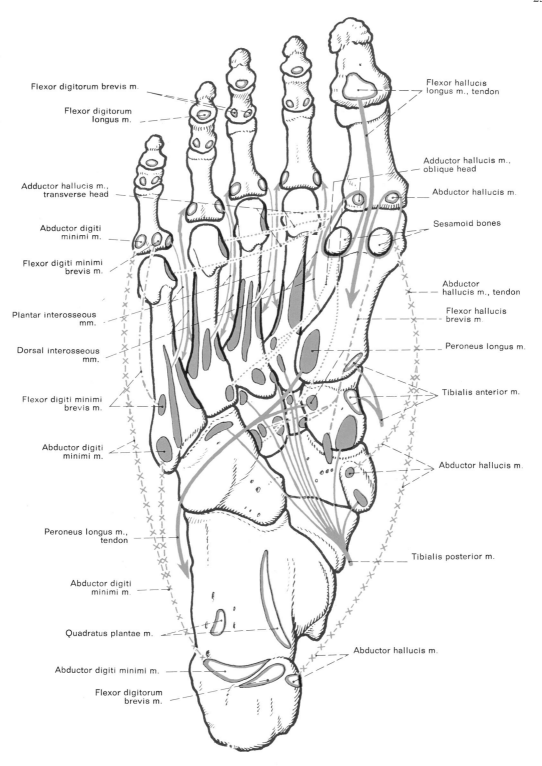

Flexor digitorum brevis m.

Flexor digitorum
longus m.

Adductor hallucis m.,
transverse head

Abductor digiti
minimi m.

Flexor digiti minimi
brevis m.

Plantar interosseous
mm.

Dorsal interosseous
mm.

Flexor digiti minimi
brevis m.

Abductor digiti
minimi m.

Peroneus longus m.,
tendon

Abductor digiti
minimi m.

Quadratus plantae m.

Abductor digiti minimi m.

Flexor digitorum
brevis m.

Flexor hallucis
longus m., tendon

Adductor hallucis m.,
oblique head

Abductor hallucis m.

Sesamoid bones

Abductor
hallucis m., tendon

Flexor hallucis
brevis m.

Peroneus longus m.

Tibialis anterior m.

Abductor hallucis m.

Tibialis posterior m.

Abductor hallucis m.

**Fig. 354.**   Muscle origins and insertions mapped out on the sole of the right foot.

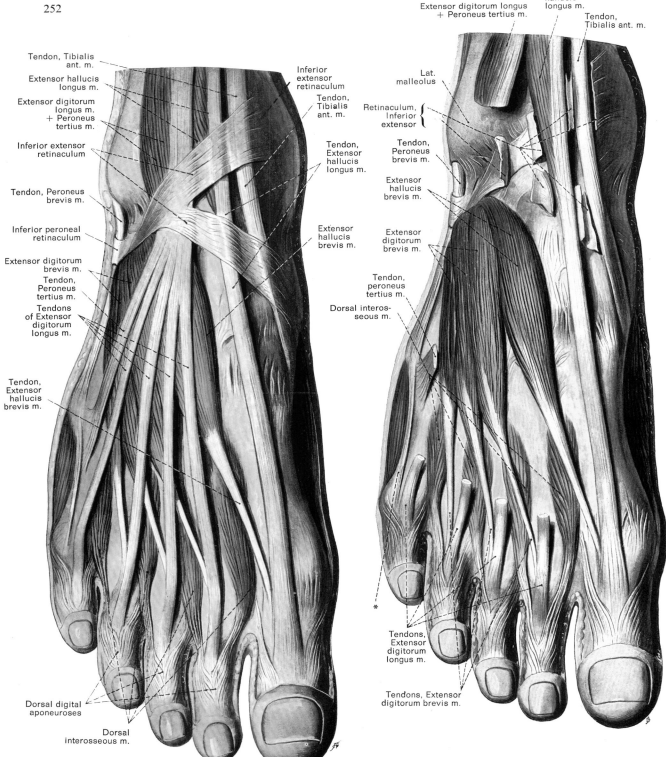

252

Tendon, Tibialis ant. m.

Extensor hallucis longus m.

Extensor digitorum longus m. + Peroneus tertius m.

Inferior extensor retinaculum

Tendon, Peroneus brevis m.

Inferior peroneal retinaculum

Extensor digitorum brevis m.

Tendon, Peroneus tertius m.

Tendons of Extensor digitorum longus m.

Tendon, Extensor hallucis brevis m.

Dorsal digital aponeuroses

Dorsal interosseous m.

Inferior extensor retinaculum

Tendon, Tibialis ant. m.

Tendon, Extensor hallucis longus m.

Extensor hallucis brevis m.

Extensor digitorum longus + Peroneus tertius m.

Extensor hallucis longus m.

Tendon, Tibialis ant. m.

Lat. malleolus

Retinaculum, Inferior extensor {

Tendon, Peroneus brevis m.

Extensor hallucis brevis m.

Extensor digitorum brevis m.

Tendon, peroneus tertius m.

Dorsal interosseous m.

*

Tendons, Extensor digitorum longus m.

Tendons, Extensor digitorum brevis m.

**Fig. 355.** Superficial muscles and the tendons of the dorsum of the foot.

**Fig. 356.** Muscles and tendons of the dorsum of the foot. The retinaculum of the Inferior extensor muscle has been split.
* The continuation of the tendon of the Peroneus (fibularis) brevis muscle on the small toe (var.).

## Muscles of the Dorsum of the Foot  (Figs. 355-357)

| Name | Origin | Insertion |
|------|--------|-----------|
| **Extensor digitorum brevis m.** | Lateral and dorsal surface of the calcaneus | Dorsal aponeurosis of 3 middle toes (3 thin tendons) |
| **Extensor hallucis brevis m.** | Dorsal surface of calcaneus | Base of 1st phalanx of big toe |

*Nerve:*   Deep peroneal (fibularis) nerve (L 5; S 1)

*Action:*   Extension of the toes (dorsiflexion)

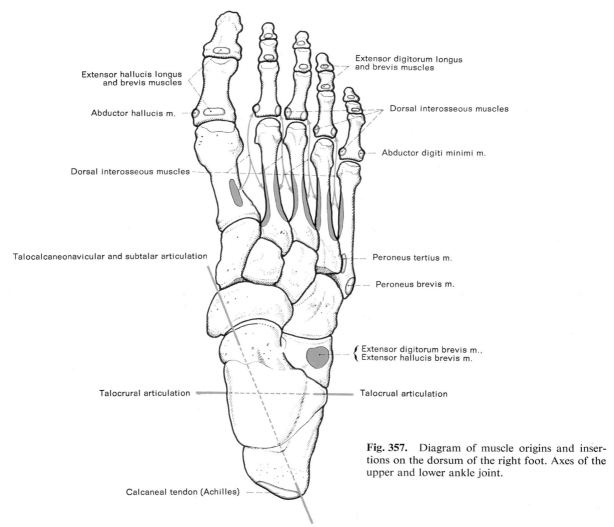

Fig. 357.  Diagram of muscle origins and insertions on the dorsum of the right foot. Axes of the upper and lower ankle joint.

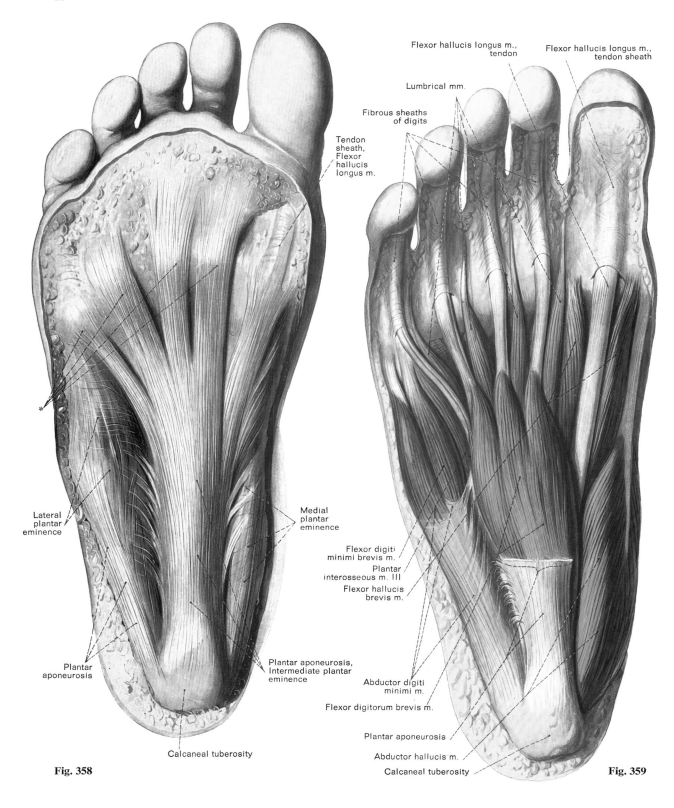

Flexor hallucis longus m.,
tendon

Flexor hallucis longus m.,
tendon sheath

Lumbrical mm.

Fibrous sheaths
of digits

Tendon
sheath,
Flexor
hallucis
longus m.

Lateral
plantar
eminence

Medial
plantar
eminence

Flexor digiti
minimi brevis m.

Plantar
interosseous m. III

Flexor hallucis
brevis m.

Plantar
aponeurosis

Plantar aponeurosis,
Intermediate plantar
eminence

Abductor digiti
minimi m.

Flexor digitorum brevis m.

Plantar aponeurosis

Abductor hallucis m.

Calcaneal tuberosity

Calcaneal tuberosity

**Fig. 358**

**Fig. 359**

### Muscles of the Sole of the Foot *(planta pedis)* **(Figs. 354, 359-361)**

| Name | Origin | Insertion |
|---|---|---|
| **Flexor digitorum brevis muscle** Plantar muscle forms the intermediate plantar eminence | Medial process, tuberosity of calcaneus; medial part of plantar aponeurosis | By 4 thin tendons (perforated by tendons of the Flexor digitorum longus muscle) on the middle phalanges of the 4 lateral toes |

*Nerve:*    Medial plantar nerve (L 4, 5)

*Action:*    Flexes middle phalanges of the toes

| | | |
|---|---|---|
| **Quadratus plantae muscle** *(Flexor accessorius m.)* | Two heads from plantar surface of calcaneus; long plantar ligament | Lateral margin of tendon of Flexor digitorum longus muscle |

*Nerve:*    Lateral plantar nerve (S 1, 2)

*Action:*    Supports action of the Flexor digitorum longus muscle and corrects oblique direction of pull of its tendons

Note: The muscle pattern on the sole of the foot is formed by 3 muscular eminences: Lateral, intermediate, and medial. In between are 2 longitudinal grooves: The medial and lateral plantar sulci which contain the lateral and medial plantar vessels and nerves having the same name (Fig. 358). There is an abductor and flexor for the toe in its corresponding compartment.

The medial plantar eminence (compartment for the big toe) contains the belly of the Abductor hallucis muscle and the Flexor hallucis longus and brevis muscles. The intermediate plantar eminence (central compartment for the sole of the foot) is the thickest and contains the belly of the Flexor digitorum brevis, which is covered by the plantar aponeurosis. The lateral plantar eminence (compartment for the small toe) contains the Abductor digiti minimi and Flexor digiti minimi brevis muscles.

**Fig. 358.**    The plantar aponeurosis of the right foot.  * Radiation of the digital slips of the plantar aponeurosis to the toes.

**Fig. 359.**    The superficial musculature of the sole of the right foot. Part of the plantar aponeurosis is removed with the exception of the posterior part.

256

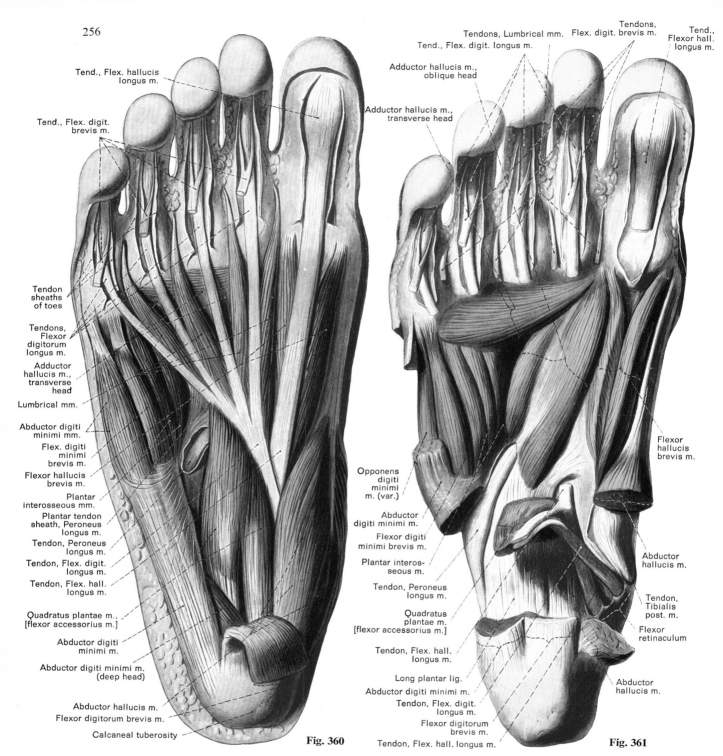

Tend., Flex. hallucis longus m.

Tend., Flex. digit. brevis m.

Tendon sheaths of toes

Tendons, Flexor digitorum longus m.

Adductor hallucis m., transverse head

Lumbrical mm.

Abductor digiti minimi mm.

Flex. digiti minimi brevis m.

Flexor hallucis brevis m.

Plantar interosseous mm.

Plantar tendon sheath, Peroneus longus m.

Tendon, Peroneus longus m.

Tendon, Flex. digit. longus m.

Tendon, Flex. hall. longus m.

Quadratus plantae m., [flexor accessorius m.]

Abductor digiti minimi m.

Abductor digiti minimi m. (deep head)

Abductor hallucis m.

Flexor digitorum brevis m.

Calcaneal tuberosity

Fig. 360

Tendons, Lumbrical mm.

Tend., Flex. digit. longus m.

Tendons, Flex. digit. brevis m.

Tend., Flexor hall. longus m.

Adductor hallucis m., oblique head

Adductor hallucis m., transverse head

Flexor hallucis brevis m.

Opponens digiti minimi m. (var.)

Abductor digiti minimi m.

Flexor digiti minimi brevis m.

Plantar interosseous m.

Tendon, Peroneus longus m.

Quadratus plantae m. [flexor accessorius m.]

Tendon, Flex. hall. longus m.

Long plantar lig.

Abductor digiti minimi m.

Tendon, Flex. digit. longus m.

Flexor digitorum brevis m.

Tendon, Flex. hall. longus m.

Abductor hallucis m.

Tendon, Tibialis post. m.

Flexor retinaculum

Abductor hallucis m.

Fig. 361

**Fig. 360.**  The middle layer of the musculature of the sole of the foot. Most of the Flexor digitorum brevis was removed.

**Fig. 361.**  Deep layer of the musculature of the sole of the foot. The following were transected: the tendons of the Flexor digitorum brevis and longus, the Quadratus plantae [Flexor accessorius], Abductor digiti minimi, Abductor hallucis, and Flexor hallucis longus muscles. The tendon sheath of the Peroneus (fibularis) longus muscle has been split for its entire length.

## Muscles of the Great Toe  (Figs. 359-361)

| Name | Origin | Insertion |
|---|---|---|
| **1. Abductor hallucis muscle**<br>Plantar muscle united to the medial plantar eminence | Medial process of tuberosity of calcaneus and plantar aponeurosis | Base of proximal phalanx of great toe (Fig. 354) |
| **2. Flexor hallucis brevis muscle** | Plantar surface of cuboid and lateral cuneiform bones; tendon of Tibialis posterior m. | Two heads on medial and lateral sides of proximal phalanx of big toe; sesamoid bones (Fig. 354) |
| **3. Abductor hallucis muscle**<br>*Oblique head* | Bases of metatarsal bones 2 to 4; sheath of tendon of Peroneus longus muscle | Lateral side of base of proximal phalanx of great toe; sesamoid bones (Fig. 354) |
| *Transverse head* | Metatarsophalangeal ligaments of the 3 lateral toes; deep transverse metatarsal ligament | |

*Nerve:*   For No. 1 and No. 2, the medial plantar nerve; No. 3 (and sometimes No. 2) lateral plantar nerve (S 1, 2)

*Action:*   As the name implies: abducts, flexes, adducts big toe: above all, however, gives effective transverse and longitudinal tension to the plantar arch

## Muscles of the Small Toe  (Figs. 354, 359-361)

| Name | Origin | Insertion |
|---|---|---|
| **1. Abductor digiti minimi muscle**<br>(Plantar m. united with lateral plantar eminence) | Medial and lateral process of tuberosity of calcaneus; plantar aponeurosis | Lateral side of proximal phalanx of small toe (and often into tuberosity of the 5th metatarsal bone) |
| **2. Flexor digiti minimi brevis muscle** | Base of 5th metatarsal bone; sheath of Peroneus longus tendon | Proximal phalanx of small toe |
| **3. Opponens digiti minimi muscle**<br>(inconstant)<br>(omitted by NA) | | Lateral margin of 5th metatarsal |

*Nerve:*   Lateral plantar nerve

*Action:*   As the name implies: abducts, flexes and opponed the small toe; above all, however, gives effectiv tension to the plantar arch

The *Lumbrical muscles* of the foot arise from the tendons of the Flexor digitorum longus. The first one by a single head from the medial ridge of the first tendon (2nd toe) and the other three by two heads. They join the dorsal aponeurosis of the toes in the region of the metatarsophalangeal joints from the medial side. Most small bursa of the lumbricals are found at their insertion. The medial plantar nerve (L 4, 5) supplies the first lumbrical and the other three lumbricals are supplied by the lateral plantar nerve (S 1, 2).

*Action:* Flexes proximal phalanges, as in the hand.

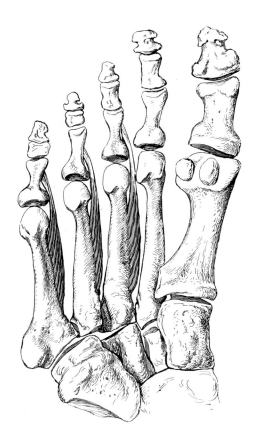

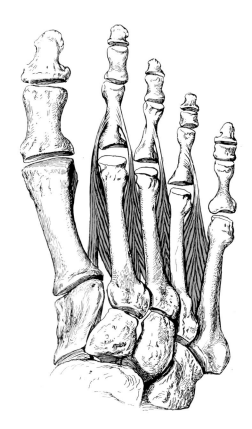

**Fig. 362.** The Plantar interossei muscles.

**Fig. 363.** The Dorsal interossei muscles.

The *Interosseus muscles* of the foot are arranged somewhat like those of the hand: There are four dorsal and three plantar muscles. The latter are relatively strong (stronger than the dorsal muscles of the foot) in contrast to those of the hand. All three Plantar muscles act in the same direction and arise from the medial border of the metatarsals III, IV, V, and all three are inserted in the dorsal aponeuroses of the toes of the same side. The relatively weak dorsal interosseus muscles arise by two heads as in the hand. The tendons (as in the hand) do not go in the same direction: I and II go to the second toe.

*Nerve:* The lateral plantar nerve.

*Action:* Similar to the muscles of the hand: Abduction, or else adduction and flexion.

259

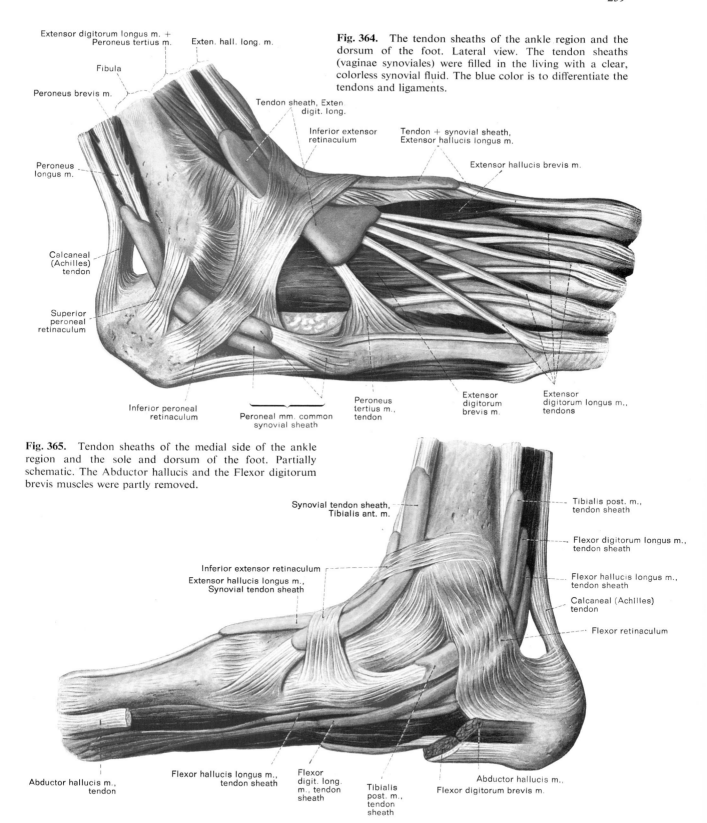

Extensor digitorum longus m. +
Peroneus tertius m.

Exten. hall. long. m.

Fibula

Peroneus brevis m.

Peroneus
longus m.

Calcaneal
(Achilles)
tendon

Superior
peroneal
retinaculum

Tendon sheath, Exten
digit. long.

Inferior extensor
retinaculum

Tendon + synovial sheath,
Extensor hallucis longus m.

Extensor hallucis brevis m.

**Fig. 364.** The tendon sheaths of the ankle region and the dorsum of the foot. Lateral view. The tendon sheaths (vaginae synoviales) were filled in the living with a clear, colorless synovial fluid. The blue color is to differentiate the tendons and ligaments.

Inferior peroneal
retinaculum

Peroneal mm. common
synovial sheath

Peroneus
tertius m.,
tendon

Extensor
digitorum
brevis m.

Extensor
digitorum longus m.,
tendons

**Fig. 365.** Tendon sheaths of the medial side of the ankle region and the sole and dorsum of the foot. Partially schematic. The Abductor hallucis and the Flexor digitorum brevis muscles were partly removed.

Synovial tendon sheath,
Tibialis ant. m.

Tibialis post. m.,
tendon sheath

Flexor digitorum longus m.,
tendon sheath

Flexor hallucis longus m.,
tendon sheath

Calcaneal (Achilles)
tendon

Flexor retinaculum

Inferior extensor retinaculum

Extensor hallucis longus m.,
Synovial tendon sheath

Abductor hallucis m.,
tendon

Flexor hallucis longus m.,
tendon sheath

Flexor
digit. long.
m., tendon
sheath

Tibialis
post. m.,
tendon
sheath

Abductor hallucis m.,
Flexor digitorum brevis m.

# Subject Index

(All numbers refer to the numbers of pages)

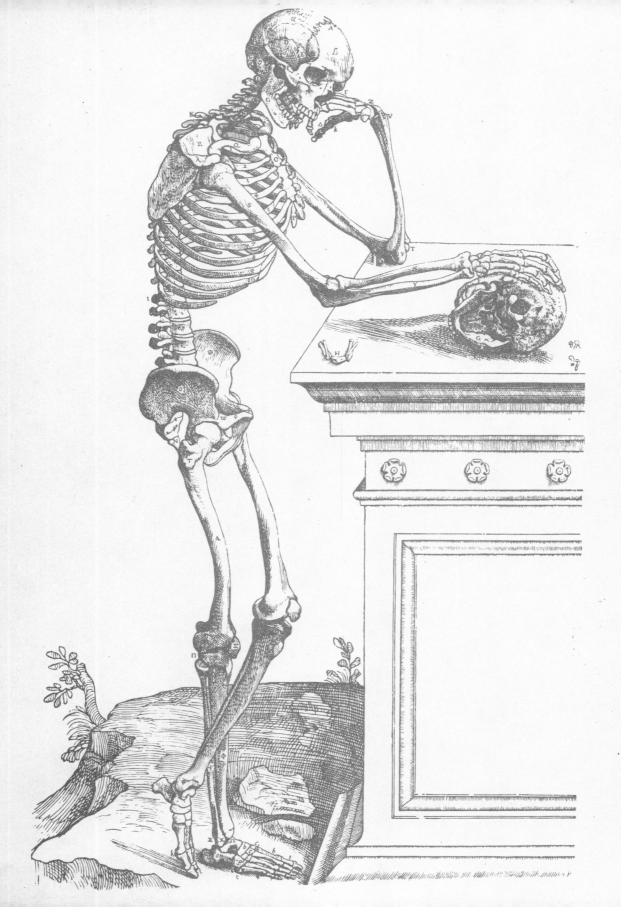